02 MAR 2005

D0452508

CRITICAL CARE

KEY TOPICS IN

CRITICAL CARE

Second Edition

Edited by

Tim Craft MB BS FRCA
Consultant in Anaesthaesia and Intensive Care Medicine
Royal United Hospital
Bath
UK

Jerry Nolan MB BS FRCA
Consultant in Anaesthaesia and Intensive Care Medicine
Royal United Hospital
Bath
UK

Mike Parr
MB BS FRCP FRCA FANZCA FJFICM
Consultant in Intensive Care Medicine
Liverpool Hospital
Lecturer in Intensive Care, Anaesthesia and Emergency Medicine
University of New South Wales
Sydney
Australia

Taylor & Francis
Taylor & Francis Group

LONDON AND NEW YORK

A MARTIN DUNITZ BOOK

© 2004 Taylor & Francis, an imprint of the Taylor & Francis Group

First edition published in the United Kingdom in 1999 by
BIOS Scientific Publishers Limited

Second edition published by Taylor & Francis, an imprint of the Taylor & Francis Group,
2 Park Square, Milton Park, Abingdon, Oxfordshire OX14 4RN

Tel.:   +44 (0) 20 7583 9855
Fax.:   +44 (0) 20 7842 2298
E-mail: info@dunitz.co.uk
Website: http://www.dunitz.co.uk

Although every effort has been made to ensure that all owners of copyright material have
been acknowleged in this publication, we would be glad to acknowledge in subsequent
reprints or editions any omissions brought to our attention.

A CIP record for this book is available from the British Library.

Library of Congress Cataloging-in-Publication Data

Data available on application

ISBN 1 85996 229 7

Distributed in the North and South America by

Taylor & Francis
2000 NW Corporate Blvd
Boca Raton, FL 33431, USA

Within Continental USA
Tel: 800 272 7737;   Fax: 800 373 3401
Outside Continental USA
Tel: 561 994 0555;   Fax: 561 361 6018
E-mail: orders@crcpress.com

Distributed in the rest of the world by
Thomson Publishing Services
Cheriton House
North Way
Andover, Hampshire SP10 5BE, UK
Tel.: +44 (0) 1264 332424
E-mail: saleorder.tandf@thomsonpublishingservices.co.uk

Production editor: Julian Evans
Composition by Wearset Ltd, Boldon, Tyne and Wear
Printed and bound in Great Britain by TJ International Ltd, Padstow, Cornwall

Contents

Contributors

Tim Cook MB BS BA FRCA
Consultant in Anaesthesia and Intensive Care Medicine, Royal United Hospital, Bath, UK

Giorgia Ferro MD MDM
Registrar in Intensive Care, Liverpool Hospital, Sydney, Australia

Stephen Fletcher MB BS MRCP FRCA FFICANZCA
Consultant in Anaesthesia and Intensive Care, Bradford Royal Infirmary, Bradford, UK

Claire Fouque MB BS FRCA
Consultant in Anaesthesia and Intensive Care Medicine, Southmead Hospital, Bristol, UK

Alex Goodwin MB BS FRCA
Consultant in Anaesthesia and Intensive Care Medicine, Royal United Hospital, Bath, UK

Kim Gupta MB ChB FRCA
Consultant in Anaesthesia and Intensive Care Medicine, Royal United Hospital, Bath, UK

Jonathan Hadfield MB BS FRCA
Consultant in Anaesthesia and Intensive Care Medicine, Bristol Royal Infirmary, Bristol, UK

Jeff Handel MB BS MRCP FRCA
Consultant in Anaesthesia and Intensive Care Medicine, Royal United Hospital, Bath, UK

S. Kim Jacobson MB ChB MSc MRCP MRCPath
Consultant Medical Microbiologist, Royal United Hospital, Bath, UK

Myrene Kilminster MB BS FANZCA FFICANZCA
Consultant in Intensive Care, Lismore Hospital, New South Wales, Australia

Stephen Laver MB ChB
Staff Doctor in Anaesthesia and Intensive Care Medicine, Royal United Hospital, Bath, UK

James Low MB BCh DCH FRCA DICM
Consultant in Anaesthesia and Intensive Care Medicine, Derbyshire Royal Infirmary, Derby, UK

Rachel Markham MB ChB FRCA
Registrar in Intensive Care, Liverpool Hospital, Sydney, Australia

Caleb McKinstry BM MRCP FRCA
Advanced Trainee in Intensive Care Medicine, Royal United Hospital, Bath, UK

Tim Murphy MA MB BS FRCA
Specialist Registrar in Anaesthesia, Frenchay Hospital, Bristol, UK

Susan Murray PhD FRCPath
Clinical Microbiologist, Royal United Hospital, Bath, UK

Cathal Nolan MB BCh BAO FFARCSI
Registrar in Intensive Care, Liverpool Hospital, Sydney, Australia

Matt Oram MB BCh FRCA DICM (UK)
Specialist Registrar in Anaesthesia and Intensive Care Medicine, Royal United Hospital, Bath, UK

Andrew Padkin MB ChB BSc MRCP FRCA
Consultant in Anaesthesia and Intensive Care Medicine, Royal United Hospital, Bath, UK

Richard Protheroe MB BS MRCS MRCP FRCA
Consultant in Anaesthesia and Intensive Care Medicine, Hope Hospital, Manchester, UK

Martin Schuster-Bruce MB BS BSc MRCP FRCA
Consultant in Anaesthesia and Intensive Care Medicine, Royal Bournemouth Hospital, Bournemouth, UK

Jas Soar BA MB BCh MA FRCA
Consultant in Anaesthesia and Intensive Care Medicine, Southmead Hospital, Bristol, UK

Anthony Stewart MB BS FANZCA
Consultant in Intensive Care, Liverpool Hospital, Sydney, Australia

Victor Tam MB BS
Senior Registrar in Intensive Care Medicine, Liverpool Hospital, Sydney, Australia

Minh Tran MB BS BSc FANZCA
Consultant in Anaesthesia, Liverpool Hospital, Sydney, Australia

Jenny Tuckey MB ChB DCH FRCA
Consultant in Anaesthesia, Royal United Hospital, Bath, UK

Cynthia Uy MB BS
Consultant in Palliative Medicine, Hope Healthcare, North Sydney, Australia

Nicky Weale BM BS FRCA
Specialist Registrar in Anaesthesia, Frenchay Hospital, Bristol, UK

Abbreviations

ACE	angiotensin-converting enzyme
ACT	activated clotting time
ACTH	adrenocorticotrophic hormone
ADH	anti-diuretic hormone
AF	atrial fibrillation
AICD	automatic implantable cardioverter defibrillator
AIS	Abbreviated Injury Scale
ALF	acute liver failure
ALI	acute lung injury
ALS	advanced life support
APACHE	acute physiology and chronic health evaluation
APC	activated protein C
APPT	activated partial thromboplastin time
APS	Acute Physiology Score
ARDS	acute respiratory distress syndrome
AST	aspartate amino-transferase
ATN	acute tubular necrosis
AVM	arteriovenous malformation
BE	base excess
BiPAP	bilevel positive airway pressure
BLS	basic life support
CABG	coronary artery bypass graft
CBF	cerebral blood flow
CES	compression elastic stockings
CHF	congestive heart failure
$CMRO_2$	cerebral metabolic rate for oxygen
CNS	central nervous system
COPD	chronic obstructive pulmonary disease
CPAP	continuous positive airway pressure
CPK	creatine phosphokinase
CPP	cerebral perfusion pressure
CPR	cardiopulmonary resuscitation
CSF	cerebrospinal fluid
CT	computed tomography
CTPA	computed tomographic pulmonary angiography
CVP	central venous pressure
CVS	cardiovascular system
CVVH	continuous venovenous haemofiltration
CVVHD	continuous venovenous haemodialysis
CVVHDF	continuous venovenous haemodiafiltration
CXR	chest X-ray
DDAVP	d'-8-amino arginine vasopressin or desmopressin
DI	diabetes insipidus
DIC	disseminated intravascular coagulation

DKA	diabetic ketoacidosis
DPL	diagnostic peritoneal lavage
DVT	deep venous thrombosis
ECCO$_2$R	extracorporeal CO_2 removal
ECF	extracellular fluid
ECMO	extracorporeal membrane oxygenation
ESBL	extended spectrum beta-lactamase
EVLW	extravascular lung water
FBC	full blood count
FDPs	fibrin degradation products
FEV$_1$	forced expiratory volume in one second
FFP	fresh frozen plasma
FiO$_2$	Fractional inspired concentration of oxygen
FOB	fibreoptic bronchoscopy
FRC	functional residual capacity
GALT	gut associated lymphoid tissue
GBS	Guillain–Barré syndrome
GCS	Glasgow Coma Scale
GDT	goal-directed therapy
GFR	glomerular filtration rate
GI	gastrointestinal
GTN	glyceryl trinitrate
GvHD	graft versus host disease
HDU	high dependency unit
HFJV	high-frequency jet ventilation
HFOV	high-frequency oscillation ventilation
HFV	high-frequency ventilation
HHS	hyperglycaemic hyperosmolar state
HITTS	heparin-induced thrombocytopenia and associated thrombosis syndrome
HLA	human leukocyte antigen
IABP	intra-aortic balloon pump
IAP	intra-abdominal pressure
ICF	intracellular fluid
ICP	intracranial pressure
ICU	intensive care unit
IDDM	insulin dependent diabetes mellitus
IHD	intermittent haemodialysis
IMV	intermittent mandatory ventilation
INR	international normalised ratio
IPC	intermittent pneumatic compression
ISF	interstitial fluid
ISS	Injury Severity Score
ITBV	intrathoracic blood volume
IVC	inferior vena cava
LDH	lactate dehydrogenase
LMA	laryngeal mask airway

LMWH	low molecular weight heparin
LODS	Logistic Organ Dysfunction Score
LP	lumbar puncture
LRTI	lower respiratory tract infection
LV	left ventricular
LVEDP	left ventricular end diastolic pressure
MAP	mean arterial pressure
MH	malignant hyperthermia
MI	myocardial infarction
MILS	manual in-line cervical stabilisation
MODS	multiple organ dysfunction syndrome
MOF	multiple organ failure
MPM	Mortality Probability Models
MRI	magnetic resonance imaging
MRSA	methicillin resistant *Staphylococcus aureus*
MRTB	multi-resistant *Mycobacterium tuberculosis*
NGT	nasogastric tube
NIDDM	non-insulin dependent diabetes mellitus
NIPPV	non-invasive positive pressure ventilation
NIV	non-invasive ventilation
NSAID	non-steroidal anti-inflammatory drug
PAFC	pulmonary artery flotation catheter
PAOP	pulmonary artery occlusion pressure
PCA	patient controlled analgesia
PCI	percutaneous intervention
PCP	*Pneumocystis carinii* pneumonia
PD	peritoneal dialysis
PDT	percutaneous dilatational tracheostomy
PE	pulmonary embolism
PEEP	positive end-expiratory pressure
PEEPi	intrinsic positive end-expiratory pressure
PEF	peak expiratory flow
PEG	percutaneous gastrostomy
pHi	intramucosal pH
PLV	partial liquid ventilation
PND	paroxysmal nocturnal dyspnoea
PSV	pressure support ventilation
PT	prothrombin time
PTSD	post-traumatic stress disorder
ROSC	return of spontaneous circulation
RRT	renal replacement therapy
RTA	road traffic accident
RVEDV	right ventricular end diastolic volume
SAGM	saline, adenine, glucose and mannitol
SAH	subarachnoid haemorrhage
SaO_2	oxygen saturation of haemoglobin in arterial blood
SAPS	Simplified Acute Physiology Score

SDD	selective decontamination of the digestive tract
SIADH	syndrome of inappropriate antidiuretic hormone
SIMV	synchronised intermittent mandatory ventilation
SIRS	systemic inflammatory response syndrome
SLE	systemic lupus erythematosus
SMR	standardised mortality ratio
SOFA	Sequential Organ Failure Assessment
SVC	superior vena cava
SVR	systemic vascular resistance
TBW	total body water
TED	thromboembolism deterrent
TENS	transcutaneous electrical nerve stimulation
TIA	transient ischaemic attack
TISS	Therapeutic Intervention Scoring System
TNF	tumour necrosis factor
TOE	transoesophageal echocardiography
t-PA	tissue plasminogen activator
TURP	transurethral resection of the prostate
UFH	unfractionated heparin
UTI	urinary tract infection
V/Q	ventilation/perfusion
VAD	ventricular assist device
VAS	visual analogue scale
VAP	ventilator-associated pneumonia
VF	ventricular fibrillation
VRE	vancomycin resistant enterococcus
VT	ventricular tachycardia
VTE	venous thromboembolism
WFNS	World Federation of Neurological Surgeons Scale

Preface to the first edition

Critical care in acute hospitals is developing perhaps faster than any other clinical speciality. The pace of change is driven both by an ever increasing ability of medicine to offer the chance of survival from critical illness and the expectations of our patients. At the same time we have a responsibility to ensure that our critical care resources are directed only at those patients who will benefit from them. The importance of critical care medicine is recognised, too, by many of the Royal Colleges in their exam structure. Critical care now forms a part of the examinations for Fellowship of the Royal College of Anaesthetists, Membership of the Royal College of Physicians, and Fellowship of the Royal Colleges of Surgeons, amongst others.

Key Topics in Critical Care provides a framework for candidates of postgraduate medical examinations as well as a footing for all those expected to care for critically ill patients. Care of the critically ill involves clinicians working together as teams across some of the more traditional professional boundaries. *Key Topics in Critical Care* has been written by clinicians from a variety of different backgrounds working in two different continents. As usual with the Key Topics format, each topic presents a succinct overview of its subject and is referenced with current publications for further reading. Wherever possible, these references are to major review articles in widely available journals.

TM Craft, JP Nolan, MJA Parr
(Bath and Sydney, 1999)

Preface to the second edition

High-quality critical care medicine is a crucial component of advanced health care. Since the first edition of *Key Topics in Critical Care*, this importance has been underlined by clinical and political initiatives. The desire for the best possible outcomes for our patients, despite increased cost and demand, means we must be able to justify our practice and increasingly, adopt an evidence-based approach. These aspects of care are reflected in the succinct review style of *Key Topics in Critical Care*. This new text has been expanded to accommodate new important topics, and there is increased emphasis on recent reviews and landmark papers, as well as referral to websites that provide reference information, and which will also provide future updates. We hope this book will continue to prove invaluable to clinicians pursuing a career in critical care medicine.

TM Craft, JP Nolan, MJA Parr
(Bath and Sydney 2004)

Admission and discharge criteria

Critical care is a service for patients with potentially recoverable conditions who can benefit from more detailed observation and invasive treatment than can safely be provided in general wards. Identification of the patients who are most likely to benefit from admission to a critical care unit can be very difficult. These resources are scarce and expensive. Patients who are not ill enough to require critical care and those unlikely to benefit because they are too ill must be excluded. In 1996, the United Kingdom Department of Health's publication 'Guidelines on admission to and discharge from Intensive Care and High Dependency Units' provided useful advice. Since then, the concept of extending care to ill patients outside the walls of the critical care unit (Outreach Services) has led to a new classification of critically ill patients, which describes the level of care required (Level 0–4) instead of the location. A recent publication by the Intensive Care Society defines the criteria for these levels of care.

Criteria for levels of care

Level 0 criteria
- Needs can be met through normal ward care.

Level 1 criteria
- Patients recently discharged from a higher level of care.
- Patients in need of additional monitoring, clinical input or advice, e.g. observations needed at least every 4 hours.
- Patients requiring critical care outreach support, e.g. abnormal vital signs.
- Patients requiring staff with special expertise and/or additional facilities for at least one aspect of critical care delivered in a ward environment, e.g. epidural analgesia, tracheostomy care.

Level 2 criteria
- Patients needing single organ system support (see below). Patients in need of advanced respiratory support satisfy criteria for level 3.
- Patients needing preoperative optimisation, e.g. need for invasive monitoring.
- Patients needing extended postoperative care, e.g. major elective surgery, emergency surgery in high-risk patient. This includes patients needing short-term ventilation (<24 h).
- Patients needing a greater degree of observation and monitoring, e.g. invasive monitoring.
- Patients with major uncorrected physiological abnormalities, e.g. respiratory rate > 40 breaths min^{-1}, heart rate > 120 beats min^{-1}, temperature < 35°C for > 1 h, systolic blood pressure < 80 mmHg for > 1 h, GCS < 10 and at risk of deterioration.

Level 3 criteria
- Patients needing advanced respiratory monitoring and support, e.g. positive pressure ventilation. Patients needing short-term postoperative ventilation who are otherwise well (e.g. fast-track cardiac surgery) are excluded.

- Patients needing monitoring and support for two or more organs, one of which may be basic, or advanced respiratory support.
- Patients with chronic impairment of one or more organ systems sufficient to restrict daily activities (co-morbidity) and who require support for an acute reversible failure of another organ system, e.g. severe ischaemic heart disease and major perioperative bleeding.

Categories of organ system monitoring and support

1. Advanced respiratory support:

    1.1. Mechanical ventilatory support (excluding mask continuous positive airway pressure (CPAP) or non-invasive ventilation).
    1.2. The possibility of a sudden deterioration in respiratory function requiring immediate tracheal intubation and mechanical ventilation.

2. Basic respiratory monitoring and support:

    2.1. The need for more than 50% oxygen by fixed performance mask.
    2.2. The possibility of progressive deterioration to the point of needing advanced respiratory support.
    2.3. The need for physiotherapy to clear secretions at least 2-hourly.
    2.4. Patients recently extubated after a prolonged period of intubation and mechanical ventilation.
    2.5. The need for mask CPAP or non-invasive ventilation.
    2.6. Patients who are intubated to protect the airway, but not needing ventilatory support.

3. Circulatory support:

    3.1. The need for vasoactive drugs.
    3.2. Support for circulatory instability due to hypovolaemia from any cause and which is unresponsive to modest volume replacement.
    3.3. Patients resuscitated following cardiac arrest where intensive or high-dependency care is considered clinically appropriate.
    3.4. Intra-aortic balloon counterpulsation.

4. Neurological monitoring and support:

    4.1. Central nervous system depression sufficient to prejudice the airway and protective reflexes.
    4.2. Invasive neurological monitoring.

5. Renal support:

    5.1. The need for acute renal replacement therapy.

Critical care staffing

The provision of level 3 critical care typically requires:

- A designated area where there is a minimum nurse-to-patient ratio of 1:1, together with a nurse-in-charge, throughout 24 h.
- Twenty-four hour cover by resident medical staff.
- The ability to support organ system failures.

The provision of level 2 critical care typically requires:

- A designated area where there is a minimum nurse-to-patient ratio of 1:2, together with a nurse-in-charge, throughout 24 h.
- Continuous availability of medical staff.
- Appropriate monitoring and other equipment.

Admission to a critical care unit

Referral
When considering referral for critical care, where possible, it is essential to consult with the patient and the patient's family and to determine their wishes. The referral should be on a consultant-to-consultant basis, although this may not always be possible.

Reversibility of illness
The potential benefits of critical care will depend on whether or not the patient's acute condition is reversible. This is not always easy to determine and in some cases it is necessary to admit the patient and assess the response to a trial of treatment. The potential benefit of critical care, in terms of quality and length of life, should be discussed with the patient (where possible) and with the patient's family.

Co-morbidity
Co-morbidity is a chronic impairment of one or more organs sufficient to restrict daily activities. Intensive care cannot reverse chronic ill health and significant co-morbidity will weigh against a patient's admission to a critical care unit. However, patients often adapt to their co-morbidity and accept a quality of life that others would find unacceptable. Thus, denying critical care admission to a patient with significant co-morbidity may not be in their best interests.

Discharge from critical care
A patient should be discharged from the critical care unit when the condition that led to the admission has been reversed adequately or when the patient is no longer benefiting from the treatment available. If it is clear that there is no chance of survival with a quality of life that would be acceptable to the patient, it may be appropriate to limit or withdraw aggressive therapy. The Intensive Care Society and the General Medical Council have published guidelines on this subject. Unless a patient's death is

imminent, it is appropriate to transfer the patient to another area of the hospital and allow death with dignity.

Bed management policies should prevent patients being detained inappropriately in a critical care unit. This ideal is becoming increasingly difficult to achieve as acute general hospitals run on the absolute minimum number of ward beds. When well enough, level 3 patients may be discharged to level 2 facilities or to the general ward, as appropriate.

Further reading

Department of Health NHS Executive. *Guidelines on Admission to and Discharge from Intensive Care and High Dependency Units*. Department of Health, 1996.

Cohen SL, Bewley JS, Ridley S, Goldhill D and members of the ICS Standards Committee. *Guidelines for Limitation of Treatment for Adults Requiring Intensive Care*. Intensive Care Society, 2003.
www.ics.ac.uk/downloads/LimitTreatGuidelines2003.pdf

Council of the Intensive Care Society. *Levels of Critical Care for Adult Patients, 2002*.
www.ics.ac.uk/downloads/icsstandards-levelsofca.pdf

General Medical Council. *Withholding and Withdrawing Life-Prolonging Treatments: Good Practice in Decision-Making*.
www.gmc-uk.org

Acute respiratory distress syndrome

Tim Cook

Acute respiratory distress syndrome (ARDS) is a syndrome of respiratory failure associated with severe hypoxia and low respiratory compliance. The characteristic radiological changes are of widespread pulmonary infiltrates. Pulmonary artery occlusion pressure measurements may be low or normal. The plasma oncotic pressure is usually normal. The reported annual incidence of ARDS is variable: 5:100000 being quoted in the UK, but 75:100000 in the USA. This reflects differing thresholds for diagnosis. Genomic polymorphism of the angiotensin-converting enzyme influences the incidence and outcome from ARDS.

The clinical disorders causing ARDS can be divided into those associated with direct injury to the lung, such as pneumonia, fat embolism, aspiration or smoke inhalation, and, more commonly, those that cause indirect lung injury as part of the systemic inflammatory response syndrome (SIRS). Sepsis and trauma are the commonest causes of ARDS. Other causes of indirect lung injury include haemorrhage with hypotension, transfusion, obstetric emergencies, cardiopulmonary bypass and pancreatitis. Onset of the disease is rapid; most cases develop within 24 h of the initial insult. The clinical presentation is with tachypnoea, laboured breathing and cyanosis.

The pathophysiological features of ARDS are initially due to epithelial injury and include a severe protein-rich alveolar oedema with inflammatory infiltrates (principally neutrophils), although ARDS may occur in the neutropenic patient. Surfactant denaturation by protein leaking into the alveolus leads to atelectasis, a reduced functional residual capacity (FRC) and hypoxia. Type I alveolar cells are damaged and type II cells proliferate. Later, fibroblast infiltration and collagen proliferation lead, in some cases, to an accelerated fibrosing alveolitis, and microvascular obliteration. This disease process does not affect the lung in a uniform fashion; there may be considerable functional variation between different lung regions.

Diagnosis

There are strict definitions for the diagnosis of acute lung injury (ALI) and ARDS. The triad of hypoxia, low lung compliance and widespread infiltrates on chest X-ray (CXR) should be accompanied by a known precipitant of the syndrome and a normal left atrial pressure (PAOP). A $PaO_2/FIO_2 \leq 300$ mmHg (~40 kPa) defines ALI and a $PaO_2/FIO_2 \leq 200$ mmHg (~27 kPa) defines ARDS.

Prognosis

The reported mortality for ARDS is variable. This is related in part to lack of consistency in diagnosis. Sepsis is associated with the greatest mortality at any stage of the disease whilst fat embolism alone is associated with a low mortality (90% survival). ARDS associated with bone marrow transplant or liver failure has negligible survival. Over 80% of deaths in ARDS are attributable to sepsis and multiple organ failure rather than respiratory failure. Recent studies show that the mortality rate has fallen in the past decade from 60–70% to 35%.

Treatment

Treatment is supportive, but control of infection is vital. Bacteriological specimens should be cultured and every effort made to prevent nosocomial infection. Maintain patients in a 30–45° head-up position to reduce the incidence of microaspiration and nosocomial pneumonia. Nursing and medical hygiene must be scrupulous. Positive blood cultures should be followed by an extensive search for the site of infection.

Ventilation

The principles of mechanical ventilation are to provide adequate oxygenation and CO_2 removal while minimising the risk of barotrauma and volutrauma. Cyclic overdistension and collapse of alveoli induces damaging shear forces and increases levels of systemic inflammatory cytokines. The use of low tidal volumes and moderate positive end-expiratory pressure (PEEP) will reduce these shear forces and minimise damage. A protective ventilation strategy using low tidal volume and low inspiratory plateau pressure improves survival in patients with ARDS. The use of low tidal volumes may cause hypercarbia; $PaCO_2$ is allowed to rise to 10 kPa or higher providing renal compensation minimises the accompanying acidosis (permissive hypercarbia).

The ARDS network (ARDSNet) demonstrated improved survival in ARDS patients ventilated with an initial tidal volume of 6 ml kg^{-1} predicted body weight and a plateau pressure ≤ 30 cmH$_2$O compared with those ventilated with 12 ml kg^{-1} and a plateau pressure ≤ 50 cmH$_2$O. The study has been criticised because of the comparatively high tidal volumes used in the control group and some experts believe that tidal volumes as low as 6 ml kg^{-1} could even be harmful. A popular, pragmatic approach is to use tidal volumes of 6–8 ml kg^{-1} predicted body weight and to keep the plateau pressure ≤ 35 cmH$_2$O. If chest wall compliance is poor – for example, in the presence of severe oedema or abdominal distension – it is appropriate to allow the plateau pressure to increase. This is because the amount of stretch applied to the lungs is dependent on the transpulmonary pressure and not simply the inspiratory pressure.

Recruitment manoeuvres, such as continuous positive airway pressure of 40 cmH$_2$O applied for 40 s, will inflate collapsed dependent alveoli (recruitment) and a PEEP of 5–18 cmH$_2$O will help to maintain inflation. Prolonged inspiratory times (i.e. inverse ratio ventilation) will increase intrinsic PEEP (PEEPi) and oxygenation; however, there is a risk of overinflation of the lungs and the impairment to venous return can reduce cardiac output dramatically. Prolonged use of high inspired O$_2$ concentrations is thought to induce lung injury. The inspired oxygen concentration (FiO$_2$) should be reduced to ≤ 0.5 as soon as possible by setting targets for acceptable hypoxaemia (e.g. oxygen saturation [SaO$_2$] $> 88\%$). The optimum level of PEEP in relation to the FiO$_2$ is unknown. In the early stages of ARDS, ventilation in the prone position will improve oxygenation in two-thirds of cases. Although extracorporeal membrane oxygenation (ECMO) with CO_2 removal is of benefit in infantile ARDS, its use to treat refractory hypoxaemia in adults remains controversial and a randomised controlled trial is ongoing.

Measurement of cardiac output using a pulmonary artery flotation catheter (PAFC) or non-invasive technique may help to guide fluid resuscitation and inotropes. Measurement of mixed venous saturation from a PAFC, or central venous oxygen saturation, and lactate or base deficit may help to determine the adequacy of oxygen delivery. Extravascular lung water may be controlled by judicious administration of fluids to prevent high left atrial pressures. The choice between colloid and crystalloid is controversial, but most critical care physicians use both.

Specific treatment

Steroid therapy may be beneficial during the fibrosing stage of ARDS (late steroid rescue). This benefit is limited to a narrow therapeutic window of between 7 and 15 days after the onset of ARDS.

Nitric oxide

Nitric oxide (NO) is a potent vasodilator. When it is inhaled it enters only ventilated areas of the lung and causes appropriate vasodilatation, thus improving ventilation–perfusion matching and oxygenation. This is in contrast to intravenous vasodilators that tend to do the converse and so increase shunt. NO has a great affinity for haemoglobin (15 000 times that of carbon monoxide) and combines rapidly with it on entering the bloodstream; thus, NO does not cause systemic vasodilatation. The delivery of NO must be monitored carefully and when delivery is stopped rebound pulmonary hypertension can be a significant problem. Use of NO does not improve outcome from ARDS and its use in the treatment of adults is now uncommon.

Epoprostenol

Nebulised epoprostenol $2-10\,\text{ng}\,\text{kg}^{-1}\,\text{min}^{-1}$ will improve oxygenation as effectively as NO and is easier to monitor and deliver. It may be useful as a means of improving oxygenation in patients unresponsive to prone ventilation.

Survivors

The outlook for survivors is good. At 1 year, 50% of survivors have abnormal lung function and some functional respiratory disability. Many recover completely. Late deaths in ARDS are secondary to pulmonary fibrosis (55%) and sepsis/multiple organ failure (69%).

Further reading

Bernard GR, Artigas A, Brigham KL, *et al.* Report of the American-European Consensus Conference on ARDS: definitions, mechanisms, relevant outcomes and clinical trial coordination. *Intens Care Med* 1994; **20**: 225–32.

Herringe MS, Cheung AM, *et al*. One-year outcome in survivors of the acute respiratory distress syndrome. *N Engl J Med* 2003; **348**: 683–93.

The Acute Respiratory Distress Syndrome Network. Ventilation with lower tidal volumes as compared with traditional tidal volumes for acute lung injury and the acute respiratory distress syndrome. *N Engl J Med* 2000; **342**: 1301–8.

Tobin MJ. Advances in mechanical ventilation. *N Engl J Med* 2001; **344**: 1986–96.

Ware LB, Matthay MA. The acute respiratory distress syndrome. *N Engl J Med* 2000; **342**: 1334–49.

Wyncoll DLA, Evans TW. Acute respiratory distress syndrome. *Lancet* 1999; **354**: 497–501.

Related topics of interest

Pneumonia – hospital acquired (p. 227)
Respiratory support – invasive (p. 260)
SIRS, sepsis and multiple organ failure (p. 276)
Weaning from ventilation (p. 331)

Adrenal disease

The adrenal cortex produces glucocorticoid, mineralocorticoid and sex hormones (mainly testosterone). Cortisol, the principal glucocorticoid, modulates stress and inflammatory responses. It is a potent stimulator of gluconeogenesis and antagonises insulin.

Aldosterone is the principal mineralocorticoid. It causes increased sodium reabsorption, and potassium and hydrogen ion loss at the distal renal tubule. Adrenal androgen production increases markedly at puberty, declining with age thereafter. Androstenedione is converted by the liver to testosterone in the male and oestrogen in the female. Cortisol and androgen production are under the diurnal pituitary control of adrenocorticotrophic hormone (ACTH) secreted by the anterior pituitary gland. Aldosterone is released in response to increased circulating angiotensin II, itself produced following renal renin release and subsequent pulmonary conversion of angiotensin I to angiotensin II.

Clinical diseases result from relative excess or lack of hormones. The conditions below are relevant to critical care.

Adrenocortical excess

1. **Cushing's syndrome** may result from steroid therapy, adrenal hyperplasia, adrenal carcinoma or ectopic ACTH.
2. **Cushing's disease** is due to an ACTH-secreting pituitary tumour.

Clinical features of adrenocortical excess include moon face, thin skin, easy bruising, hypertension (60%), hirsutism, obesity with a centripetal distribution, buffalo hump, muscle weakness, diabetes (10%), osteoporosis (50%), aseptic necrosis of the hip, and pancreatitis (especially with iatrogenic Cushing's syndrome).

Problems
- Control of blood sugar (insulin may be required).
- Hypokalaemia, resulting in arrhythmias, muscle weakness and postoperative or post critical illness respiratory impairment.
- Hypertension, polycythaemia and congestive heart failure.

Adrenocortical insufficiency

1. **Primary adrenocortical insufficiency** is commonly due to an autoimmune adrenalitis (Addison's disease) and may be associated with other autoimmune disorders. Females are affected more often than males. Other causes include adrenal infiltration with tumour, leukaemia, infection (TB, histoplasmosis) and amyloidosis.
2. **Secondary adrenocortical insufficiency** is caused by a deficiency of ACTH; it may occur as a result of administration of corticosteroid in sufficient dose to suppress ACTH release, or as a consequence of hypothalamic or pituitary dysfunction.

Adrenocortical insufficiency may present as either an acute disease or a slowly progressive chronic condition:

1. **Acute deficiency (Addisonian crisis)** may follow sepsis, pharmacological adrenal suppression or adrenal haemorrhage associated with anticoagulant therapy or meningococcal sepsis (Waterhouse–Friderichsen syndrome). Postpartum pituitary infarction (Sheehan's syndrome) may also present as acute adrenocortical insufficiency. Clinical features include apathy, hypotension, coma and hypoglycaemia. Circulatory failure and shock may be present, as may a history of recent infection. The diagnosis should be considered in all shocked patients in whom the cause is not immediately apparent. Adrenocortical insufficiency may be more common in the critically ill than previously suspected.
2. **Chronic deficiency** may follow surgical adrenalectomy or autoimmune adrenalitis, or be secondary to pituitary dysfunction. Clinical features include fatigue, weakness, weight loss, nausea and hyperpigmentation. Hypotension, hyponatraemia, hyperkalaemia, eosinophilia and occasionally hypoglycaemia may also occur.

Investigations
- Biochemistry to assess hyponatraemia, hypochloraemia, hyperkalaemia, hypercalcaemia, hypoglycaemia and a raised blood urea.
- Haematology may reveal an elevated haematocrit (dehydration) and possible eosinophilia.
- Endocrine investigations: a low cortisol level supports the diagnosis. An ACTH assay will differentiate between primary and secondary disease, being high in the former and low or normal in the latter. A raised baseline cortisol does not exclude insufficiency as it may accumulate in the presence of renal failure.
- Arterial blood gas analysis may show a metabolic acidosis with an additional respiratory contribution in the presence of severe muscle weakness.
- Immunology may reveal autoantibodies.

Management
Patients presenting with an acute crisis should be admitted to a critical care unit to enable invasive monitoring of circulatory pressures and arterial blood gases. Circulatory shock is treated in the usual way with initial attention to the critical elements covered by the ABC scheme of assessment/treatment. Large volumes (6–8 litres in 24h) of isotonic saline and inotropic support may be required in the first few hours of treatment.

Corticosteroids are given without waiting for confirmatory laboratory results. Hydrocortisone is administered as an intravenous bolus (100–200 mg), followed by 50 mg every 6 h.

Infection is treated with appropriate antibiotics.

Investigation and determination of the precipitating cause will guide further management.

Steroid withdrawal
Withdrawal of corticosteroid therapy may cause an acute Addisonian-type crisis. Patients who have been taking steroids (more than 10 mg daily) for periods in excess of 1 year are at particular risk, though the critically ill may show similar signs after much shorter treatment periods. Withdrawal of steroids should thus be gradual. If there is doubt about a patient's ability to restore normal adrenocortical function an ACTH stimulation test (Synacthen test) should be performed:

- Administer tetracosactrin (synthetic 1-24-ACTH (Synacthen)) 250 μg i.m.
- Measure baseline level and blood cortisol levels at 30 and 60 min following injection.

Diminished or absent cortisol response (peak value $<20\,\mu g\,dl^{-1}$) indicates insufficient endogenous adrenocortical activity.

Hyperaldosteronism – primary (Conn's syndrome)

This is caused by an adenoma in the zona glomerulosa secreting aldosterone. Clinical features include hypokalaemia, muscle weakness and hypertension.

Problems
- Hypokalaemia may result in cardiac arrhythmias, postoperative muscle weakness and ventilatory impairment.
- Hypertension.
- Hormone replacement required following adrenalectomy.

Steroid therapy in the critically ill

Steroids have important immunomodulatory effects (e.g. reducing transcription of proinflammatory genes) and contribute to the control of vascular tone. Acute illness normally provokes an increase in cortisol levels. However, critically ill patients may develop relative adrenal insufficiency, in which cortisol levels are raised but are still inadequate to control the inflammatory response. The diagnosis of relative adrenal insufficiency in critical illness is problematic but, following 250 μg tetracosactrin, an increase in serum cortisol of less than $9\,\mu g\,dl^{-1}$ from baseline is abnormal and is associated with an increased risk of death. A low-dose (1 μg) tetracosactrin test may be more sensitive for the diagnosis of relative adrenal insufficiency but this requires further validation. Patients with relative adrenal insufficiency should be given hydrocortisone 50 mg intravenously every 6 h. This will reduce the requirement for vasopressors and may increase survival. Therapy is often started before the results of a tetracosactrin test are available. The hydrocortisone should be stopped if the results do not indicate the presence of adrenal insufficiency; this therapy may be harmful in those with a normal adrenal response.

Adrenal medullary excess (phaeochromocytoma)

Phaeochromocytomata are rare chromaffin cell tumours of the sympathetic nervous system. They secrete catecholamines and the majority arise in the adrenal glands (10% are extra-adrenal and 10% are malignant). Patients present with the symptoms of catecholamine excess (tachycardia, sweating, hypertension, anxiety and autonomic dysfunction). Treatment is surgical but only after careful preoperative control of blood pressure (alpha-blockade, and, later, beta-blockade if required), fluid replacement (patients are centrally dehydrated following chronic vasoconstriction) and potassium and magnesium replacement. Postoperative admission to a critical care unit may be required to ensure a smooth transition from a state of catecholamine excess and hypotensive therapy to a normal blood pressure and hydration.

Further reading

Abraham E, Evans T. Corticosteroids and septic shock. *JAMA* 2002; **288**: 886–7.
Breslow MJ, Ligier B. Hyperadrenergic states. *Crit Care Med* 1991; **19**: 1566–78.
Cooper MS, Stewart PM. Corticosteroid insufficiency in acutely ill patients. *N Engl J Med* 2003; **348**: 727–34.

Related topics of interest

SIRS, sepsis and multiple organ failure (p. 276)

AIDS

Cynthia Uy

The 1993 Centers for Disease Control surveillance case definition for AIDS includes all HIV-infected persons who have a CD4 T-lymphocyte count $<200\,\text{ml}^{-1}$ of blood or a CD4 T-lymphocyte percentage of total lymphocytes below 14. Indicator diseases of AIDS include: *Pneumocystis carinii* pneumonia (PCP), pulmonary tuberculosis, extrapulmonary cryptococcosis, cryptosporidiosis, infection with cytomegalo and herpes simplex virus, coccidioidomycosis, toxoplasmosis, candidiasis, salmonella (nontyphoid) septicaemia, non-Hodgkin's lymphoma, Kaposi sarcoma, HIV encephalopathy and HIV wasting syndrome.

HIV can be transmitted by sexual contact (homosexual or heterosexual), blood or blood products (e.g. haemophiliacs and intravenous drug users) and by mother-to-child intrapartum, perinatally or through breast milk. There is a small risk of HIV transmission among health care workers who work with HIV-infected specimens. Needlestick and surgical knife accidents are the likeliest causes of seroconversion and data from several studies suggest that the risk of HIV infection following a percutaneous injury with an HIV-contaminated needle is approximately 0.3%. Infection of health care workers after exposure of broken skin or mucous membranes to HIV-infected materials has also been reported. At present, the risk of transmission from an infected health care worker to a patient is too low to be measured.

Since AIDS was first reported in 1981, there has been an exponential rise in the number of people infected with HIV worldwide. Currently, an estimated 34 million people are infected with the virus and, notably, women and children represent an increasing proportion of the AIDS patient population. Since 1996, death rates in developed nations have decreased and this is attributed to better prevention efforts, improved prophylaxis and treatment of opportunistic infection, and the use of highly active antiretroviral therapy.

With the rise in the number of cases of AIDS, there has been increasing use of critical care resources by HIV-infected patients. Initially, poor survival rates raised concerns that the intensive care of patients with AIDS was futile, unethical and not cost-effective; however, subsequent studies in the early 1990s have shown improvement in both survival rate and cost per life saved in these patients, for reasons which are unclear.

Despite the decreasing incidence of PCP, the commonest reason for HIV-infected patients to be admitted to a critical care unit is for ventilatory support for respiratory failure secondary to PCP. Other causes for admission are respiratory failure secondary to non-specific interstitial pneumonitis, bacterial pneumonia, ARDS, cardiac arrhythmia, congestive heart failure, hypotension due to sepsis or adrenal insufficiency, seizures, neurological disease, gastrointestinal disease, upper airway obstruction, drug toxicity and suicide attempts.

Pneumocystis carinii pneumonia

Presentation

This usually includes a prolonged prodromal illness, fever, dry cough and a characteristic pleuritic, retrosternal pain. Shortness of breath on exertion, lethargy and weight loss are seen in more advanced cases. Findings on examination are minimal. The CXR is either normal or, as severe PCP resembles ARDS, can show a faint bilateral interstitial infiltrate.

Laboratory evaluation

This is usually unhelpful. Studies of oxygen saturation and diffusing capacity for carbon monoxide are sensitive but not specific for PCP. A definitive diagnosis is made when the organism is identified in samples obtained from induced sputum, bronchoalveolar lavage or transbronchial or open lung biopsy. Serum lactate dehydrogenase (LDH) elevation is also frequently seen in patients with PCP.

Complications

Pneumothorax occurs in approximately 2% of cases, more so in patients who have had previous episodes of PCP or who have received prophylactic nebulised pentamidine. The mortality of PCP associated with pneumothorax is 10%. Sclerotherapy or surgical intervention may be indicated.

Treatment

Treatment is chiefly with intravenous co-trimoxazole or pentamidine isetionate. The main problem with therapy is the high incidence of side effects, exceeding 50% in most series. Adverse reactions to co-trimoxazole include nausea, vomiting, diarrhoea, rashes, glossitis, erythema multiforme, epidermal necrolysis, pancreatitis, blood dyscrasias, pseudomembranous colitis, jaundice and hepatic necrosis. Adverse reactions to pentamidine isetionate include hypoglycaemia, pancreatitis, cardiac arrhythmias, renal dysfunction, hypocalcaemia, blood dyscrasias, hyperglycaemia, rashes, bronchoconstriction and orthostatic hypotension.

Patients on treatment do not begin to improve until the end of the first week. Some patients clinically deteriorate during the first few days of treatment, presumably due to the deaths of large numbers of organisms in the lung resulting in increased capillary permeability and oedema formation.

Glucocorticoids used as adjuvant therapy with standard antipneumocystis treatment have been shown to reduce the risk of respiratory failure and death in patients with AIDS, when instituted within 24–72 h of treatment. They are indicated in AIDS patients with a $PaO_2 < 9.3$ kPa or an arterial/alveolar gradient > 4.66 kPa. Further studies on the use of steroids in this setting are needed before definitive recommendations can be made on dose and duration of treatment.

CPAP has been successful in improving arterial oxygenation in patients with PCP-associated respiratory failure. If full mechanical ventilation is needed, generally high respiratory rates by assist control or intermittent mandatory ventilation (IMV) modes are needed. PEEP can modestly increase oxygenation.

Advanced directives while the patient is capable of making informed decision should be encouraged, either as a living will or by designating a person with durable power of attorney.

Prevention

Universal precautions

Universal precautions, which assume that all patients may be infected, are recommended to minimise the chances of transmission of HIV. Guidelines include:

- The use of gloves when there is any risk of contact with infective body fluids.
- The wearing of masks and protective eyewear, when infective fluids may become airborne and the wearing of gowns made of impervious material if there is any chance of being splashed.
- Open or exudative wounds should be covered and contact with potentially infective fluids avoided. If any contact with body fluids occurs, the affected part should be washed immediately.
- Needles must not be resheathed or passed from one person to another. In the event of a needlestick injury, the wound should be washed and confidential advice, including the role of prophylactic drug therapy, should be sought.
- Contaminated waste must be segregated, placed in a suitable leakproof container and contained at the place it is generated before being disposed of in an appropriate manner.
- It is advisable, given the high prevalence of hepatitis B and pulmonary tuberculosis in HIV patients, for staff to be immunised/vaccinated.

Additional precautions

In addition, to protect other patients:

- All blood and blood products should be screened for antibodies to HIV. Transmission can occur in the 3-month 'window period' between infection and seroconversion, or due to clerical errors in reporting results or labelling blood. This risk is less than one in a million per transfused unit of blood.
- Disposable equipment should be used for infected patients. Reusable devices used in invasive procedures must be disinfected and sterilised.
- In HIV-infected patients with undiagnosed respiratory illness, tuberculosis must be considered and patients nursed in a single room. Mechanical ventilators should be fitted with exhaled gas scavenging systems and a filter.
- The isolation of seropositive patients is not appropriate unless the patient is bleeding or requires isolation due to immunosuppression or a contagious secondary infection. HIV-infected individuals should not carry out procedures where their hands are not completely visible.

Further reading

Afessa B, Green B. Clinical course, prognostic factors and outcome prediction for HIV patients in the ICU. *Chest* 2000; **118**: 138–45.

De Palo VA, Millstein BH, Mayo PH, *et al.* Outcome of intensive care in patients with HIV infection. *Chest* 1995; **107**: 506–10.

Huang L, Zimmerman L. Critical care of patients with HIV. HIV InSite Knowledge Base Chapter, Feb 1998. University of California, San Francisco.
http://hivinsite.ucsf.edu/InSite

Related topics of interest

Analgesia in critical care – basic

The International Society for the Study of Pain defines pain as 'an unpleasant sensory and emotional experience associated with actual or potential tissue damage or described in terms of such damage'.

Problems

1. Assessment of pain is difficult in critical care patients. Injury, intoxication or sedation may impair their conscious state. Intubated and paralysed patients cannot respond verbally. There may be multiple foci for pain from injury, surgery, invasive monitors and indwelling catheters. It may be difficult to distinguish pain from anxiety; the two will often coexist.
2. Haemodynamic instability, renal failure and hepatic failure will influence the pharmacodynamics and pharmacokinetics of analgesic strategies. Coagulopathy will preclude the use of regional catheter techniques.
3. The need for sedation (and sometimes paralysis) coexists with the need for analgesics.
4. Prolonged infusion of opioids leads to tolerance, dependence and accumulation of the drug and its metabolites, especially in renal or hepatic failure.
5. Misunderstanding of the importance of analgesia may lead to underprescribing and underdosing of drugs. A majority of patients discharged from critical care units (60–70%) recall being in pain. Patients suffering ischaemic cardiac pain may minimise and under-report their pain. The early administration of effective analgesia to patients with abdominal pain does not interfere with diagnosis.

Pain assessment

It is difficult to make an objective measure of a subjective experience. Tools of assessment include adjective, numeric or behaviour and physiological parameters:

1. **Adjective scale.** None, mild, moderate, severe, intolerable.
2. **Visual analogue scale (VAS).** Pain is indicated on a 10cm scale continuum or expressed as a numeric value from 0 to 10.
3. **Happy and sad faces.** A qualitative scale for paediatric patients.
4. **Poker chips.** A quantitative measure in paediatric patients expressed in number of chips (between 1 and 4).
5. **Observer scale.** For non-communicative or intubated patients. This scores a series of behavioural and physiological parameters, including vital signs, non-vocal communication, facial expression, posture and agitation.

Pain assessment must be continuous and should include the response to an intervention and subsequent adjustments in therapy.

Non-pharmacological pain management

- Attention to aspects of nursing with repositioning and pressure area care. Positioning of catheters and invasive monitors so that they don't drag. Elevation of limbs assists venous drainage and prevents stasis oedema. Circulatory assessment of covered limbs. Relief of urinary retention. Correct posture for optimal ventilation.
- Physiotherapy, both passive and active.
- Relaxation techniques reduce distress and use of analgesic medication and increase comfort. Cognitive–behavioural interventions are time consuming but may have a positive effect on pain management and, despite pragmatic considerations, should not be considered invalid.
- Psychological support is important: talking to and explaining procedures, even to sedated or unconscious patients, may reduce overall stress. Involvement of relatives and friends.
- Transcutaneous electrical nerve stimulation (TENS): see Analgesia in critical care – advanced (p. 22).

Pharmacological pain management

Non-steroidal anti-inflammatory drugs (NSAIDs)

Paracetamol

Paracetamol is an analgesic and antipyretic. It inhibits central and peripheral prostaglandin synthesis. It is a poor anti-inflammatory. It has few irritant side effects and is excreted by the kidney following hepatic conjugation. Paracetamol has a ceiling effect and is used for mild pain. It is given orally (or by NGT) or rectally. A parenteral form is available in some countries. It should be given regularly if it is to have an opioid sparing effect.

Other NSAIDs

These non-opioids are reversible inhibitors of cyclo-oxygenase, or COX (the enzyme responsible for prostaglandin synthesis), reducing levels of prostaglandin, prostacyclin and thromboxane A_2 pain mediators. There are two COX enzymes: COX-1 regulates physiological function in the gut, including the production of protective prostaglandins in the stomach, and kidney; COX-2 is induced in inflammation and repair. Both enzymes are inhibited by non-specific NSAIDs. COX-2 inhibitors have little effect on COX-1 activity and so do not inhibit prostaglandin synthesis. COX-2 inhibitors should provide the same analgesic efficacy as the non-selective NSAIDs with fewer gastrointestinal adverse reactions. COX-2 inhibitors include rofecoxib and celecoxib. Parecoxib is an injectable COX-2 inhibitor.

NSAIDs have both a central and peripheral role in blocking the prostaglandin-mediated lowering of pain receptor thresholds and are useful for the management of mild-to-moderate pain. They can be used in combination with opioids and regional analgesic techniques. Salicylates are non-reversible inhibitors of prostaglandins.

Side effects of NSAIDs

Gastrointestinal effects.   Gastrointestinal erosions are due to local irritation, reduced gastric blood flow and increased acid secretion mediated by prostaglandin inhibition. Rectal and parenteral routes may lessen the risk. H_2 antagonists and proton pump inhibitors may reduce the risks also.

Blood disorders. Platelet aggregation homeostasis is mediated by a balance between the platelet-derived thromboxane A_2 (promotes aggregation) and endothelial-derived prostacyclin (a vasodilator which inhibits aggregation). Aspirin-induced inhibition of platelet function is irreversible, prolonging bleeding time for the life of the platelet (8–11 days). Other NSAIDs will affect bleeding time for five times the half-life of the drug.

Asthma. Aspirin-induced asthma may occur in some adult asthmatics. Cross-sensitivity with other NSAIDs does exist.

Renal effects. Renal failure may be precipitated when prostaglandin-dependent intrarenal blood flow is reduced in patients with reduced intravascular volume. In volume-depleted states, compensatory humoral and sympathetic homeostatic responses will reduce renal blood flow in an effort to conserve water and sodium. The only remaining vasodilatory mechanism that maintains renal blood flow is prostaglandin dependent. Prostaglandin inhibition by NSAIDs, alone or in combination with the administration of other renal toxins (aminoglycoside antibiotics, contrast media) or pre-existing renal impairment, may precipitate acute tubular necrosis. NSAIDs may promote sodium, potassium and water retention, causing oedema.

Opioid analgesics

Opioids are those analgesics with morphine-like actions. They may be opiates: derivatives of the opium poppy *Papaver somniferum* (morphine and codeine) or synthetic analogues (pethidine, fentanyl, methadone). They are agonists at opioid receptors in the central and peripheral nervous systems.

Opioid receptors are subclassed as mu, kappa and delta. Opioid analgesics are primarily mu receptor agonists. They produce both excitatory and inhibitory phenomena, including analgesia, respiratory depression, euphoria, bradycardia, pruritus, meiosis, nausea and vomiting (via the chemoreceptor trigger zone) and inhibition of gut motility.

In equianalgesic doses, and in most patients, the incidence of side effects is similar regardless of the opioid used.

Side effects of opioids

Respiratory effects. Respiratory depression, with direct depression of the respiratory centre in the medulla, causes reduced respiratory rate and tidal volume and reduced sensitivity to hypercapnoea. Suppression of cough reflex reduces sputum clearance and may risk airway soiling. The best early sign of opioid-induced respiratory depression is sedation. Decreased respiratory rate is a late and unreliable sign. Sedation may be due to the combined effect of opioid and elevated $PaCO_2$. Thus, respiratory depression can coexist with a normal respiratory rate and, if the patient is receiving supplemental oxygen, a normal PaO_2 does not preclude hypoventilation.

Cardiovascular side effects. These are due to direct arterial and venous smooth muscle relaxation and histamine release (morphine, diamorphine, pethidine and codeine) causing vasodilatation. Postural hypotension may occur. Significant supine hypotension suggests hypovolaemia that is unmasked by opioids. Vagally mediated bradycardia can occur. Pethidine, however, has atropine-like effects and mediates tachycardia.

Pruritus. This may be histamine or non-histamine mediated. Mast cell histamine release localised to the site of injection or along the vein of injection may cause localised or generalised pruritus and is not indicative of opioid allergy. Centrally mediated pruritus is possibly mu receptor mediated and is more commonly associated with epidural or intrathecal opioid, especially morphine. Pruritus may be treated with antihistamines or naloxone.

Bowel motility. This is reduced by local and central mechanisms and causes constipation and aggravates ileus. Sphincter of Oddi spasm and urinary retention can be reversed by naloxone.

True opioid allergy is not common. It is mediated by the immune system, resulting in rash, urticaria, bronchoconstriction, CVS collapse and angio-oedema.

In general, dosage varies inversely with age (not size). There is still a ten-fold variation in dose requirements between individuals of the same age. The initial dose should be based on patient age and subsequent doses titrated to suit the individual with respect to renal and hepatic function and cardiorespiratory function.

Equianalgesic doses
Equianalgesic doses of opioids are given in Table 1.

Table 1 Equianalgesic doses of opioids

Opioid	i.m./i.v. (mg)	Oral (mg)	Elimination half life $t_{1/2}\beta$ (h)
Morphine	10	30–60	2–3
Pethidine	100	400	3–4
Fentanyl	0.1	N/A	3–4
Alfentanil			
Codeine[a]	130	200	3–4
Oxycodone	15	10–20	2–3
Diamorphine	5	60	0.5 (rapidly hydrolysed to morphine)
Methadone	10	20	15–40

[a]The metabolic conversion of codeine to morphine is subject to wide pharmacogenetic variation. It is a poor choice of analgesic in critical care.

Adjuvant therapy
Anxiolysis. Hypnotic medication providing sedation will reduce distress and form adjuvant therapy to analgesics.

Antidepressants. Useful during long-term critical care admissions for mood elevation. They can be weaned following recovery. Tricyclic antidepressants are commonly used.

Drug tolerance and withdrawal
Tolerance results when, over time, more drug is needed to produce the same effect. It occurs with long-term administration of opioids. It may be due to altered drug receptor affinity and may be minimised by using the lowest dose possible to achieve analgesia.

Withdrawal phenomena will be experienced when drugs to which the patient is tolerant are ceased abruptly. Such drugs should be withdrawn slowly. Substitution with drugs with a long half-life may be of benefit.

Addiction is a behavioural phenomenon and occurs rarely in a clinical setting. Addicts demonstrate tolerance and suffer withdrawal.

Further reading

www.nice.org.uk/pdf/coxiifullguidance.pdf

Related topics of interest

Analgesia in critical care – advanced (p. 22)

Analgesia in critical care – advanced

Epidural analgesia

Infusion of a combination of local anaesthetics and/or an opioid into the epidural space will block and modify the conduction of pain impulses.

Benefits
- Selective sensory nerve blockade.
- High-quality analgesia.
- The reduced or absent systemic plasma concentration of opioid reduces or avoids opioid-related side effects.
- The quality of comfort is beneficial for physiotherapy, positioning and nursing.
- Weaning from ventilation is assisted by the absence of opioid-related sedation and respiratory depression.

Disadvantages and complications
- Expertise required to site the epidural catheter.
- Hypotension due to sympathetic nerve blockade.
- Risk of infection in the epidural space increases with the duration of catheter placement.
- Small risk of nerve root or cord damage, epidural haematoma, infection with neurological sequelae (transient: $\sim 1:4000$, permanent: $\sim 1:35000$).
- Catheter misplacement into subarachnoid space causing massive subarachnoid block with bradycardia, hypotension and loss of consciousness.
- Catheter misplacement into a vessel causing systemic local anaesthetic toxicity with CNS and then CVS collapse.
- Dural puncture headache which may be confused with meningism.

Drug actions
Local anaesthetics
Local anaesthetics block sodium channels, preventing neural transmission. Higher concentrations are required to block motor nerves which have the thickest myelin sheath. Unmyelinated and lightly myelinated C and A delta pain and temperature fibres are blocked at low concentrations. Autonomic nerves are also blocked; thus, vasodilatation and hypotension are side effects. Intravenous fluid loading and vasopressors are used to combat hypotension. Blockade at the level of cardioaccelerator fibres $T_1–T_4$ will cause bradycardia and hypotension.

Opioids
Opioids act at opioid receptors in the dorsal horn to provide analgesia. Highly lipid-soluble fentanyl will act near the site of absorption across the dura. Less lipid-soluble morphine has a longer half-life in the CSF, and may circulate up to the medulla, causing respiratory depression. This risk persists for 18–24 h. Morphine and fentanyl do not block sensory autonomic or motor nerves.

Extensive cover is provided by larger volumes or by simultaneous epidurals at two levels (lumbar and thoracic).

Contraindications to epidural analgesia
- Patient refusal.
- Infection at the site of insertion.
- Coagulopathy (risk of epidural haematoma).
- Septicaemia is a relative contraindication (theoretical risk of epidural abscess).

Patient-controlled analgesia (PCA)

Some patients receiving critical care may be sufficiently orientated and motivated to utilise PCA. A drug delivery system (syringe driver) delivers a bolus of opioid upon demand by the patient. The patient should be reassured about addiction and over-dosage. They should be instructed to anticipate pain (e.g. prior to physiotherapy) and advised to use regular dosing rather than allow severe pain to develop.

Transcutaneous electrical nerve stimulation (TENS)

Low-frequency pulses of electricity from electrodes placed over the dermatome of pain stimulate large nerve fibres, which in turn transmit to the dorsal horn substantia gelatinosa cells. Input from large fibres produces negative feedback in the substantia gelatinosa, preventing onward transmission of nociceptive signals.

Ketamine

This phencyclidine derivative may be used in conjunction with benzodiazepines for short painful procedures. It provides good analgesia without respiratory depression at subanaesthetic concentrations; its unpleasant psychological sequelae are minimised by concomitant benzodiazepines.

Clonidine

An imidazoline derivative that is a centrally acting antihypertensive, clonidine also has analgesic actions and is given by continuous epidural infusion for the control of intractable cancer pain. Clonidine is most commonly used in critical care patients to provide sedation, especially in those experiencing drug or alcohol withdrawal. Its analgesic actions may also be of benefit, though it is more likely to help with neuro-pathic pain than with somatic or visceral pain.

Related topics of interest

Anaphylaxis

Adverse immunological responses may be anaphylactic (IgE mediated) or anaphylactoid (non-IgE mediated and often following first exposure to the trigger agent). Anaphylactic reactions occur following 'classical' pathway complement activation. Previous exposure to the antigen with antibody formation is required. 'Alternative' pathway activation occurs when the trigger activates the cascade directly; previous exposure to the antigen is not necessary (e.g. reactions to drugs, dextrans or contrast media). Reactions to drugs may also occur as a consequence of direct activation of mast cells by the drug (pharmacological histamine release) and do not involve complement activation (e.g. after administration of certain muscle relaxants).

The manifestations and management of severe anaphylactic and anaphylactoid reactions are similar. The distinction is thus less important in the acute phase, though it may aid follow-up management.

Clinical signs and symptoms

Typically, patients present with angio-oedema, urticaria, dyspnoea and hypotension. Features include:

- Cardiovascular collapse due to vasodilatation and loss of plasma from the circulating compartment. It is present in 90% of patients and is the only feature in 10%.
- Bronchospasm, present in 50% and the only feature in 3%.
- Acute upper airway obstruction due to laryngeal oedema.
- Skin erythema (urticaria), conjunctivitis, rhinitis.
- Gastrointestinal symptoms, including nausea, vomiting, abdominal pain and diarrhoea.

Anaphylactic reactions vary in severity and progression. The onset may be rapid, slow or (unusually) biphasic.

Treatment considerations

1. Adrenaline (epinephrine) is the most important drug for the treatment of severe reactions. Its alpha-adrenoceptor agonism reverses peripheral vasodilatation and reduces oedema. Its beta-adrenoceptor activity dilates the airways, increases the force of myocardial contractility and suppresses release of mediators such as histamine and leukotrienes. Adrenaline works best when given shortly after the onset of a reaction. Its use is not without risk, however, especially when given intravenously. Rarely, adrenaline may fail to reverse the signs of a severe reaction, especially if given late or to a patient already being treated with beta-blockers. Under such circumstances aggressive volume replacement may be life-saving.
2. Anti-H_1 antihistamines should be given to all patients suffering an anaphylactic reaction. They help combat histamine-mediated vasodilatation and control symptoms such as urticaria.
3. Corticosteroids are slow-onset drugs whose action may take 4–6h to develop,

even after intravenous administration. They are not life-saving drugs in anaphylaxis. They may be useful, however, in preventing recurrent or shortening protracted reactions and thus should be given to all victims of a severe reaction.

Management

A. Airway. 100% oxygen by facemask.
B. Breathing. Bag and mask ventilation if assistance needed. Intubate if there is serious airway obstruction or in cardiac arrest.
C. Circulation. Intramuscular adrenaline requires an effective circulation. Give intravenous fluids.

Adrenaline (epinephrine)
Give adrenaline intramuscularly to all patients with signs of shock, airway swelling or breathing difficulty.

Adults
Give 0.5 ml of a 1:1000 solution of adrenaline i.m. (i.e. 500 μg).
In the critical care unit it is more appropriate to titrate 0.5–1 ml of a 1:10 000 solution of adrenaline intravenously, i.e. 50–100 μg. Intravenous adrenaline should not be given without continuous ECG monitoring.

It should be repeated after 5 min if there are no signs of improvement or the patient deteriorates.

Caution. Patients receiving monoamine oxidase inhibitors should be given only 25% of the dose of adrenaline at a time due to a potentially dangerous interaction.

Children
>11 years	up to 500 μg i.m. (0.5 ml 1:1000 solution)
6–11 years	250 μg i.m. (0.25 ml 1:1000 solution)
2–5 years	125 μg i.m. (0.125 ml 1:1000 solution)
<2 years	62.5 μg i.m. (by additional dilution of 1:100 solution)

If anaphylaxis is thought to have been precipitated by a drug or infusion, stop giving it immediately.

Antihistamine
Give an antihistamine (e.g. chlorpheniramine 10–20 mg).

Hydrocortisone
Give hydrocortisone (100–500 mg i.m. or by slow i.v. injection) for severe attacks especially in asthmatics.

β_2-Agonists
Give inhaled β_2-agonists to patients with persisting bronchospasm (see Asthma, p. 38).

Investigation

Once the patient has recovered from the immediate life-threatening reaction, they should be investigated for the cause.

Non-specific tests

Take blood samples for measurement of complement and tryptase. An elevated blood C3 and C4 complement level indicates an immune-mediated response. Elevation of C3 alone suggests alternative pathway activation. Total IgE antibody levels may also be measured. Blood histamine levels may be elevated for a short time only, but its metabolite methylhistamine has a longer half-life and is measurable in urine up to 2–3 h following a reaction. Tryptase, a mast cell-specific protease released during degranulation, may also remain in the blood for about 3 h.

Specific tests

Drug-specific antibodies may be quantified using labelled anti-human IgE antibody by a radioallergosorbent test (RAST).

Skin testing

These tests should be performed only where full resuscitation facilities are immediately available. The optimum time for testing is 6 weeks following a reaction. The patient should not be taking drugs that may interfere with the response (e.g. corticosteroids, antihistamines).

Intradermal testing utilises dilute solutions of potential antigens. Solutions of the test agents are diluted to 1:1000 and 1:100 and a control solution (e.g. saline) prepared. A 1 mm weal of each solution is then raised on the forearm of the patient. A positive result occurs when a weal > 10 mm persists for more than 30 min.

Skin prick testing is safer, quicker and easier to perform (the test agent does not require dilution). A drop of solution is placed on the skin and a puncture made through it (< 1 mm). A wheal > 3 mm after 15 min is considered a positive result.

Further reading

Brown AFT. Anaphylactic shock: mechanisms and treatment. *J Accident Emerg Med* 1995; **12**: 89–100.

Project Team of The Resuscitation Council (UK). *The Emergency Medical Treatment of Anaphylactic Reactions for First Medical Responders and for Community Nurses.* London: Resuscitation Council (UK), 2002.

Working Party of the Association of Anaesthetists of Great Britain and Ireland. *Suspected Anaphylactic Reactions Associated with Anaesthesia,* 3rd edn, 2003.
http://www.aagbi.org/pdf/ Anaphylaxis.pdf

Related topics of interest

Arterial blood gases – acid–base physiology

Alex Goodwin

A biochemical milieu maintained within a narrow range is required for the normal function of enzymes within the cells of the body. The concentration of hydrogen ions (H^+) is low but crucial for normal enzyme function.

The following definitions are essential to the understanding of acid–base physiology:

Acid	Proton donor
Base	Proton acceptor
Strong acid	Fully dissociates in solution
Weak acid	Partially dissociates in solution
Buffer	A chemical substance that prevents large changes in H^+ concentration when an acid or base is added to a solution
Acidaemia	Decrease in pH
Acidosis	Increase in H^+ concentration

The normal plasma concentration of sodium is $140\,mmol\,l^{-1}$, whereas that of H^+ is $0.00004\,mmol\,l^{-1}$. Thus, H^+ concentration is represented as pH, which is the negative $\log_{10}$ of the H^+ concentration. The normal extracellular pH is 7.4, venous blood 7.35, red blood cells 7.2, muscle cells 6.8–7.0 (in anaerobic metabolism 6.40) and that of CSF 7.32.

Aerobic metabolism produces 1400 mmol of carbon dioxide per day. This is termed volatile acid because it is excreted via the lungs. Amino acid metabolism produces approximately 80 mmol per day of non-volatile acid. Anaerobic metabolism produces lactic acid and the abnormal metabolism of fats produces keto acids (e.g. diabetic ketoacidosis).

The body's defence against an H^+ load involves the following compensatory mechanisms:

Dilution

Acid produced in cells is diluted in total body water because it diffuses into the extra-cellular fluid and into other cells. Each ten-fold dilution increases the pH by 1 unit.

Buffers

An acid–base buffer is a solution of two or more chemical compounds that prevents marked changes in H^+ concentration when an acid or a base is added. The pK of a buffer system defines the pH at which the ionised and unionised forms are in equilibrium. It is also the pH at which the buffer system is most efficient.

Important buffer systems are plasma and cells (including blood).

The Henderson–Hasselbalch equation considers the relationship of a buffer system to pH:

$$pH = pKa + \log_{10} base/acid$$

For the bicarbonate system:

$$pH = 6.1 + \log_{10} HCO_3^-/PaCO_2$$

Hence, at plasma bicarbonate of $24\,\text{mmol}\,l^{-1}$ and a $PaCO_2$ of $5.3\,\text{kPa}$ the equation becomes:

$$pH = 6.1 + \log_{10} 24/(2.3 \times 5.3)$$

where 2.3 = solubility coefficient of carbon dioxide $(\text{mmol}\,\text{kPa}^{-1})$

$$pH = 7.4$$

Respiratory compensation

The respiratory system is able to regulate pH. An increase in CO_2 concentration leads to a decrease in pH and a decrease in CO_2 leads to a rise in pH. If the metabolic production of CO_2 remains constant, the only factor that affects CO_2 concentration is alveolar ventilation. The respiratory centre in the medulla oblongata is sensitive to H^+ concentration and changes alveolar ventilation accordingly. This affects H^+ concentration within minutes. Thus, the respiratory system is a 'physiological buffer'.

Renal control

The kidneys control acid–base balance by controlling the secretion of H^+ relative to the amount of filtered bicarbonate.

Tubular secretion of hydrogen ions

Hydrogen ions are secreted throughout most of the tubular system. There are two distinct methods of secretion:

- Secondary active transport of H^+ occurs in the proximal tubule, thick segment of the ascending loop of Henle, and the distal tubule. Within the epithelial cell, carbon dioxide combines with water under the influence of carbonic anhydrase to form carbonic acid. This then dissociates into a H^+ and bicarbonate. The H^+ is secreted into the tubular lumen by a mechanism of sodium/hydrogen counter-transport.
- Primary active transport occurs in the latter part of the distal tubules all the way to the renal pelvis. This transport system accounts for less than 5% of the total H^+ secreted. However, it can concentrate H^+ 900-fold compared with four-fold for secondary active transport. The rate of H^+ secretion changes in response to alterations in extracellular H^+ concentration.

Interaction of bicarbonate and hydrogen ions in the tubules

The bicarbonate ion does not diffuse into the epithelial cells of the renal tubules readily because it is a large molecule and is electrically charged. However, it combines with a secreted H^+ to form carbon dioxide and water and is, effectively, 'reabsorbed'. The CO_2 diffuses into the epithelial cell and combines with water to form carbonic acid, which immediately dissociates to bicarbonate and H^+. The bicarbonate ion then diffuses into the extracellular fluid.

The rate of H^+ secretion is about $3.5\,mmol\,min^{-1}$ and the rate of filtration of bicarbonate is $3.46\,mmol\,min^{-1}$. Normally, the H^+ and bicarbonate titrate themselves. The mechanism by which the kidney corrects either acidosis or alkalosis is by incomplete titration. An excess of H^+ in the urine can be buffered by phosphate and ammonia.

The liver

The liver assists in acid–base balance by regulating ureagenesis. Amino acid metabolism leads to the generation of bicarbonate and ammonia. These combine to form urea, CO_2 and water:

$$2NH_4^+ + 2HCO_3^- \leftrightharpoons NH_2\text{–}CO\text{–}NH_2 + CO_2 + 3H_2O$$

The lungs remove the CO_2 and there is no net acid or base production. The liver is able to regulate the metabolism of ammonia and bicarbonate to urea. In alkalosis, ureagenesis increases, consuming bicarbonate. In acidosis, ureagenesis decreases, increasing available bicarbonate. The liver also affects acid–base balance by carbon dioxide production from complete oxidation of substrates (carbohydrates and fats), metabolism of organic acid anions (lactate, ketones and amino acids) and the production of plasma proteins, especially albumin.

Bone

Extracellular H^+ can exchange with cations from bone and cells (e.g. sodium, potassium, magnesium and calcium). This is a slow process and may take hours or days.

The Stewart approach to acid–base balance

The concept of acid–base balance has historically been expressed in terms of the balance between respiratory and non-respiratory (metabolic) systems. Stewart's physicochemical approach is similar to the traditional empirical approach in its classification and measurement of acid–base disturbances. The difference lies in the explanation and interpretation of acid–base disturbances and control mechanisms. Stewart's approach is conceptually simple and elegant but is operationally complicated and unwieldy.

The biochemistry of aqueous solutions is complex. All human solutions contain water, which is an inexhaustible supply of H^+. Hydrogen ion concentration is determined by the dissociation of water. The laws of physical chemistry, particularly electroneutrality and conservation of mass, determine the dissociation of water. In plasma, the determinants of H^+ concentration can be reduced to three: strong ion difference (SID), partial pressure of carbon dioxide (PCO_2) and total weak acid concentration (A_{TOT}). Neither H^+ concentration nor bicarbonate ion concentration can change unless there is a change in one or more of these variables. The principle of conservation of mass shows that strong ions can neither be destroyed nor created to satisfy electroneutrality, but H^+ are generated or consumed by changes in water dissociation.

Saline administration

$$\text{Strong ion difference} = (Na^+ + K^+ + Ca^+ + Mg^+) - (Cl^- + lactate^-)$$

From the above equation, sodium and chloride are the principal tools in altering SID.

An increase in sodium with respect to chloride increases the SID and increases the pH. The reverse occurs with an increase in chloride relative to sodium. An increase in SID leads to a reduction in water dissociation and hence a reduction in plasma H^+. As sodium is controlled to maintain tonicity, it appears that chloride is the principal tool in altering SID and hence plasma pH. Loss of strong anions, e.g. in conditions associated with nasogastric aspirates, will cause an increase in SID.

A decrease in SID may be brought about by the addition of strong anions (lactate or chloride). When saline is given to a patient, the relative excess of chloride reduces the SID and increases the dissociation of water and, therefore, the plasma H^+.

Stewart's approach provides an alternative method for assessing acid–base abnormalities. In particular, it provides a useful explanation for the aetiology of hyperchloraemic acidosis, which is seen commonly in critically ill patients.

Further reading

Gluck SL. Acid–base. *Lancet* 1998; **352**: 474–9.

Kellum JA. Acid–base physiology in the post-Copernicum era. *Curr Opin Crit Care* 1999; **5**: 429–36.

Related topics of interest

Arterial blood gases – analysis (p. 31)

Arterial blood gases – analysis

Alex Goodwin

An understanding of arterial blood gases (ABGs) is fundamental to the management of critically ill patients. Having processed an arterial blood sample, the blood gas analyser typically will display the following information:

PaO_2 – partial pressure of oxygen in arterial blood

This is measured directly. The PaO_2 is always less than the PAO_2 because of shunt. The relationship between the PAO_2 and the fractional inspired oxygen concentration (FIO_2), is described by the alveolar gas equation:

$$PAO_2 = FIO_2 (P_b - P_{H_2O}) - PACO_2/RQ$$

PAO_2 = Alveolar oxygen pressure	FIO_2 = Inspired oxygen fraction
P_b = Atmospheric pressure	PA_{H_2O} = Water vapour pressure
$PACO_2$ = Alveolar CO_2 pressure	RQ = Respiratory quotient

When breathing air at an atmospheric pressure of 100kPa (760mmHg), the partial pressure of inspired oxygen is 20.9kPa (158mmHg). Having become fully saturated with water in the upper respiratory tract the partial pressure of oxygen falls to 19.5kPa (148mmHg). At the alveolus, oxygen is taken up and replaced by CO_2, which reduces the PaO_2 to 14kPa (106mmHg). Because of shunt, the arterial oxygen pressure is always slightly lower than that in the alveolus. Shunt increases with age. When breathing air, the normal PaO_2 is 12.5kPa (92mmHg) at the age of 20 years and 10.8kPa (82mmHg) at 65 years.

$PaCO_2$ – partial pressure of carbon dioxide in arterial blood

This is measured directly and is normally 5.3kPa (40mmHg).

pH

This is the negative $\log_{10}$ of the hydrogen ion concentration and is measured directly. The normal pH is 7.35–7.45.

Standard bicarbonate

This is calculated from the CO_2 and pH using the Henderson–Hasselbalch equation. It is the concentration of bicarbonate in a sample equilibrated to 37°C and $PaCO_2$ 5.3kPa. Thus, the metabolic component of acid–base balance can be assessed. The normal value is 21–27 mmol l^{-1}.

Actual bicarbonate

This reflects the contribution of both the respiratory and metabolic components. The normal value in venous blood is $21–28\,mmol\,l^{-1}$.

Base excess and base deficit

This is a measure of the amount of acid or base that needs to be added to a sample, under standard conditions (37°C and $PaCO_2$ 5.3 kPa), to return the pH to 7.4. It is traditionally reported as 'base excess'. The normal range is $+2\,mmol\,l^{-1}$ to $-2\,mmol\,l^{-1}$.

Interpretation of blood gas data

When evaluating respiratory and acid–base disorders, arterial blood gas data must be considered within the context of the wider clinical picture. Having noted the FIO_2 and PaO_2, the ABG results should be assessed as follows:

1. Assess the hydrogen ion concentration:
   pH > 7.45 – alkalaemia
   pH < 7.35 – acidaemia
   7.35–7.45 – no disturbance or mixed disturbance
2. Assess the metabolic component:
   $HCO_3^- > 33\,mmol\,l^{-1}$ – metabolic alkalosis
   $HCO_3^- < 23\,mmol\,l^{-1}$ – metabolic acidosis
3. Assess the respiratory component:
   $PaCO_2 > 5.9\,kPa$ – respiratory acidosis
   $PaCO_2 < 4.6\,kPa$ – respiratory alkalosis
4. Combine the information from 1, 2 and 3 and determine if there is any metabolic or respiratory compensation.
5. Consider the anion gap. This indicates the presence of non-volatile acids (lactic acid, keto acids and exogenous acids). The normal anion gap is $10–18\,mmol\,l^{-1}$ and can be estimated using the following equation:

$$([Na^+] + [K^+]) - ([Cl^-] + [HCO3^-])$$

Disorders of acid–base balance are divided into acidosis and alkalosis and into those of metabolic and respiratory origin. They can be subdivided by the presence or absence of an abnormal anion gap.

Pre-analytical sources of error include air bubbles, time delays, heparin, leucocytosis, halothane and labelling. When blood is cooled, CO_2 becomes more soluble; hence PCO_2 falls. With every degree centigrade fall in temperature, pH increases by 0.015. Haemoglobin accepts more hydrogen ions when cooled.

Disorders of acid–base balance

1. Metabolic acidosis (with a normal anion gap)
- Increased gastrointestinal bicarbonate loss (e.g. diarrhoea, ileostomy, ureterosigmoidostomy).

- Increased renal bicarbonate loss (e.g. acetazolamide, proximal renal tubular acidosis (type 2), hyperparathyroidism, tubular damage, e.g. drugs, heavy metals, paraproteins).
- Decreased renal hydrogen secretion (e.g. distal renal tubular acidosis (type 1), type 4 renal tubular acidosis (aldosterone deficiency)).
- Increased HCl production (e.g. ammonium chloride ingestion, increased catabolism of lysine).

2. Metabolic acidosis with abnormal anion gap
Accumulation of organic acids. A useful memory aid is the acronym KUSMEL: Ketones, Uraemia, Salicylate, Methanol, Ethylene glycol, Lactate.

- Lactic acidosis
  L-lactic acid – Type A (anaerobic metabolism, hypotension/cardiac arrest, sepsis, poisoning – ethylene glycol, methanol). Type B (decreased hepatic lactate metabolism, insulin deficiency, metformin accumulation, haematological malignancies, rare inherited enzyme defects).
  D-lactic acid (fermentation of glucose in the bowel, e.g. in blind loops).
- Ketoacidosis (e.g. insulin deficiency, alcohol excess, starvation).
- Exogenous acids (e.g. salicylates).

3. Metabolic alkalosis
- Loss of acid (e.g. hydrogen ion loss from GI tract – vomiting, nasogastric suction, hydrogen loss from kidney – diuretics, hypokalaemia, excess mineralocorticoid, low chloride states – diuretic therapy).
- Addition of alkali (e.g. sodium bicarbonate (paradoxical intracellular acidosis), addition of substance converted to bicarbonate – citrate, lactate, acetate).

4. Respiratory acidosis
- Respiratory depression (e.g. drugs, cerebral injury).
- Muscle weakness (e.g. Guillain–Barré syndrome, myasthenia, polio, muscle relaxants).
- Trauma (e.g. flail chest, lung contusion).
- Pulmonary insufficiency (e.g. pulmonary oedema, pneumonia, ARDS).
- Airway obstruction.
- Artificial ventilation (e.g. inadequate minute volume, excessive PEEP).

5. Respiratory alkalosis
- Excessively high minute volume.
- Hypoxaemia.
- Pulmonary embolism.
- Asthma (early).
- Impairment of cerebral function (e.g. head injury, meningo-encephalitis).
- Respiratory stimulants (e.g. salicylate overdose – early)
- Sepsis (early).
- Parenchymal pulmonary disorder (e.g. oedema).

6. Mixed disorders

- Metabolic acidosis and respiratory acidosis (e.g. cardiac arrest, respiratory failure with anoxia).
- Metabolic alkalosis and respiratory alkalosis (e.g. CCF and vomiting, diuretics and hepatic failure, diuretic therapy and pneumonia).
- Metabolic alkalosis and respiratory acidosis (e.g. COPD and diuretics, COPD and vomiting).
- Metabolic acidosis and respiratory alkalosis (e.g. salicylate overdose, septic shock, sepsis and renal failure, CCF and renal failure).
- Metabolic alkalosis and metabolic acidosis (e.g. diuretics and ketoacidosis, vomiting and renal failure, vomiting and lactic acidosis).

Simple arithmetic related to acid–base disorders

- If $pH = 7.ab$ and $[H^+] = cd$ nmol/l, then $ab + cd = 83$; e.g. $pH = 7.23$, $[H+] = 83 - 23 = 60$
- For a 1.6 kPa (12 mmHg) change in PCO_2 there will be a 0.1 change in pH and a 6 mmol change in base excess.
- $PCO_2 \times$ ventilation = constant.

Further reading

Armstrong RF. The interpretation of arterial blood gases. *Current Anaesthesia Intensive Care* 1994; **5**: 74–80.

Related topics of interest

Arterial blood gases – acid–base physiology (p. 27)

Arterial cannulation

Peripheral arterial cannulation is a common procedure performed in critical care units. The radial artery at the wrist is the most popular site but there are a number of other suitable arteries: the ulnar, dorsalis pedis and posterior tibial arteries are, like the radial artery, relatively small distal vessels, but each has a collateral vessel. The brachial, femoral and axillary arteries do not have collaterals but are much larger and less likely to thrombose.

Indications

1. Continuous monitoring of arterial blood pressure:
   (a) Where haemodynamic instability is anticipated:
   - Major surgical procedures, e.g. cardiac, vascular.
   - Large fluid shifts, e.g. major trauma.
   - Medical problems, e.g. heart valve disease.
   - Drug therapy, e.g. inotropes.
   (b) For neurosurgical procedures.
   (c) Where non-invasive blood pressure monitoring is not possible, e.g. burns.
2. Sampling:
   - Blood gases.
   - Repeated blood sampling (to prevent the need for multiple punctures).

Contraindications

- Local infection.
- Coagulopathy is a relative contraindication.

Technique

A modified Allen's test may be performed to assess the adequacy of collateral blood flow to the hand before cannulating the radial artery. However, ischaemia may occur despite a normal result and an abnormal result does not reliably predict this complication. Consequently, most clinicians have discarded the Allen's test; if there is any doubt about the perfusion of the hand after radial cannulation, remove the cannula immediately. A 20 guage arterial cannula may be inserted under local anaesthesia in the same way as a venous cannula, although on occasions it can be easier to transfix the vessel first.

Alternatives to radial artery cannulation

Ulnar artery
The ulnar artery can be cannulated using the position and technique described above. If multiple attempts at cannulation of the radial artery have been unsuccessful, do not attempt to cannulate the ipsilateral ulnar artery.

Brachial artery

The brachial artery may be cannulated just proximal to the skin crease of the ante-cubital fossa, medial to the biceps tendon and lateral to pronator teres.

Dorsalis pedis

If perfusion to the foot is satisfactory, the dorsalis pedis or posterior tibial arteries may be cannulated safely with a 20 gauge catheter.

Femoral artery

The femoral artery may be cannulated 1–2 cm distal to the inguinal ligament at the midpoint of a line drawn between the superior iliac spine and the symphysis pubis. Insert an 18 gauge central venous cannula into the artery using a Seldinger technique. A standard 20 gauge arterial cannula is too short for reliable femoral access.

Sources of error

An overdamped trace will under-read the systolic pressure and over-read the diastolic pressure. Causes of overdamping include a kinked cannula, partial obstruction of the cannula by blood clot or by the vessel wall, and air bubbles in the manometer line or transducer. An underdamped trace will over-read the systolic and under-read the dia-stolic pressure. The usual cause of this is resonance in long manometer lines. The mean arterial pressure should remain accurate even in the presence of damping or resonance.

Complications

The most significant complications are ischaemia and infection but, overall, the inci-dence of serious complications is low. Thrombosis is more likely to occur when the cannula is large relative to the artery, particularly if it is left in place for longer than 72 h. In some series, 50% of radial artery cannulations have resulted in thrombosis but few of these cause ischaemia. Thrombi at the catheter tip can embolise peripherally. Flushing the arterial catheter can cause retrograde emboli of thrombus or clot. Dis-connection can cause extensive haemorrhage, and bleeding around the catheter site can cause haematomas, particularly in patients with a coagulopathy.

Infection is extremely rare in patients who have arterial catheters solely for intra-operative monitoring, but it is a significant risk in the critical care unit, particularly after about 4 days. An arterial catheter should be removed immediately there is any local inflammation. Accidental injection of drugs may cause distal gangrene. Aneurysm and pseudoaneurysm formations are rare, late complications.

Further reading

Cohen NH, Brett CM. Arterial catheterization. In: Benumof JL (ed.), *Clinical Procedures in Anesthesia and Intensive Care*. Philadelphia: JB Lippincott, 1992, pp. 375–90.

Related topics of interest

Asthma

Asthma is a chronic disease characterised by increased responsiveness of the tracheo-bronchial tree to various stimuli (e.g. inhaled allergens, infection, exercise, anxiety, cold or drugs). It manifests as widespread airway narrowing with mucosal oedema and a cellular infiltrate. Reversibility of airway obstruction is characteristic and distinguishes asthma from the fixed obstruction of chronic bronchitis and emphysema. The severity of airflow obstruction varies widely over short periods but airway resistance may be normal for long periods. Acute severe asthma may be a life-threatening condition, especially when combined with one or more adverse psychosocial factors (psychiatric illness, alcohol or drug ingestion, unemployment, etc.).

Features of acute severe asthma

1. Peak expiratory flow (PEF) $<50\%$ of predicted.
2. Unable to complete sentences in one breath.
3. Respiratory rate >25 breaths min^{-1}.
4. Pulse rate >110 beats min^{-1}.

and in children

5. Too breathless to talk or too breathless to feed.

Features of life-threatening asthma

1. PEF $<33\%$ of predicted, $SpO_2<92\%$, $PaO_2<8\,kPa$.
2. Silent chest, cyanosis or feeble respiratory effort.
3. Bradycardia, dysrhythmia or hypotension.
4. Exhaustion, confusion or coma.

Features of near-fatal asthma

Raised $PaCO_2$ and/or requiring mechanical ventilation with raised inflation pressures.

Treatment – immediate

1. Oxygen. High concentration.
2. β_2-agonist via oxygen driven nebuliser (salbutamol 5 mg or terbutaline 10 mg – halve doses in very young children). Intravenous β_2-agonists should be reserved for those patients in whom inhaled therapy cannot be used reliably. Their use may have a role in ventilated patients but there is little evidence to support this.
3. Steroids. Prednisolone 30–60 mg orally or hydrocortisone 200 mg i.v. or both. (Prednisolone 1–2 mg kg^{-1} to a maximum of 40 mg in children.)
4. NO SEDATION.
5. Chest X-ray to exclude a pneumothorax or consolidation.

If acute severe or life-threatening asthma or in those with a poor initial response

6. Add ipratropium (0.5 mg 4–6 hourly) to nebulised β_2-agonist (0.25 mg in children or 0.125 mg in the very young).
7. Patients with acute severe asthma will be hypomagnesaemic. Consider a single dose of i.v. magnesium sulphate (2 g infused over 20 min).
8. Intravenous aminophylline is not likely to result in any additional bronchodilatation in acute asthma compared with treatment with β_2-agonists and steroids. Side effects such as palpitation, arrhythmias and vomiting are increased if i.v. aminophylline is used.
9. There is no published study of the use of leukotriene receptor antagonists in the management of acute asthma.
10. Antibiotics are not indicated routinely for acute asthma. Where an infection precipitates an exacerbation of asthma, it is likely to be viral.

Monitoring treatment

- Repeat measurement of PEF 15–30 min after starting treatment.
- Maintain $SpO_2 > 92\%$.
- Repeat blood gas measurement if initial $PaO_2 < 8\,kPa$, $PaCO_2$ normal or raised, or there is any possibility that the patient may have deteriorated.

Transfer the patient to a critical care unit accompanied at all times by a doctor prepared to intubate if there is:

- Exhaustion, feeble respirations, confusion or drowsiness.
- Deteriorating PEF, worsening or persisting hypoxia or hypercapnoea.
- Coma or respiratory arrest.

Mechanical ventilation of a patient with acute severe asthma

This is a procedure of last resort. It should be considered only when maximal medical therapy has failed to improve the patient. Serious life-threatening complications of ventilation are not uncommon under such circumstances. The decision to ventilate should be based on the patient's degree of exhaustion.

Dehydration is common in the asthmatic *in extremis*. Oral fluid intake will have been low, the patient may have been sweating and tachypnoea will have increased fluid loss. High positive intrathoracic pressures during mechanical ventilation will reduce venous return to the right heart. Before induction of anaesthesia and intubation, intravenous fluid should be infused rapidly. Hypokalaemia can be caused or exacerbated by β_2-agonist and/or steroid treatment and must be corrected.

Ventilator settings must be optimised for individual patients. The appropriate settings will vary considerably over time. It is important not to overventilate or aim for normocarbia. Permissive hypercarbia should be tolerated, providing pH is > 7.2. This will help limit inspiratory pressures and thus barotrauma and cardiovascular depression. A slow inspiratory flow rate may be optimal for low intrathoracic pressures but may not deliver an adequate tidal volume or allow sufficient time for expiration. As much time as possible should be allowed for expiration. Dynamic hyperinflation is common. Peak inspiratory pressures should be kept as low as possible and muscle relaxation in addition to sedation may be required to prevent the patient from coughing.

The patient and a current chest X-ray should be examined regularly for evidence of extensive alveolar rupture (mediastinal emphysema, subcutaneous emphysema or pneumothorax). Maximal medical therapy should be continued throughout the period of ventilation. Volatile anaesthetics can be added to the ventilator gas mixture to provide further bronchodilatation.

Further reading

http://www.brit-thoracic.org.uk/sign/index.html
  (The web address for the guidelines on the management of asthma produced by the British Thoracic Society and the Scottish Intercollegiate Guidelines Network (SIGN).)
The British Thoracic Society Guidelines on Asthma Management. *Thorax* 2003; **58(suppl 1)**.

Related topics of interest

Anaphylaxis (p. 24)
Chronic obstructive pulmonary disease (p. 114)

Blood and blood products

Myrene Kilminster

Improvements in the safety of the blood supply have been achieved but cost has increased substantially.

Screening

All donors are screened carefully and those considered to be at risk are excluded from donating. In the UK, those who have been transfused blood since 1980 are now excluded from donating. International blood screening varies but it is now common practice to screen for the following:

- ABO and Rhesus (Rh) D blood groups.
- Red cell antibodies.
- HIV 1 and 2 antibodies and RNA.
- Hepatitis B surface antigen.
- Hepatitis C antibody and hepatitis C RNA.
- CMV.
- HTLV I/II antibody (Australia).
- Syphilis serology.

Collection and storage

Approximately 430 ml of whole blood is collected into a closed triple pack containing CPD-A (citrate, phosphate, dextrose-adenine) anticoagulant. Platelets and plasma are separated and the remaining red cells are resuspended in optimal additive (e.g. SAGM (saline, adenine, glucose and mannitol)). The shelf life of SAGM blood is 35 days.

Continuing metabolic activity causes the following biochemical and cellular changes:

- Depletion of 2,3-diphosphoglycerate (2,3-DPG), adenosine triphosphate (ATP), PO_4^{2-}, platelets and factors V and VIII.
- Accumulation of CO_2, H^+, activated clotting factors, denatured and activated proteins, microaggregates of platelets, white cells and fibrin.
- The $Hb–O_2$ dissociation curve is shifted to the left by acidosis and reduced 2,3-DPG.
- The P_{50} is less than 2.4 kPa after 1 week.
- A reduction in red cell membrane integrity causes an increase in extracellular K^+, increased osmotic fragility and an increase in free haemoglobin.

Blood components

Blood

Fresh blood is less than 5 days old. It is rich in clotting factors and platelets. It is inefficient to store blood as whole blood because most patients require only red cells, and the separation of platelets and plasma enables these products to be given to other patients. The shelf life of whole blood is shorter than SAGM blood. There is more microaggregate formation and a higher risk of haemolysis and graft-versus-host-disease (GVHD) because of larger amounts of plasma and white cells. SAGM blood has a haematocrit of 50–70%. Following theoretical concerns about the transmission of prions in white cells, all donated blood in the UK, and several other countries, is now leukocyte depleted. Frozen red cells are used for rare blood groups or autologous storage in large amounts.

Platelets

One unit-equivalent of platelet concentrate will increase the platelet count by approximately $7 \times 10^9 \, l^{-1}$. The shelf life is up to 7 days, but they need to be stored on a horizontal shaker. The presence of some red cells can result in sensitisation if ABO-Rh incompatible platelets are transfused. This can cause Rhesus sensitisation in Rhesus-negative females, low-grade haemolysis and a positive Coombs test.

Fresh frozen plasma

The fractionated volume of fresh frozen plasma (FFP) is approximately 200 ml. It can be spun further into cryoprecipitate and supernatant. FFP contains all the clotting factors and components of the fibrinolytic and complement systems.

Large volumes (4–8 units) are required to produce clinically important increases in serum levels of clotting factors. It carries infectious risks, and donor plasma leucocyte antibodies can cause transfusion-related acute lung injury (TRALI). There are methods of reducing the infectious risk:

- Photochemical inactivation with methylene blue is applied to single units of plasma and is effective against enveloped viruses (hepatitis B, hepatitis C and HIV) and partially effective against non-enveloped viruses (hepatitis A, parvoviruses). It is unlikely to be effective against prions. Approximately 70–80% of clotting factor activity is retained.
- Detergent methods require pooling of up to 360 l and are not effective against non-enveloped viruses.

In the UK, from 2004, FFP given to children will be sourced from the United States and will be methylene blue treated.

Cryoprecipitate

Cryopreciptate is prepared from FFP. It contains factor VIII (FVIII:C), fibrinogen, factor XIII, von Willebrand's factor and fibronectin. It is indicated in fibrinogen deficiency/depletion, particularly in disseminated intramuscular coagulation (DIC) and massive transfusion.

Preoperative autologous donation

In an attempt to avoid the hazards of homologous transfusion, patients undergoing elective procedures that are likely to require transfusion can pre-donate their own blood. Collections can occur weekly for up to 4 weeks pre-surgery. This autologous blood is subject to the same screening tests as the homologous supply. The process is relatively expensive because unused autologous blood cannot be returned to the homologous blood bank. The risk of administrative errors is the same as for homologous blood. For these reasons, the technique of preoperative autologous blood donation is becoming less popular.

Perioperative red cell salvage

Salvage techniques are used widely in trauma, cardiothoracic, vascular and orthopaedic surgery. Postoperatively, cardiac surgical patients can receive both re-transfused pump blood and blood from thoracic drains. Intraoperative cell saver blood consists of washed red cells without platelets or clotting factors. Problems with these techniques include traumatic haemolysis, air emboli, microemboli, infusion of irrigants and hyperkalaemia.

Other plasma products

Albumin, immunoglobulins and factor VIII are all derived from large plasma pools. Recipients are thus exposed to multiple donors. The sterilisation processes for albumin and immunoglobulin products may not be sufficient to inactivate non-enveloped viruses, but are thought to be safe for enveloped viruses. The theoretical risk of prion transmission led the Department of Health in the UK to source all albumin from the United States.

Albumin
Albumin is made by cold fractionation followed by heating to 60°C for 10h to inactivate viruses. It is supplied as 4–5% or 20% albumin solution, each with varying constituents. Current evidence indicates that albumin infusion does not improve outcome in critically ill patients.

Factor VIII
The current sterilisation processes for factor VIII are thought to inactivate viruses completely. However, transfusion of human factor VIII exposes each recipient to 20000 donors. In the UK, the theoretical risk of disease transmission has invoked legislation dictating the use the genetically engineered factor VIII in new haemophilia patients and those under the age of 16. Recombinant factor VIII is derived from genetically engineered Chinese hamster ovary cells. It is indicated for bleeding in patients with haemophilia A, but is not useful in von Willebrand's disease.

Red cell substitutes

Several red cell substitutes are at advanced stages of investigation. They can be divided into two groups: haemoglobin-based oxygen carriers and perfluorocarbons.

Haemoglobin-based oxygen carriers

Haemoglobin based oxygen carriers (HBOCs) can be produced from three sources: out-of-date human blood, animal blood or by recombinant techniques. The short intravascular half-life of free haemoglobin has been increased by polymerisation or linkage to large molecules. Most of the HBOCs cause some degree of vasoconstriction and increase in blood pressure because of nitric oxide uptake by the haemoglobin. They lack 2,3-DPG and thus have a low P_{50} (the partial pressure at which 50% of the haemoglobin is saturated). It may be possible to affect oxygen-carrying characteristics of HBOCs by means other than the concentration of 2,3-DPG. Diaspirin cross-linked haemoglobin (DCLHb) was withdrawn after a clinical study in trauma patients demonstrated increased mortality in the DCLHb group. A glutaraldehyde polymerised bovine HBOC has been licensed for clinical use in South Africa and an application has been submitted to the Food and Drug Administration (FDA) in the United States. The P_{50} of bovine haemoglobin is determined by chloride rather than 2,3-DPG and the P_{50} of this bovine HBOC is a very favourable 4.9 kPa (37 mmHg). Development of a genetically engineered recombinant haemoglobin solution has recently been stopped.

Perfluorocarbons

Perfluorocarbons (PFCs) are hydrocarbons with F^- ions replacing H^+ ions. This increases the solubility for oxygen. They are chemically inert and immiscible in water, but can be emulsified with surfactant. Fluosol-DA 20% can carry 1–2 ml O_2 per 100 mmHg (three times that of plasma). It requires a high FiO_2 for efficacy, which has severely restricted any useful clinical application. A new generation PFC, perflubron, has undergone phase III trials but has yet to be licensed for general clinical practice.

Further reading

Goodenough LT, Brecher ME, Kanter MH, AuBuchon JP. Transfusion medicine. Blood transfusion. *N Engl J Med* 1999; **340**: 438–47.

McClelland DBL. *Handbook of Transfusion Medicine* 3rd edn. Norwich: The Stationary Office, 2001.

Related topics of interest

Blood coagulation

Coagulation failure is common in critically ill patients. Normal haemostasis requires equilibrium between the fibrinolytic system and the clotting cascade, the vascular endothelium and platelets. There are many reasons for coagulation failure in the critically ill:

- Surgical and non-surgical vessel trauma.
- Acquired deficiencies of clotting factors (e.g. major trauma, massive transfusion, disseminated intravascular coagulation (DIC), extracorporeal circuits, liver disease).
- Thrombocytopenia: (e.g. drug-induced, antiplatelet antibodies (idiopathic thrombocytopenic purpura (ITP), heparin-induced thrombotic thrombocytopenic syndrome (HITTS), sepsis).
- Hypothermia, which impairs clotting factor activity.
- Anticoagulants (e.g. heparin, warfarin, aspirin, thrombolytics).
- Congenital coagulation factor deficiency.

Coagulation tests

Prothrombin time (PT) tests the extrinsic pathway, with vitamin K-dependent factors (II, VII and X). Factor VII is the first to decrease with warfarin therapy. A normal time is 12–14 s for clot formation; the test sample should clot within 3 s of the control. Prolonged PT occurs in factor VII deficiency, liver disease, vitamin K deficiency or oral anticoagulant therapy.

Activated partial thromboplastin time (APTT) tests the intrinsic pathway (factors XII, XI, IX, VIII and X) activated by kaolin or cephaloplastin. The normal time is 39–42 s and samples that clot more than 6 s beyond the control are abnormal. APPT is prolonged in the presence of heparin, the haemophilias, von Willebrand's disease, severe fibrinolysis and DIC.

Activated clotting time (ACT) is measured after whole blood is activated with diatomaceous earth. Clot formation normally occurs 90–130 s later. It tests predominantly the intrinsic pathway and is used as a bedside test for the action of heparin, but is also prolonged by thrombocytopenia, hypothermia, fibrinolysis and high-dose aprotinin.

Thrombin time: both the PT and the APTT include the final common pathway in their tests. This is tested specifically by the addition of thrombin to plasma (thrombin time). A normal time is 9–15 s. Unlike a reptilase test, it is affected by heparin and fibrin degradation products (FDPs).

Bleeding time (normal range: 3–9 min) tests primary haemostasis of platelets and vessels. A blood pressure cuff is inflated to 40 mmHg and a standardised skin incision is made distal to it. If bleeding stops within 9 min, this is considered normal.

Platelet count (normal range: $150–400 \times 10^9 \, l^{-1}$): specific platelet function tests are rarely used in practice but thromboelastography allows some functional assessment.

All factors can be assayed, but factor VII components and fibrinogen are the ones most commonly measured. Normal fibrinogen level is 2–4.5 g. Factor Xa assays are used to monitor the anticoagulant effect of low molecular weight heparins that do not affect APTT.

D-dimers and FDPs released by plasminolysis can be assayed and are often measured to confirm DIC. Levels of 20–40 µg ml^{-1} occur following surgery and trauma and may also accompany sepsis, DVT and renal failure. Assay of the D-dimer fragments is more specific but less sensitive for fibrinolysis. Minor elevations of D-dimer may also occur post-surgery, trauma, sepsis, venous thrombosis and renal impairment. High D-dimer levels suggest excessive fibrinolysis (e.g. DIC).

Euglobulin lysis time (ELT): ELT reflects the presence of plasminogen activators. With fibrinolytic activation the ELT time is shortened (normal range > 90 min).

Specific problems

Haemophilias
Haemophilia A (classical haemophilia) is a sex-linked disorder due to a deficiency of factor VIII. Haemophilia B or Christmas disease is due to factor IX deficiency, and is less common than haemophilia A. Treatment is with factor VIII and IX respectively.

Von Willebrand's disease
This disease is autosomal dominant and the commonest hereditary coagulation disorder. Prophylactic infusion of DDAVP 0.3 µg kg^{-1} augments release of factor VIII and von Willebrand's factor and reduces the risk of haemorrhage. Cryoprecipitate and fresh frozen plasma (FFP) will also correct the defects.

Haemostatic failure associated with liver disease
Cholestatic liver disease is associated with deficiencies of the vitamin K-dependent coagulation factors (II, VII, IX and X). This is reversed rapidly with vitamin K therapy. In the presence of extensive hepatocellular damage, vitamin K may be ineffective. Liver disease is also associated with thrombocytopenia secondary to splenomegaly.

Oral anticoagulant agents
Oral anticoagulants cause deficiencies of vitamin K-dependent clotting factors (II, VII, IX and X). FFP will provide short-term reversal of anticoagulation (factor VII has a half-life of around 7 h) while vitamin K provides long-term antagonism of warfarin.

Heparin
Heparin potentiates the action of antithrombin III, which inhibits coagulation and can be measured by prolongation of APTT. Protamine sulphate is a direct antagonist of heparin and 1 mg protamine will neutralise 100 units of heparin. In overdose protamine is anticoagulant and it must be given slowly to avoid hypotension caused by pulmonary vasoconstriction. The low molecular weight heparins do not affect APPT; anti-Xa levels can be used for monitoring; their effect may not be fully reversed by protamine.

Antiplatelet agents
Aspirin and other non-steroidal anti-inflammatory drugs (NSAIDs) have platelet-

inhibitory effects. Platelet function effects are largely irreversible, lasting up to 10 days after administration. Platelet transfusion may be required despite a normal platelet count.

Drotrecogin alfa (activated)

Drotrecogin alfa (activated) is a recombinant version of the natural plasma-derived activated protein C (APC), which is an important regulator of coagulation. It limits thrombin formation by inactivating factors Va and VIIIa and has antithrombotic, profibrinolytic and anti-inflammatory properties. It has been licensed recently for the treatment of severe sepsis. Patients receiving drotrecogin alfa (activated) are at increased risk of bleeding and it should be discontinued 2h before the start of any procedure that may cause bleeding. It can be started 12h after completion of invasive procedures.

Disseminated intravascular coagulopathy (DIC)

Disseminated intravascular coagulopathy occurs when a powerful or persisting trigger activates haemostasis. The release of free thrombin leads to widespread deposition of fibrin and a secondary fibrinolytic response.

The major problem and presenting feature of acute DIC is bleeding. Thrombotic, haemorrhagic or mixed manifestations in various organ systems may also coexist. DIC is associated with numerous underlying problems:

- Sepsis (bacterial, especially Gram-negative organisms, viral, protozoal, especially malaria).
- Shock, burns and trauma. Snake bite. Heat stroke.
- Eclampsia, placental abruption, amniotic fluid embolism, retained products of conception, puerperal sepsis.
- Hepatic failure and autoimmune diseases.
- Malignancy (promyelocytic leukaemia and mucin-secreting adenocarcinomas).
- Surgery (cardiac, vascular neurosurgery, prostatic).
- Incompatible blood transfusion.
- Extensive intravascular haemolysis.
- Extracorporeal circuits.

Diagnosis

The diagnosis is usually based on the clinical picture with a supportive pattern of laboratory tests. A prothrombin time >15s, a prolonged APPT, fibrinogen level <160mgdl^{-1} and platelet count $<150000 \times 10^9 l^{-1}$ with high levels of FDPs (D-dimers) are confirmatory although they may not be present in all cases. The blood film may show fragmentation of the red cells (microangiopathic haemolytic anaemia), which is more commonly seen in chronic DIC associated with malignancy.

Management

- Treatment of the precipitating cause.
- Replacement of deficient clotting factors and platelets.
- Heparin may be useful in theory but is rarely used in practice.

Thrombocytopenia

Thrombocytopenia results from decreased production, increased consumption or extracorporeal loss of platelets. All of these factors play a role in the thrombocytopenia associated with sepsis.

1. Decreased production. Leukaemias, drug-induced thrombocytopenia (thiazides, quinine, antituberculis drugs, carbamazepine, chloroquine, chlorpropamide, gold salts, methyldopa, chloramphenicol, high-dose penicillin, chemotherapy agents), marrow depression or infiltration by malignancy.

2. Increased consumption. Sepsis. ITP due to antiplatelet IgG autoantibodies, thrombotic thrombocytopenic purpura (TTP), haemolytic uraemic syndrome (HUS), shock, DIC, hypersplenism due to splenomegaly, HITTS.

3. Extracorporeal loss. Due to haemorrhage and haemodilution, extracorporeal circuits (cardiopulmonary bypass, renal replacement therapy, plasmaphoresis).

Treatment is directed at the underlying cause. Platelet transfusion if count is < 10–$20 \times 10^9 l^{-1}$. Prophylactic platelets are given prior to surgery or an invasive procedure.

Aprotinin

Aprotinin is a naturally occurring serine protease inhibitor with a half-life of 2 h. Aprotinin given during cardiopulmonary bypass preserves platelet function and reduces perioperative blood loss. It may have a role in other situations such as repeat neurosurgery and multitrauma. The loading dose is 2 million units followed by $500\,000\,IU\,h^{-1}$.

Bleeding related to thrombolysis

With increasing use of thrombolytic agents, haemorrhagic complications are more common. The majority of haemorrhage occurs from cannula sites or the urinary or gastrointestinal tract. Less than 1% of bleeding complications are intracranial but the mortality rate is high. The risk of bleeding increases with dose and is increased if heparin is also administered. In the presence of serious bleeding, stop the infusion of thrombolytic agents and correct clotting by giving FFP and platelets.

Recombinant factor VIIa (rFVIIa)

The vitamin K-dependent glycoprotein rFVIIa facilitates haemostasis by complexing with tissue factor (TF) lipoprotein found in vessel intima. This complex forms an integral part of the extrinsic pathway and the rFVIIa converts factor X to Xa, which converts prothrombin to thrombin. The glycoprotein rVIIa was originally reserved for use in haemophilia patients with inhibitors to factors VIII or IX, but is being used increasingly after conventional therapy has failed to stop severe bleeding in a variety of settings, particularly trauma. Dosages of 35–$200\,\mu g\,kg^{-1}$ repeated up to three times have been used and appear to produce impressive anecdotal results. Formal trials and clear guidelines on indications and dosage are awaited.

Management of abnormal bleeding

- Prevent hypovolaemia and hypoxia, and correct hypothermia and acidosis.
- Exclude surgical bleeding: large vessel bleeding and external haemorrhage may be controlled initially by pressure but usually require surgical haemostasis. Use non-surgical haemostasis where appropriate (e.g. fracture immobilisation, vessel embolisation).
- Take blood samples for coagulation studies and platelet count.
- Give blood to maintain adequate circulating haemoglobin.
- Give FFP to replace lost coagulation factors.
- Give platelets to maintain a platelet count of $>50–100 \times 10^9 l^{-1}$ in the presence of active bleeding.
- In the absence of active bleeding a platelet count of $>20 \times 10^9 l^{-1}$ is tolerated in most patients.
- Give platelets to those patients who are bleeding with known recent aspirin or NSAID use.
- Give cryoprecipitate to replace fibrinogen.
- Give other specific clotting factors as indicated (e.g. VIII, IX for the haemophilias).
- Give vitamin K in liver failure and to reverse the effects of warfarin: 1 mg of vitamin K will reverse warfarin effects within 12 h while 10 mg will saturate liver stores and impair warfarin anticoagulation for weeks.
- Give protamine to reverse the effects of heparin.
- Consider the use of aprotinin or alternative agents such as epsilon-aminocaproic acid and rFVIIa.

Further reading

Cobas M. Preoperative assessment of coagulation disorders. *Int Anesthesiol Clin* 2001; **39**: 1–15.

Dahlback B. Blood coagulation. *Lancet* 2000; **355**: 1627–32.

Douglas S. Coagulation history, Oxford 1951–53. *Br J Haematol* 1999; **107**: 22–32.

Lusher JM. Screening and diagnosis of coagulation disorders. *Am J Obstet Gynecol* 1996; **175**: 778–83.

Mannucci PM. Haemostatic drugs. *N Engl J Med* 1998; **339**: 245–53.

Parker RI. Etiology and treatment of acquired coagulopathies in the critically ill adult and child. *Crit Care Clin* 1997; **13**: 591–609.

Stammers AH, Bruda NL, Gonano C, Hartmann T. Point-of-care coagulation monitoring: applications of the thromboelastography. *Anaesthesia* 1998; **53(Suppl 2)**: 58–9.

Related topics of interest

Blood transfusion and complications (p. 50)

Blood transfusion and complications

Myrene Kilminster

Several institutions have recently published guidelines on transfusion practices in an attempt to minimise the incidence of adverse reactions and reduce costs. In the UK and Ireland, the Serious Hazards of Transfusion (SHOT) enquiry has been established to monitor the adverse effects of blood transfusion.

Exposure to homologous blood and blood products should be minimised and autologous blood should be used where possible. The cause of anaemia must be sought aggressively and treated. Blood restoration should be optimised with the use of iron supplementation, folic acid, vitamin B_{12}, vitamin C, erythropoietin (EPO) and adequate nutrition.

Causes of anaemia in the critically ill

ICU patients become anaemic for many reasons:

- Overt or occult bleeding may occur from within the GI tract, intra-abdominal or intrathoracic cavities or the pelvis. Orthopaedic injuries may continue to bleed into tissues.
- Frequent blood sampling.
- Anaemia of critical illness:
  - Bone marrow suppression.
  - Reduced EPO production by impaired kidneys.
  - Inhibition of marrow response to EPO.
  - Altered iron metabolism.

Inflammatory mediators, many of which work via inducible nitric oxide synthase (iNOS) pathways, probably induce these responses.

Compatibility testing

Clerical error remains the most common cause for an ABO incompatible transfusion reaction. The risks of immunological reaction are small if ABO-compatible blood is used. There are more than 30 common antigens and hundreds more rare antigens, but apart from ABO and Rhesus (Rh) D they rarely cause problems with matching.

Donor and recipient blood is grouped using direct antiglobulin testing with the addition of A, B and RhD antisera to a suspension of donor red cells. This determines the ABO and RhD status and takes 5 min. There are two types of cross-match:

- An immediate spin cross-match involves the addition of recipient serum to donor cells and observing for immediate agglutination. It confirms ABO compatibility and will take about 5 min to perform. It will not reliably detect unexpected antibodies.

- A full cross-match requires incubation of donor cells and recipient sera for at least 15 min and observing for agglutination. A Coombs' test is then performed to detect antibody on donor red cells. The full cross-match test takes about 45 min.

An antibody screen may be performed in conjunction with a cross-match or as part of a 'type and screen'. The recipient's serum is added to red cells from several normal group O blood samples expressing known antigens. Once a blood sample has been typed and screened, if, later on, blood is required urgently, it can be released following just a spin cross-match to confirm ABO compatibility. Thus, fully compatible blood is available in just 15 minutes.

The risk of a major incompatible reaction varies with the extent of compatibility testing undertaken:

- Randomly selected (untyped donor and recipient)   35.6%
- Group O   0.8%
- ABO-compatible   0.6%
- ABO and Rhesus compatible   0.2%
- ABO, Rhesus and negative antibody screen   0.06%
- Complete compatibility testing   0.05%

In an emergency, group O positive for males and postmenopausal females and group O negative for premenopausal females (to reduce the risk of sensitisation to RhD antigen) have been established to be safe. Patients who are group O are most at risk for an incompatible transfusion reaction due to the presence of anti-A and anti-B in their plasma; they are implicated in 70% of incompatible reactions while representing only 45% of the population. Patients who receive large transfusions of group O cells should undergo full cross-matching before receiving blood of their original group; they may have received a large amount of anti-A and anti-B in the sera of the previous transfusions.

Blood transfusion triggers

The safe lower limit of haemoglobin concentration in critically ill patients is controversial. There is no doubt that anaemia is tolerated considerably better than hypovolaemia. However, patients with fixed perfusion defects of vital organs and serious co-morbidity are far less likely to tolerate such a dramatic reduction in oxygen delivery without adverse consequences.

With restoration of an adequate circulating volume there are a variety of mechanisms to compensate for acute anaemia and maintain oxygen delivery. Cardiac output is increased as a result of lower viscosity, lower SVR and autoregulation in regional capillary beds. Most tissues (except the myocardium and renal medulla) can increase oxygen extraction substantially. Tolerance to reduced oxygen content will depend on the individual's ability to compensate, and maintain a favourable oxygen supply to oxygen demand. This will vary from patient to patient and organ to organ. Blood transfusion may not always improve oxygen delivery; increased viscosity may reduce cardiac output and in combination with a reduced P_{50}, any increase in O_2 content may be negated.

Critically ill patients have increased O_2 demand due to a catabolic state, pain, fever, increased work of breathing, use of inotropes and sepsis. Their ability to compensate may be impaired by myocardial dysfunction, respiratory failure, renal failure, coronary artery, cerebrovascular or renovascular disease, and co-morbidity.

There is no single criterion to trigger transfusion. The decision must be based on:

- Haemoglobin concentration.
- Likelihood of continuing blood loss.
- Chronicity of anaemia.
- Presence of fixed perfusion defects in vital organs.
- Cardiopulmonary reserve (which declines at extremes of age).
- Catabolic state.
- Evidence of impaired tissue oxygenation.

A haemoglobin of $7\,g\,dl^{-1}$ may be tolerated in a fit young postoperative patient without anticipated further blood loss, whereas a haemoglobin $>10\,g\,dl^{-1}$ may be required for a patient with severe coronary artery disease. A multicentre, randomised controlled trial supports a more restrictive practice for red cell transfusion in the critically ill. This demonstrated that maintaining a haemoglobin of 7–$9\,g\,dl^{-1}$ was as effective and possibly superior to a liberal transfusion strategy of maintaining a haemoglobin of 10–$12\,g\,dl^{-1}$.

Control of haemorrhage

Control of haemorrhage may require surgical or radiological intervention, cessation or reversal of anticoagulation. Antifibrinolytics (e.g. tranexamic acid) may be indicated in patients who have received recent fibrinolytic therapy. Correction of clotting abnormalities and thrombocytopenia may be enough to control the bleeding and reduce the need for ongoing transfusion.

Massive transfusion

Packed cells and resuspended cells are deficient in platelets and factors V and VIII. During massive transfusion, coagulation and platelet counts must be assessed. Indications for their replacement are described on p. 49.

Complications of blood transfusions

Immediate immune reactions

- Acute haemolytic transfusion reaction is usually due to an ABO, Lewis, Kell or Duffy incompatible transfusion. IgM complement-mediated cytotoxicity or IgG-mediated lysis of red cells results in liberation of anaphylotoxins, histamine and coagulation activation. There may be fevers, rigors, chest pain, back pain, dyspnoea, headache, urticaria, cyanosis, bronchospasm, pulmonary oedema and cardiovascular collapse. Acute renal failure (secondary to hypotension, microvascular thrombosis and haemoglobin plugging of tubules) is common. The transfusion must be ceased while appropriate organ support is started. Investigations include a Coombs' test, LDH and haptoglobin, LFTs, baseline coagulation studies, electrolytes, urea, creatinine and FBC.

- Febrile non-haemolytic transfusion reactions (NHFTR) account for 75% all reactions (1–5% of all transfusions) and are due to recipient antibody to donor white cell/platelet human leukocyte antigen (HLA). Patients may require washed or leukocyte-depleted red cells subsequently.
- Allergy is more common after whole blood or plasma transfusions. The reaction is usually mild but can be severe with hypotension, angio-oedema, bronchospasm, urticaria and fever.
- Transfusion-related acute lung injury (TRALI) is non-cardiogenic pulmonary oedema caused by recipient antibody to donor leucocyte HLA. It happens usually within 6 h and can occur with minimal volumes. FFP is the commonest cause of TRALI.

Delayed immune reactions
Delayed haemolytic transfusion reactions (4–14 days after transfusion) are due to undetected antibody. They can be similar to acute reactions but are generally more benign. Alloimmunisation to cellular or protein antigens is common, and rarely affects the patient until the next time they need a blood transfusion. Graft-versus-host disease is due to donor lymphocytes in blood products that react against host tissue. It is more likely in immunocompromised individuals, or those with some shared HLA (family member donors).

Non-immune immediate reactions
- The risk of microbial contamination of blood is related directly to the length of storage. The most commonly implicated organism is *Yersinia enterocolitica* but a number of other organisms have been described.
- There is considerable evidence that homologous transfusion has an immunosuppressive effect and increases the risk of infection that is independent of bacterial contamination. Whether blood transfusion increases the risk of recurrence of cancer is still controversial.
- Volume overload is more likely with a normovolaemic transfusion in the elderly and those with impaired cardiac function.
- Haemolysis due to red cell trauma, osmotic lysis and senescent red cells can occur but is rarely of great clinical significance.
- Microaggregates of white cells, platelets and fibrin are associated with lung sequestration and acute lung injury and the potential for ARDS.
- Massive transfusion (>10 units or >1 blood volume) may cause a coagulopathy, hypothermia, DIC, hyperkalaemia, hypoalbuminaemia and acidosis. The coagulopathy of massive transfusion is multifactorial (deficiencies of factors V and VIII and platelets, DIC, hypothermia). FFP and platelets should be given empirically after 10 bags if non-surgical bleeding is a problem.
- Metabolic abnormalities resulting from a storage lesion are rarely a clinical problem except in rapid administration or massive transfusion. It is more likely with older blood. Hyperkalaemia, metabolic acidosis and metabolic alkalosis (citrate metabolism) may occur. Citrate toxicity, resulting in hypocalcaemia, is exceedingly rare.

Non-immune delayed reactions
- Viral infections. The current estimated infection risks (per unit transfused) associated with voluntary donor programmes are approximately: HIV 1:1 000 000,

hepatitis B 1:100000, hepatitis C 1:100000, CMV 1:2. The risk of transmitting non-A, non-B, non–C hepatitis is unknown.
- Iron overload is a complication of multiple transfusions over a long period of time. It results in haemosiderin deposition with myocardial and hepatic damage.

Further reading

Goodenough LT, Brecher ME, Kanter MH, AuBuchon JP. Transfusion medicine. Blood transfusion. *N Engl J Med* 1999; **340**: 438–47.
Hebert PC, Wells G, Blajchman MA, *et al.* A multicenter, randomized, controled clinical trial of transfusion requirements in critical care. *N Engl J Med* 1999; **340**: 409–17.
McClelland B (ed.). *Handbook of Transfusion Medicine*, 3rd edn. Blood Transfusion Services of the United Kingdom. London: Norwich: The Stationary Office, 2001.
http://www.arcbs.redcross.org.au Site for The Transfusion Medicine Manual (2003).

Related topics of interest

Blood and blood products (p. 41)
Blood coagulation (p. 45)

Brain death and organ donation

Brain death is defined as the irreversible cessation of brain function, but not necessarily the physical destruction of the brain. In the UK (as with many other countries), it has been agreed that brain stem death = death (i.e. despite the presence of a beating heart). Prior to the diagnosis of brain death it is necessary to consider certain preconditions and exclusions. Head injury and intracranial haemorrhage account for approximately 80% of cases. Brain death has been the subject of two joint Royal College reports.

Preconditions

1. Apnoeic coma requiring ventilation.
2. Irreversible brain damage of known cause.

Exclusions

1. Hypothermia (temperature $< 35°C$).
2. Drugs (no depressant or muscle relaxant drugs present).
3. Acid–base abnormality.
4. Metabolic/endocrine disease, e.g. uncontrolled diabetes mellitus, uraemia, hyponatraemia, Addison's disease, hepatic encephalopathy, thyrotoxicosis.
5. Markedly elevated $PaCO_2$.
6. Severe hypotension.

The brain death tests

These tests should be performed by two doctors but not necessarily at the same time. Neither should belong to the transplant team and both should have been registered for 5 years or more. One must be a consultant. More than 6h should have elapsed since the event that caused the suspected brain death. Two sets of tests must be performed. They may be carried out by the doctors separately or together. The tests are often repeated to eliminate observer error, although this is not required by law. Careful records should be kept.

1. Pupillary responses. There are no direct or consensual reactions to light. This tests the 2nd cranial nerve and the parasympathetic outflow.

2. Corneal reflex. No response to lightly touching the cornea. This tests the 5th and 7th cranial nerves.

3. Painful stimulus to the face. No response in the cranial nerve distribution. This tests the 5th and 7th cranial nerves.

4. Caloric tests. After visualising both ear drums (wax may need to be removed first), 30ml of ice cold water is injected into each external auditory canal. No response should be seen. Nystagmus occurs if the vestibular reflexes are intact. (Tests 8th, 3rd and 6th cranial nerves.)

5. Gag reflex. Tests the 9th and 10th cranial nerves.

6. Apnoea test. The patient is ventilated with 100% O_2 and then disconnected from the ventilator, while observing for respiratory effort. A tracheal catheter supplies $61min^{-1}$ of O_2 by insufflation. The patient is left disconnected for 10 min or until the $PaCO_2$ is >6.65 kPa. If marked bradycardia or haemodynamic instability occur, the test is discontinued. The SpO_2 should not fall below 90%. It may help the patient's relatives come to terms with the concept of brain death if they witness the apnoea test.

Other tests

Doll's eyes movement. The head is moved rapidly from side to side. If the brain stem is dead the eyes remain in a fixed position within the orbit. This is the oculocephalic reflex and tests the 8th cranial nerve. If the cortex is dead but the brain stem is intact, the eyes appear to move to the opposite side and then realign with the head. It does not form part of the legally required brain death tests.

Some countries require other tests for the diagnosis of brain death. These include EEG, 'four vessel' cerebral angiography, radioisotope scanning and transcranial Doppler ultrasound. There is no evidence that these tests increase the accuracy of diagnosis. Their use may be limited but they may be helpful in situations where the clinical testing described above cannot be undertaken (e.g. local cranial nerve injuries, an inability to perform the apnoea test because of severe hypoxia).

Potential problems

1. Spinal reflexes may be present. However, decerebrate posturing means some brain stem activity exists.
2. The presence of drugs or other unresponsive states may lead to a false diagnosis of brain death.
3. Communication with relatives. The discussion of a 'hopeless prognosis' being misinterpreted as brain death. A subsequent survival may then be ascribed to an incorrect diagnosis of brain death.
4. Death of the cortex leading to a vegetative state is not brain death.
5. Elective ventilation. A patient who is dying should not commence assisted ventilation simply to allow organ donation where this ventilation is of no therapeutic benefit to the dying patient.

Organ donation

The question of organ donation is often raised with relatives after the first set of brain death tests. This process may be eased if the potential donor had already registered with the NHS Organ Donor Register as an individual willing to donate. If consent is given, blood should be sent for tissue typing, HIV, hepatitis B and CMV testing. In

1993 the United Kingdom Transplant Support Authority divided the UK into a number of zones for the retrieval and allocation of donor organs. The local transplant coordinator should be contacted. If the second set of brain death tests confirm death and consent is obtained, then the patient is prepared for theatre. The 5-year survival after first heart transplantation is currently 64% but approximately 10% of transplanted organs fail early after transplantation from causes not related to acute rejection or infection. It is thus essential to optimise the function of donor organs in order to make optimal use of this scarce resource.

Potential complications in brain dead organ donors

- Cardiovascular instability.
- Hypoxaemia.
- Diabetes insipidus.
- Endocrine abnormalities (e.g. thyroid, adrenal or pancreatic function).
- Electrolyte imbalances.
- Acid–base disorders.
- Hypothermia.
- Hyperglycaemia.
- Coagulopathy.

Organ retrieval takes place in the operating theatre. Organ perfusion is maintained, with fluids and inotropes if necessary. High-dose inotropes are, however, detrimental to subsequent organ function. A pulmonary artery catheter may be considered for multi-organ donors. Ventilation to keep the $PaO_2 > 10\,kPa$ is continued.

Suggested minimum criteria for organ donation

- Mean arterial pressure (MAP) $> 60\,mmHg$.
- Central venous pressure (CVP) $< 12\,mmHg$.
- Pulmonary artery occlusion pressure (PAOP) $< 12\,mmHg$.
- Cardiac index $> 2.1\,l\,m^{-2}$.

Spinal reflexes require neuromuscular blockers and autonomic haemodynamic responses may require drugs for control. Once the organs have been retrieved, ventilation is stopped. The emotional needs of the relatives and staff must not be forgotten, particularly if a child is involved.

Non-heartbeating donation

The use of non-heartbeating donation (NHBD) has significantly increased the potential donor pool. Controlled NHBD occurs where potential donors indicated in life their wish to donate and the organ donation procedure (cannulation, etc.) has been discussed with and agreed by relatives prior to the donor's death. The general overriding principle of respect for the wishes of the individual in life can however, be overruled by refusal of consent for donation by the next of kin. This is one of the rare exceptions where relative's consent before a procedure (retrieval) on an incompetent adult is essential. The distress caused to living persons and the negative overall effect of the publicity on organ transplantation currently take precedence over the wishes of the deceased. It is ethically acceptable to cannulate a potential NHBD if it can be established beyond reasonable doubt that that individual has indicated their wish to donate in life and the view of the next of kin is unknown (uncontrolled NHBD).

The practical difficulties of NHBD centre around the need to act quickly to retrieve organs from the recently deceased donor. The use of such a donated organ should also be subject to the informed consent of the recipient, with explanation of the increased risk of delayed graft function and somewhat poorer overall outcome.

Further reading

Australian and New Zealand Intensive Care Society *(ANZICS). Recommendations on Brain Death and Organ Donation*, 2nd edn, 1998.
 http://www.anzics.com.au
British Transplant Society web address
 http://www.bts.org.uk
Milner QJW, Vuylsteke A, Ismail F, Ismail-Zade I, Latimer RD. ICU resuscitation of the multi-organ donor. *Br J Intens Care*, 1997; **7**: 49–54.
Working Party for the Department of Health. *A Code of Practice for the Diagnosis of Brain Stem Death*. Department of Health, March 1998.

Related topics of interest

Death certification (p. 127)
Head injury (p. 164)
Subarachnoid haemorrhage (p. 300)

Burns

Stephen Laver

The skin provides a protective barrier against physical, chemical and microbial agents. Once breached by temperatures of $>40°C$, the resulting burn may cause harm to deeper structures and systemic injury. In England and Wales, 10000 burns patients are admitted to hospital each year. Of the 500 who die, the vast majority die from smoke inhalation, the rest from burn-wound associated sepsis or pneumonia. Ten percent of the patients admitted to hospital require formal fluid resuscitation and burn excision and grafting.

Initial assessment and resuscitation

Inhalation, chemical or electrical burns are classified by body surface area (BSA) and depth.

BSA
The rule of nines enables rapid initial estimation of the burn area in adults. Lund and Browder charts are used to estimate burn area in children and to provide a more precise estimate in adults; the charts are age-specific and take into account children's disproportionate BSA, larger heads and smaller arms, legs and torso. In the early post-burn period it is often difficult to estimate the full extent and depth of burns.

Depth
A *superficial* burn affects only the epidermal layer. It is red, painful, and dry and is absent of blisters. Healing occurs within a week.

A *partial-thickness* burn involves the epidermal and dermal layers: it can be classified as shallow or deep, depending on the extent of damage to the dermis. The skin is red, blistered and painful and oedema is present. Healing occurs in 14 days with no scarring after a shallow burn and in 4 weeks with scarring after a deep burn, which may also require excision and grafting.

A *full-thickness* burn destroys all layers of the skin. Complex full-thickness burns involve subcutaneous tissues such as muscle. The burn appears white and is painless. There is no capillary return after applying pressure and pricking the skin with a needle causes no bleeding. Skin grafting is required to treat this burn.

Definition of a major burn (requiring referral to a specialist burns centre)

1. Full-thickness burn $>10\%$ total body surface area (TBSA).
2. Partial-thickness burn involving $>25\%$ TBSA in adults and $>20\%$ TBSA at the extremes of age.

3. Burns to the face, hands, perineum or feet.
4. Burns affecting a major joint.

Initial management of a major burn

History

The time the burn was sustained must be documented; fluid volumes for resuscitation are estimated from this point. The mechanism of injury is important (flame, chemical, etc.), because it will identify hazards that could potentially injure health care personnel. A victim receiving burns in an enclosed area is likely to have concurrent inhalation injury. Burns sustained after an explosion are likely to be accompanied by blast injury. A child with burns should provoke careful questioning to exclude abuse (10% of abuse cases involve burns and severe scalds).

Airway

Assessment

Look for direct burns to the face; singeing of eyebrows, eyelashes and nasal hair; swelling of the face, lips, tongue or oropharynx; a cough, wheeze or stridor; or soot in the nose, mouth or sputum. Signs of an airway burn indicate the need for intubation before gross swelling of the upper airway occurs. An awake fibreoptic intubation or inhalational induction should be considered as an alternative to intravenous induction.

Indirect lung injury

Acute respiratory distress syndrome (ARDS) occurs secondary to the systemic inflammatory response triggered by the burn wound matrix, infection and complications of burn therapy.

Carbon monoxide (CO) poisoning

CO poisoning is responsible for 80% of deaths associated with smoke inhalation. CO has an affinity that is 250 times that of O_2 for haemoglobin; it also shifts the oxy-haemoglobin (HbO_2) dissociation curve to the left. It therefore greatly reduces the amount of O_2 available for metabolism, causing tissue hypoxia and metabolic acidosis. Tissue hypoxia occurs from displacement of oxygen from haemoglobin, and the inhibition of complex IV in the respiratory chain in mitochondria. Clinical symptoms depend on the amount of CO present:

10–20% tinnitus, headaches and nausea.
20–40% weakness and drowsiness.
>40% coma, convulsions and cardiac arrest.

Only direct co-oximeters using multiwavelength spectroscopy can differentiate Hb, HbO_2 and carboxyhaemoglobin (HbCO). Pulse oximeters will indicate the oxygen saturation of HbO_2 but will give no indication of the true oxygen content of the blood because HbCO is not detected. Thus, the total haemoglobin oxygen saturation is overestimated.

Treatment is by high-concentration O_2 therapy, which will decrease the half-life of CO from 2h to 30min. Three hyperbaric oxygen (HBO) treatments given over a 24-h period reduce neurological sequelae in patients with symptomatic acute CO poisoning. Patients should be considered for HBO treatment if they are symptomatic and have an HbCO level >25%. In many countries, particularly the UK, hyperbaric facilities are scarce and, in any case, there are great technical difficulties in the transfer and administration of HBO treatment to a severely burned patient.

Cyanide (CN) poisoning

Hydrogen cyanide causes tissue asphyxia by inhibition of cytochrome oxidase, which prevents mitochondrial O_2 consumption and arrests the tricarboxylic acid cycle. The only pathway left for ATP production is anaerobic metabolism of pyruvate to lactate and, consequently, metabolic acidosis. Clinical symptoms vary with the concentration:

50 ppm – headache, dizziness, tachycardia and tachypnoea
100 ppm – lethargy, seizures and respiratory failure

Treatment is normally conservative but high CN levels and persisting metabolic acidosis should be treated with sodium thiosulphate (increases hepatic metabolism to inactive metabolites), sodium nitrites (provide methaemoglobin, which combines with CN to form inactive cyanomethaemoglobin) and dicobalt edetate (binds to CN to form an inactive complex).

Cardiovascular responses

The inflammatory reaction associated with major burns is the most intense that occurs in critically ill patients. Macrophages, neutrophils and endothelial cells release arachidonic metabolites that cause vasoconstriction, local (thromboxane A_2 (TxA_2), thromboxane B_2 (TxB_2)) and systemic effects. Failure of cell membrane Na^+/K^+ ATPase increases microvascular permeability and microvascular leak. 'Burn shock' is due to loss of plasma from the circulation and decrease in cardiac output. Systemic vascular resistance (SVR) is increased, increasing myocardial work. Prompt fluid resuscitation of a major burn reduces potential organ failure and maintains cardiac output. Oedema results from loss of plasma fluid into the interstitial space. During episodes of sepsis, vasoconstrictors or vasodilators may be needed to stabilise the cardiovascular system, the choice of therapy determined partly by the core−peripheral temperature difference.

Intensive care management

In the first 24–48 h following resuscitation, the hormonal response (increased cortisol, glucagon and catecholamines release) and inflammatory mediators (TNF, O_2 free radicals, endothelin and interleukins) cause hypermetabolism, immunosuppression and the systemic inflammatory response syndrome (SIRS), with changes to cardiac output and SVR.

Fluid and electrolyte management

Intravenous fluid resuscitation is required in adults if the burn involves more than 20% BSA or 15% with smoke inhalation. The fluid resuscitation is to avoid end-organ ischaemia, preserve viable tissue by restoring tissue perfusion and minimise tissue oedema. Crystalloid-only regimens are becoming increasingly popular because colloids, particularly albumin, have not been shown to improve outcome. The Parkland formula is lactated Ringer's solution (Hartmann's in the UK), $4\,ml\,kg^{-1}\,\%BSA^{-1}$ per burn in the first 24 h, with 50% being given in the first 8 h. Most critical care practitioners give a combination of colloid (starch or albumin) and crystalloid from the second day. Resuscitation formulae are merely guides and fluid resuscitation should be titrated against clinical response, invasive haemodynamic monitoring and urine output, aiming for at least $0.5\,ml\,kg^{-1}\,h^{-1}$ in adults and $1.0\,ml\,kg^{-1}\,h^{-1}$ in children. Hypokalaemia, hypophosphataemia, hypocalcaemia and hypomagnesaemia are common and should be treated.

Metabolism and nutrition

The increase in basal metabolic rate (BMR) is proportional to the size of the burn and the presence of infection, peaking at 7–10 days. There is an increase in core temperature of 1–2°C. This implies that a patient with a core temperature of 37°C is relatively hypothermic. An ambient temperature of 28–32°C with a high humidity is important to minimise the increase in BMR caused by heat and water loss. Provision of adequate nutrition is essential. The enteral route is preferred; TPN is associated with very high septic complication rates. Protein losses are high and difficult to assess due to wound loss, but urinary nitrogen loss is a guide. Protein needs are estimated in relation to caloric needs – 20% of total calories are administered as protein with a non-protein calorie: N_2 ratio of 100:1.

Gastrointestinal protection is best provided by immediate enteral feeding and H_2-receptor antagonist or proton pump inhibitor prophylaxis, especially if the patient is mechanically ventilated. Enteral feeding helps to maintain gut perfusion and intestinal mucosal integrity, helping to prevent bacterial translocation, and has been shown to decrease weight loss and sepsis.

Blood glucose levels above $7.8\,mmol\,l^{-1}$ increase mortality after major burns. Other research shows that tightly controlling blood glucose levels in critically ill patients improves mortality and morbidity.

Infection

Downregulation of immune responses and loss of the skin barrier render patients highly susceptible to infection. Burns are initially virtually free from bacteria, which are killed by the heat, but the dead tissue soon becomes heavily colonised by bacteria. This is not significant in superficial burns, but is the major cause of death in more major burns. The usual organisms are *Streptococcus pyogenes*, *Pseudomonas aeruginosa* and *Staphylococcus aureus*. The first line of defence against infection involves protecting the patient against microbial contaminants. This is achieved by primary excision and skin grafting (which also removes the burn matrix that fuels the inflammatory process), antisepsis with antibacterial substances such as 1% silver sulfadiazine, asepsis with regular dressing changes, isolation of patients and good ward hygiene. Antibiotic therapy and active or passive immunisation is used to prevent invasion of the tissues and bloodstream by bacteria growing on the burn. The role of selective decontamination of the digestive tract (SDD) in burns patients is controversial. When applied to large areas of burnt tissue, topical antimicrobials can cause systemic effects: silver nitrate can cause loss of chloride, silver sulfadiazine is a cause of neutropenia and mafenide acetate is painful when applied and can cause a metabolic acidosis secondary to carbonic anhydrase inhibition.

Diagnosis of sepsis is difficult, as leukocytosis, erythema, fever and a hyperdynamic state are all normal findings in a severely burned patient. Sepsis should be suspected if there is any change in mental status, new glucose intolerance, increasing base deficit or hypothermia.

Pharmacology
The changes in metabolism, cardiac output and fluid shifts will affect volume of distribution, protein binding (reduced levels of albumin but increased α_1-acid glycoprotein) and clearance of drugs. Careful plasma and clinical monitoring is essential. Blood flow (usually increased) and hepatic enzyme activity (decreased) affect hepatic elimination of drugs. In the kidney there is increased glomerular filtration but decreased tubular secretion of drugs. Drugs may also be eliminated through the burn itself.

Analgesia
In the early phases, incremental i.v. boluses of an opiate such as morphine are titrated to effect and later given either by PCA or continuous infusion, depending on the patient's functional state. When used in conjunction with a benzodiazepine, ketamine is useful for wound dressing changes.

Surgical management

Early tangential surgical excision and grafting removes the source of the inflammatory response and provides a barrier to infection. It has been shown to decrease pain, the number of operations required, blood loss, length of hospital stay and mortality rate, as well as achieving a better functional result. Excision and grafting should take place as soon as the patient is stable. Debridement and grafting will cause significant haemorrhage and hypothermia. The procedure should be stopped if the patient gets cold – it is often not possible to cover the patient up for surgery, as the good skin may be harvested to make grafts.

Massive burns (>60% BSA) provide difficulty with suitable donor sites. This can be overcome by:

1. Use of widely expanded meshed autologous skin graft, which can be overlaid with unmeshed cadaver skin.
2. Biosynthetic materials: Integra® has a non-cellular matrix material which mimics the 3D structure of the dermis and is overlaid with a silastic covering membrane to mimic the physical properties of the epidermis. It has been shown to be as effective as autologous skin grafting but is extremely expensive.
3. Cultured epithelial autograft is very expensive and has a high failure rate.
4. In the future, artificial skin may be available in the form of cultured allograft epidermal cells. If successful, this would have the advantage of being pathogen free and universally available, and would produce growth factors to enhance the healing process.

Psychological care/rehabilitation

The long-term effects of severe illness, pain, disfigurement and loss of independence have profound effects on the survivors of severe burns. Post-traumatic stress disorder may contribute to depression, agitation and sleep disturbance. A compassionate approach, with the early involvement of a multidisciplinary team of physiotherapists, psychologists, nurses, councillors and occupational therapists, is vital to help reduce long-term impairment.

Further reading

Weaver LK, Hopkins RO, Chan KJ, *et al.* Hyperbaric oxygen for acute carbon monoxide poisoning. *N Engl J Med* 2002; **347**: 1057–67.

Related topics of interest

Infection acquired in critical care (nosocomial) (p. 182)
Nutrition (p. 207)

Calcium, magnesium and phosphate

Calcium

Over 99% of body calcium is in bone, of which about 1% is freely exchangeable with extracellular fluid (ECF). Ionised calcium is crucial to many excitatory processes, including nerve and neuromuscular conduction/contraction and coagulation. Normal daily intake is of the order of 10–20 mmol and normal total serum calcium is in the range 2.25–2.7 mmol l^{-1}. Intestinal calcium absorption is enhanced by 1,25-dihydroxy-vitamin D$_3$ (1,25(OH)$_2$D$_3$). Around 40% is bound to albumin and total serum calcium decreases 0.02 mmol l^{-1} for each 1 g l^{-1} decrease in albumin. Ionised calcium is the physiologically important form and the normal level is 1.15 mmol l^{-1}.

Hypocalcaemia

Causes
Hypocalcaemia occurs when calcium is lost from the ECF (most commonly through renal mechanisms) in greater quantities than can be replaced by bone or the intestine. Common causes of hypocalcaemia are:

- Renal failure.
- Hypoparathyroidism.
- Sepsis.
- Burns.
- Hypomagnesaemia.
- Pancreatitis.
- Malnutrition.
- Osteomalacia.
- Alkalosis (reduced ionised calcium).
- Citrate toxicity (massive transfusion).

As a result of reduced absorption of dietary divalent cations or poor dietary intake, hypocalcaemia and hypomagnesaemia often coexist.

Clinical features
The symptoms of hypocalcaemia correlate with the magnitude and rapidity of the decrease in serum calcium. The main features include neuromuscular irritability evidenced by extremity and circumoral paraesthesiae, Chvostek and Trousseau signs, muscle cramps, tetany, laryngospasm and seizures. A prolonged QT is seen on ECG and may progress to VT/VF and hypotension.

Treatment
Appropriate therapy depends on the severity of the hypocalcaemia and its cause. The serum magnesium and phosphate should be checked and, if low, corrected. Chronic asymptomatic mild hypocalcaemia can be treated with oral calcium supplements. If metabolic acidosis accompanies hypocalcaemia, calcium must be corrected before the acidosis is corrected. Calcium and hydrogen ions compete for protein-binding sites, so

an increase in pH will lead to a rapid decrease in ionised calcium. In the presence of acute symptomatic hypocalcaemia, an intravenous bolus of calcium (100–200 mg or 2.5–5 mmol) should be given over 5 min. This can be followed by a maintenance infusion of 1–2 mg kg^{-1} h^{-1}. Calcium chloride 10% contains 27.2 mg Ca ml^{-1} (0.68 mmol ml^{-1}) and calcium gluconate 10% contains 9 mg ml^{-1} (0.225 mmol l^{-1}). Calcium gluconate causes less venous irritation than calcium chloride.

Calcium management following parathyroidectomy

In chronic renal failure the glomerular filtration rate (GFR) decreases and phosphate (PO$_4$) is not excreted. Phosphate levels in the blood rise and this decreases the level of the active metabolite of 1,25(OH)$_2$D$_3$. As a result, patients have hypocalcaemia and defective bone mineralisation. The low calcium stimulates the parathyroid gland to increase production of parathyroid hormone, PTH (secondary hyperparathyroidism). If the secondary hyperparathyroidism is prolonged, the secretion of PTH becomes autonomous – tertiary hyperparathyroidism. This leads to high calcium levels. High calcium and high PO$_4$ levels cause precipitation of calcium in tissues and organs. After total or partial parathyroidectomy the calcium level can fall rapidly, particularly in patients who have evidence of 'hungry bone syndrome' (high alkaline phosphatase). These patients may need large quantities of i.v. calcium replacement. Some patients have hypercalcaemia with calcification of small and medium blood vessels, leading to skin necrosis and ulcers particularly on their legs. This is called calciphylaxis and these patients' calcium levels should be kept at the lower limit of normal.

Calcium infusion after parathyroidectomy

Following parathyroid surgery, calcium infusions are best given through central intusions, as peripheral i.v. may cause necrosis. Calcium levels should be checked 4-hourly until stable, then 6-hourly. Check the patient's alkaline phosphatase level preoperatively: the higher the level, the more likely postoperative low serum calcium levels and symptoms will occur. Prescribe oral calcium medications. If the corrected calcium level is < 2.4 mmol l^{-1}, commence a calcium infusion.

Dilute 20 ml 10% calcium chloride in 100 ml 0.9% sodium chloride (Table 2). Check corrected calcium 4-hourly, and adjust rate (Table 3).

If the patient has tertiary hyperparathyroidism or calciphylaxis, choose the lower infusion rate; if they have alkaline phosphatase > 300 units/l, choose the higher infusion rate.

All patients require oral calcium, 1 g, 8-hourly, and calcitriol, 0.5–1.0 μg daily in two divided doses, as soon as they are able to drink.

Table 2 Starting rate of calcium infusion

Preoperative alkaline phosphatase (ALP) level (unit l^{-1})	Calcium chloride infusion rate (ml h^{-1})
200–400	5
400–800	10
> 800	15

Table 3 Adjusted rate of calcium infusion

Plasma corrected calcium (mmol l^{-1})	Intravenous rate (ml h^{-1})
2.0–2.4	5–10
1.8–2.0	10–15
1.7–1.8	25–30
<1.7	35–40

Hypercalcaemia

Causes
Hypercalcaemia occurs generally when the influx of calcium from bone or the intestine exceeds renal calcium excretory capacity. Common causes include:

- Hyperparathyroidism (accounts for >50% of cases).
- Neoplasms (primary with ectopic PTH secretion, secondary with bone metastases).
- Sarcoidosis (increased production of 1,25(OH)$_2$D$_3$ by granulomatous tissue).
- Drugs (thiazides and lithium).
- Immobilisation of any cause.
- Vitamin D intoxication.
- Thyrotoxicosis.
- Milk-alkali syndrome (consumption of calcium-containing antacids).

Clinical features
The symptoms associated with hypercalcaemia depend on the rate of rise as well as the absolute level of calcium. Mild hypercalcaemia is usually asymptomatic. Severe hypercalcaemia causes neurological, gastrointestinal and renal symptoms. Neurological features range from mild weakness, depression, psychosis and drowsiness but may progress to coma. Gastrointestinal effects include nausea, vomiting, abdominal pain, constipation, peptic ulceration and pancreatitis. Nephrogenic diabetes insipidus (DI), renal stones, nephrocalcinosis and ectopic calcification may occur.

Treatment
The underlying cause of hypercalcaemia must be treated. The measures taken will depend on the calcium level. Most cases of mild hypercalcaemia are caused by primary hyperparathyroidism and many will require parathyroidectomy. Patients with symptomatic moderate (serum calcium >3.0 mmol l^{-1}) or severe (>3.4 mmol l^{-1}) hypercalcaemia require intravenous saline to restore intravascular volume and enhance renal calcium excretion. Thiazide diuretics should be avoided but furosemide (frusemide) will enhance calcium excretion. Patients with severe hypercalcaemia associated with raised PTH should be referred for urgent parathyroidectomy. Bisphosphonates (e.g. etidronate, sodium pamidronate) have become the main therapy for the management of hypercalcaemia due to enhanced osteoclastic bone reabsorption. Steroids are effective in hypercalcaemia associated with haematological malignancies and in diseases related to 1,25(OH)$_2$D$_3$ excess (e.g. sarcoidosis and vitamin D toxicity).

Magnesium

Magnesium is essential for normal cellular and enzyme function. The total body magnesium store is about 1000 mmol, of which 50–60% is in bone. The normal plasma range is 0.7–1.0 mmol l^{-1} but because it is primarily an intracellular ion the plasma level does not reflect total body stores. The normal daily intake is 10–20 mmol, which is balanced by urine and faecal losses. The kidney is the primary organ involved in magnesium regulation.

Hypomagnesaemia

Hypomagnesaemia occurs in up to 65% of critically ill patients and is often associated with hypokalaemia.

Causes
Usually follows loss of magnesium from the gastrointestinal tract or kidney.

- Gastrointestinal causes include prolonged nasogastric suction or vomiting, diarrhoea, extensive bowel resection, severe malnutrition and acute pancreatitis.
- Renal losses occur with volume expanded states, hypercalcaemia, diuretic therapy, alcohol, aminoglycosides and cisplatin exposure and the polyuric phase of acute tubular necrosis.
- Other causes include phosphate depletion, hyperparathyroidism and diabetes mellitus.

Clinical features
Most of the symptoms of hypomagnesaemia are rather non-specific. The accompanying ion abnormalities such as hypocalcaemia, hypokalaemia and metabolic alkalosis account for many of the clinical features. Neurological signs include confusion, weakness, ataxia, tremors, carpopedal spasm and seizures. A wide QRS, long PR, inverted T, and U wave may be seen on ECG. Arrhythmias may occur, including severe ventricular arrhythmias (torsades de pointes), and there is increased potential for cardiac glycoside toxicity.

Treatment
The underlying cause must be addressed. Symptomatic moderate-to-severe hypomagesaemia will require parenteral therapy. In the event of an acute arrhythmia or seizure, 8–10 mmol of magnesium sulphate can be given over 5 min followed by 25 mmol over 12 h. The rate should be titrated against serum levels. Potassium should be replaced at the same time. Oral magnesium sulphate is a laxative and may cause diarrhoea.

Hypermagnesaemia

Hypermagnesaemia is usually iatrogenic (e.g. excess i.v. administration). High magnesium levels antagonise the entry of calcium and prevent excitation.

Clinical features

These include hypotension, bradycardia, drowsiness and hyporeflexia (knee jerk is a useful clinical test and is lost above $4\,mmol\,l^{-1}$). Levels $>6\,mmol\,l^{-1}$ cause coma and respiratory depression.

Treatment

Administration of magnesium should be stopped. Calcium chloride will antagonise the effect of magnesium. Diuretics increase renal loss. In severe cases dialysis may be required.

Phosphate

Total body phosphate in adults is about $700\,g$: approximately 85% is in bone and 15% is in extracellular fluid and soft tissue. Phosphate is found in adenosine triphosphate (ATP), 2,3-diphosphoglycerate (2,3-DPG) in red blood cells, phospholipids and phosphoproteins. Phosphate is essential in many cellular functions and also acts as a buffer. The normal serum level is $0.85–1.4\,mmol\,l^{-1}$.

Hypophosphataemia

Causes

Hypophosphataemia results from internal redistribution, increased urinary excretion and decreased intestinal absorption.

- Internal redistribution of phosphate may result from respiratory alkalosis, refeeding after malnutrition, recovery from diabetic ketoacidosis and the effects of hormones and other agents (insulin, glucagon, adrenaline (epinephrine), cortisol, glucose).
- Increased urinary excretion of phosphate occurs in hyperparathyroidism, vitamin D deficiency, malabsorption, volume expansion, renal tubular acidosis and alcoholism.
- Decreased intestinal absorption of phosphate occurs in antacid abuse, vitamin D deficiency and chronic diarrhoea.

Clinical features

The clinical features are usually seen when the phosphate level has fallen below $0.3\,mmol\,l^{-1}$. They are often non-specific but may include weakness (which may contribute to respiratory failure and problems with weaning from mechanical ventilation), cardiac dysfunction, paraesthesia, coma and seizures.

Treatment

The underlying cause should be corrected. Oral phosphate can be given in doses of 2–3 g daily. When needed, 10 mmol potassium phosphate can be given i.v. over 60 min and repeated depending on measured levels (a sodium phosphate preparation is also available). There is a risk of hypocalcaemia associated with i.v. replacement and serum calcium must be maintained.

Hyperphosphataemia

Causes
Renal failure is the most common cause.

- Reduced renal excretion: renal failure, hypoparathyroidism, acromegaly, bisphosphonate therapy and magnesium deficiency.
- Increased exogenous load: i.v. infusion, excess oral therapy, phosphate-containing enemas.
- Increased endogenous load: tumour lysis syndrome, rhabdomyolysis, bowel infarction, malignant hyperthermia, haemolysis and acidosis.
- Pseudohyperphosphataemia: multiple myeloma.

Clinical features
Hypocalcaemia and tetany may occur with rapid rise in level. A large rise in calcium × phosphate product causes ectopic calcification in tissues, nephrocalcinosis and renal stones.

Treatment
Aluminium hydroxide is used as a binding agent. Magnesium and calcium salts are also effective and aluminium accumulation is a risk. Dialysis may be required.

Further reading

Aguilera IM, Vaughan RS. Calcium and the anaesthetist. *Anaesthesia* 2000; **55**: 779–90.
Bushinsky DA, Monk RD. Calcium. *Lancet* 1998; **352**: 306–11.
Weisinger JR, Bellorin-Font E. Magnesium and phosphorus. *Lancet* 1998; **352**: 391–6.
Yudd M, Llach F. Current medical management of secondary hyperparathyroidism. *Am J Med Sci* 2000; **320**: 100–6.

Related topics of interest

Fluid replacement therapy (p. 156)
Potassium (p. 233)
Sodium (p. 281)

Cancer patients and critical care

Cynthia Uy

Recent advances in cancer treatment have improved life expectancy and quality of life in patients with haematologic or solid malignancies. The outcomes of cancer patients in critical care units have also been improving. Cancer patients may require admission to a critical care unit for:

- Management of complications associated with the disease and treatment.
- Administration of specific cancer therapy (usually performed in specialist units).
- Postoperative care.

To aid in decisions of offering, withholding or withdrawing therapy, studies have tried to identify factors that predict critical care mortality in this population. To date, factors associated with short-term outcome include duration of stay in a critical care unit, mechanical ventilation and number of organ system failures. If the decision to admit a patient to a critical care unit is made, potential outcomes and the possibility of withdrawing life-supportive therapy should be discussed with the patient and family.

Respiratory complications

ARDS is the most common reason for admission of patients receiving chemotherapy to a general critical care unit. On clinical grounds, it may be difficult to differentiate infection from pneumonitis. Management is empirical and supportive. Confirmatory tests to consider include computed tomography (CT) scan, bronchoalveolar lavage, bronchial brushings and biopsies.

Other causes of respiratory failure in cancer patients include alveolar haemorrhage, pulmonary embolism, airway obstruction by tumour and lysis pneumopathy.

Infections

Infections can occur due to specific immune defects, cytotoxic agents, corticosteroids and bone marrow transplantation.

Respiratory infection

Respiratory failure secondary to infection remains the most common cause of death in bone marrow transplants. The organisms implicated include cytomegalovirus, *Pneumocystis carinii*, varicella zoster, toxoplasma, Gram-positive and Gram-negative bacteria and *Candida* and *Aspergillus* spp. Antimicrobial therapy requires multiple drugs and close microbiological collaboration. Patients are often treated with a third-generation cephalosporin or extended-spectrum penicillin, an aminoglycoside, vancomycin, fluconazole, co-trimoxazole and an antiviral agent.

Neutropenia

Neutropenia (neutrophil count $<1.0 \times 10^9 l^{-1}$) following treatment with cytotoxic drugs is a risk factor for serious infection. In general, neutropenia for less than 10 days is well tolerated. At $0.5 \times 10^9 l^{-1}$, the risk becomes significant. Because of low neutrophil counts and continued immunosuppression (steroids), patients do not often show the usual signs of infection. Sepsis should be assumed in any neutropenic patient presenting with a fever (T>38.5°C) and promptly managed with screening and empiric broad-spectrum antibiotics. Debate on the optimal regimen continues; suggested therapy includes two-drug therapy with a third-generation cephalosporin or extended-spectrum penicillin and an aminoglycoside. Treatment should be refined on the basis of culture results and microbiological advice. Vancomycin should not be used unless the patient is in shock, colonised with methicillin-resistant *Staphylococcus aureus* (MRSA) or has a catheter infection in a unit with a high incidence of MRSA. Vancomycin is indicated if a Gram-positive organism resistant to other antibiotics is isolated from cultures. Antifungal treatment is usually added if fungal infection is suspected or if fever persists after 7 days. Trials are under way to clarify the role of prophylactic antibiotics in afebrile neutropenic patients as well as the outpatient management of low-risk febrile neutropenic patients. Granulocyte colony stimulating factor (GCSF) is used to stimulate stem cells after chemotherapy and before stem cell harvest. Treatment reduces the duration and severity of neutropenia. Patients at high risk of infection include those with:

- Prolonged persistent neutropenia.
- Pneumonitis.
- Severe mucositis.
- Invasive catheters (intravenous, urethral, tracheal).
- Local sepsis.

Prevention of infection

Infection arises from endogenous spread (oropharynx, gastrointestinal tract, intravenous lines) and exogenous spread (staff, other patients, food, parenteral drugs and nutrition and blood products). Methods used to reduce infection are:

- Hand washing.
- Protective isolation and reverse barrier nursing.
- Sterile technique for all procedures.
- Minimising invasive procedures.
- Screening all blood products.

Oncological and haematological emergencies

From direct tumour involvement

- Superior vena cava obstruction is seen most commonly in patients with small cell lung cancer. It can be life threatening if associated with tracheal obstruction. Treatment includes the use of corticosteroids, urgent chemotherapy or radiotherapy (depending on tumour type) and anticoagulation, as thrombus formation occurs in about half of patients.
- Spinal cord compression is seen more commonly in patients with prostate, lung and

breast cancer. Neurological compromise requires prompt treatment with high-dose corticosteroids, radiotherapy and/or neurosurgery.

- Seizures from cerebral metastases or primary brain tumour should be stabilised, then followed by specific treatment with corticosteroids and cerebral irradiation.

Metabolic complications

- Hypercalcaemia of malignancy occurs more commonly in patients with lung cancer, breast cancer, renal cancer, multiple myeloma and lymphoma. Hypercalcaemia is related to parathyroid hormone-related protein (PTHrP), abnormal vitamin D production and bony metastases. It is treated with diuresis, bisphosphonates and, if rapid effect is needed, calcitonin.
- Hyponatraemia due to syndrome of inappropriate antidiuretic hormone or SIADH (vincristine, cyclophosphamide), see p. 281.
- Tumour lysis syndrome (hyperkalaemia, hyperphosphataemia, hypocalcaemia, hyperuricaemia, lactic acidosis) results from destruction of tumour cells and release of their products into the circulation. It is more common in haematological malignancies. Hydration and allopurinol are used as prophylactic measures in high-risk patients; haemodialysis may reverse toxicity.
- Haemolytic uraemic syndrome (microangiopathic haemolytic anaemia, thrombocytopenia and acute renal failure) is associated with the use of mitomycin C, cisplatin, bleomycin and gemcitabine. It is treated supportively with transfusions, dialysis and plasmaphoresis.
- Hyperviscosity is particularly seen in multiple myeloma and may be an indicator for plasmaphoresis.

Complications of treatment

- Graft-versus-host disease (GvHD) is a common, potentially fatal complication of allogeneic bone marrow transplantion. There is frequently a rash associated with variable degrees of hepatic abnormalities and gastrointestinal (GI) failure. Therapy includes steroids, ciclosporin, antithymocyte globulin, methotrexate, thalidomide, azathioprine and psoralen plus ultraviolet A (PUVA).
- Anaphylaxis and capillary leak, with resulting hypotension, can be caused by intravenous administration of interleukin-2 (IL-2). The infusion should be ceased and the patient monitored and cared for supportively.
- Nausea and vomiting is associated with most cytotoxic agents.
- Bone marrow suppression of haematopoietic progenitor cells by chemotherapy leads to leucopaenia, anaemia and thrombocytopenia. Recovery occurs over 3–4 weeks.
- Oral mucositis can be severe and may reflect damage to the whole of the GI epithelium. Mucositis is due to the effect of chemotherapy on the GI tract mucosa, which like marrow, is a rapidly dividing cell population. This results in inflammation, necrosis and subsequent regeneration. Drugs typically causing mucositis include 5-fluorouracil, methotrexate, doxorubicin, busulfan and bleomycin.
- Constipation is frequent; rarely, a paralytic ileus may present with the use of vinca alkaloids.

- Cytotoxics such as the vinca alkaloids and anthracyclines are highly vesicant and can cause tissue damage on extravasation.
- Hypersensitivity reactions can occur with nearly all chemotherapeutic agents but are seen more frequently in agents such as docetaxel, paclitaxel, etoposide and L-asparaginase.
- Anthracyclines are implicated as causative agents in cardiomyopathy. 5-Fluorouracil is associated with coronary artery spasm and ischaemia and other agents suspected of causing cardiac toxicity include paclitaxel, bleomycin and mitomycin C.
- Bleomycin causes a dose-dependent pulmonary fibrosis. Other treatments associated with pulmonary toxicity include nitrosoureas, alkylating agents, antimetabolites, vinca alkaloids, paclitaxel, IL-2 and interferon.
- Nephrotoxicity is seen with the use of platinum agents, especially cisplatin.
- Veno-occlusive liver disease may occur early after transplantation and is associated particularly with busulfan regimens.
- Peripheral and autonomic neuropathies can result from the use of platinum drugs, taxanes and vinca alkaloids. Cerebellar toxicity is seen with the use of 5-fluorouracil.
- Ototoxicity from cisplatin may be irreversible.
- Cyclophosphamide and ifosfamide cause haemorrhagic cystitis in a dose-dependent manner.
- Second malignancies are a late complication of chemotherapy use, particularly with alkylating agents and procarbazine. The most frequently reported cancer after chemotherapy is leukaemia.

Nutritional failure

This is common because of poor nutritional status, disease of the GI tract that limits enteral nutrition and a high metabolic nutritional requirement. Whenever possible, enteral nutrition is preferred but some patients with prolonged, severe mucositis will require parenteral nutrition. The use of parenteral nutrition is a recognised risk factor for infection in these patients.

Further reading

Azoulay E, Alberti C, Bornstain C, et al. Improved survival in cancer patients requiring mechanical ventilatory support: impact of noninvasive mechanical ventilatory support. *Crit Care Med* 2001; **29**: 519–25.

Blot F, Guiguet M, Nitenberg G, et al. Prognostic factors for neutropenic patients in an intensive care unit: respective roles of underlying malignancies and acute organ failures. *Eur J Cancer* 1997; **33**: 1031–7.

Kress JP, Christenson J, Pohlman AS, et al. Outcomes of critically ill cancer patients in a university hospital setting. *Am J Respir Crit Care Med* 1999; **160**: 1957–61.

Sculier JP. Intensive care and oncology. *Support Care Cancer* 1995; **3**: 93–105.

Related topics of interest

Cardiac arrhythmias

Jas Soar

Arrhythmias are common in critically ill patients. Cardiac arrhythmias may be the primary abnormality, caused by myocardial ischaemia or infarction, or they may stem from a variety of toxic and metabolic disturbances in patients with multiple system organ failure. Arrhythmias result from disturbances in automaticity or conduction through myocardial tissue.

Tachyarrhythmias can be classified as supraventricular or ventricular. Supraventricular arrhythmias include sinus tachycardia, atrial flutter and fibrillation, ectopic atrial tachycardia, multifocal atrial tachycardia, junctional tachycardia, atrioventricular (A-V) nodal re-entrant tachycardia and accessory pathway reciprocating tachycardia. Ventricular arrhythmias include premature ventricular beats, torsades de pointes, ventricular tachycardia and ventricular fibrillation.

Assessment

Answers to the following basic questions will help to determine the correct treatment of all arrhythmias:

1. How is the patient?
2. What is the arrhythmia?

The presence or absence of certain adverse signs or symptoms will dictate the appropriate treatment for most arrhythmias:

- Evidence of low cardiac output includes sweating, cold and clammy extremities (increased sympathetic activity), impaired consciousness (reduced cerebral blood flow), and hypotension.
- Excessive tachycardia causes myocardial ischaemia. The rate at which this may occur differs between narrow complex (>200 beats min^{-1}) and broad complex (>150 beats min^{-1}) tachycardias.
- Excessive bradycardia is defined as a heart rate of <40 beats min^{-1}. Patients with a poor stroke volume may need much higher rates to maintain an adequate cardiac output.
- Pulmonary oedema (failure of the left ventricle) or raised jugular venous pressure and hepatic engorgement (failure of the right ventricle).

Treatment options

First, attempt to correct any precipitants for the arrhythmia. These can include:

- Myocardial ischaemia.

- Respiratory compromise (hypoxia, hypercarbia).
- Circulatory compromise (hypovolaemia, hypotension, hypertension, low haemoglobin, reduced cardiac output).
- Electrolyte abnormalities (especially of potassium, magnesium and calcium).
- Metabolic abnormalities (acidosis, alkalosis).
- Presence of drugs (tricyclics, monoamine oxidase inhibitors (MAOIs), cocaine, amphetamine, antiarrhythmic overdose/toxicity).
- Excessive endogenous catecholamines (inadequate sedation, pain, phaeochromocytoma).
- Exogenous catecholamines (catecholamine infusions, direct and indirect vasopressors, theophylline toxicity).
- Mechanical stimulation (pacing wire, central venous pressure (CVP) line, pulmonary artery catheter).
- Mechanical cardiac abnormalities (cardiomyopathy, valvular heart disease, pulmonary embolism, tamponade).
- Raised intracranial pressure (ICP).
- Hypothermia or hyperthermia.
- Sepsis-related myocardial dysfunction.

For example, in critically ill surgical patients, hypoxia, high cardiac filling pressures, severe physiological derangement at admission and the presence of systemic inflammatory response syndrome (SIRS) and sepsis are independent risk factors for the development of arrhythmias of which atrial fibrillation is the most common.

There are three options for the immediate treatment of arrhythmias:

1. Attempted electrical cardioversion.
2. Antiarrhythmic (and other) drugs.
3. Cardiac pacing.

In general, if a patient with adverse signs has a tachyarrhythmia other than sinus tachycardia, prompt electrical cardioversion is indicated. If the patient is stable, there is more time to establish the diagnosis and decide on the most appropriate course of treatment.

1. **Electrical cardioversion** is attempted with a synchronised shock, which can convert a tachycardia to sinus rhythm. The shock is synchronised to occur with the R wave of the electrocardiogram rather than the T wave to avoid the relative refractory period. This reduces the risk of precipitating ventricular fibrillation. Serial shocks are not appropriate for recurrent (within hours or days) paroxysms (self-terminating episodes) of atrial fibrillation. This is relatively common in critically ill patients, who may have ongoing precipitating factors for their arrhythmia (e.g. metabolic disturbance or sepsis). Conscious patients will require sedation or anaesthesia for cardioversion. Cardioversion does not prevent subsequent arrhythmias. If there are recurrent episodes, drug therapy is needed.
2. **Antiarrhythmic drugs** tend to be reserved for patients without adverse signs. All drugs that are used to treat arrhythmias can cause arrhythmias. Ideally, the aim of arrhythmia treatment is to achieve sinus rhythm. In elderly patients with atrial fibrillation, ventricular rate control can be equally good in terms of haemodynamic stability and prognosis. Antiarrhythmic drug therapy should be reviewed

once the arrhythmia has resolved. This avoids continuing drugs unnecessarily in patients where the arrhythmia was precipitated by non-cardiac problems that have been corrected (e.g. sepsis, metabolic disturbance).

3. **Cardiac pacing** using external transcutaneous pacing is simple and reliable for treating symptomatic bradycardias resistant to atropine or adrenaline (epinephrine)/isoprenaline infusion. It also buys time for transvenous pacing to be initiated.

Management of specific arrhythmias

For arrhythmias associated with cardiac arrest see p. 104.

Figures 1–3 are the treatment recommendation algorithms of the European Resuscitation Council for bradycardia, narrow complex tachycardia and broad complex

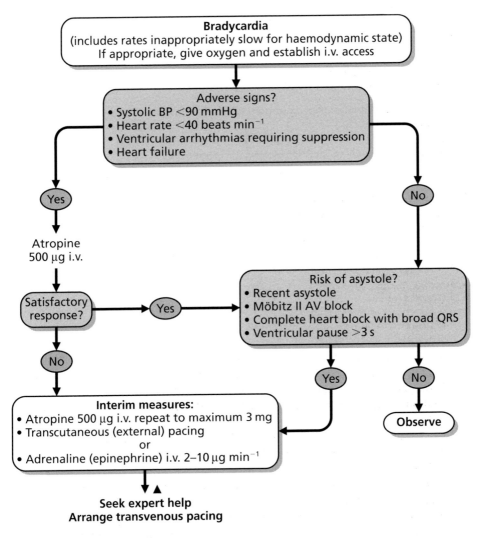

Figure 1 Bradycardia algorithm.

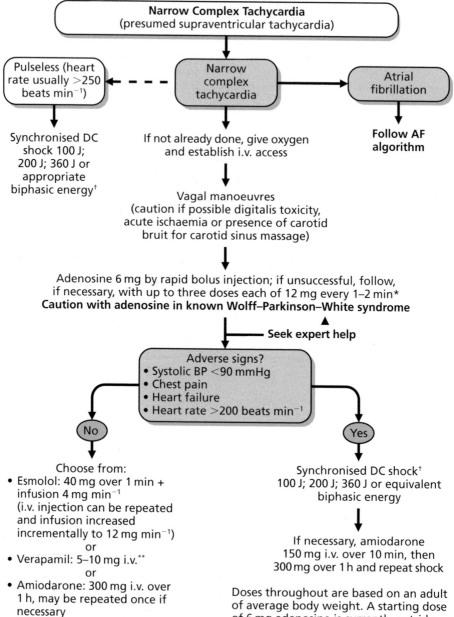

Figure 2 Narrow complex tachycardia algorithm.

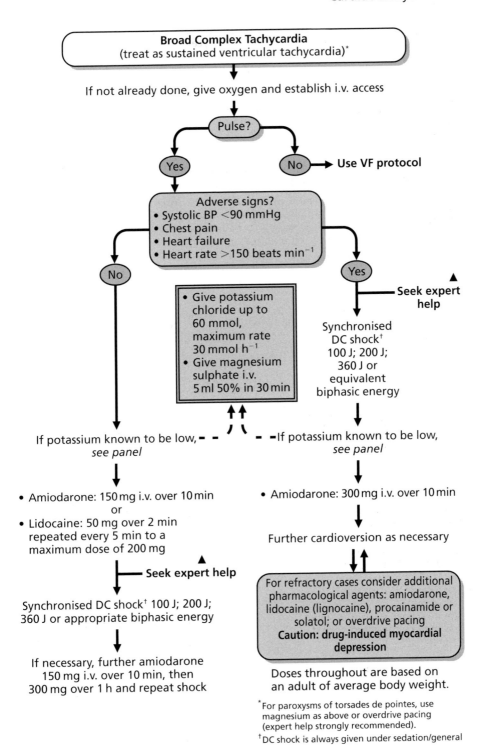

Figure 3 Broad complex tachycardia algorithm.

tachycardia, respectively. In all circumstances it is assumed that the patient is being given additional oxygen to breath and intravenous access has been established.

Further reading

Edhouse J, Morris F. ABC of clinical electrocardiography. Broad complex tachycardia Part I. *BMJ* 2002; **324**: 719–22.

Edhouse J, Morris F. ABC of clinical electrocardiography. Broad complex tachycardia Part II. *BMJ* 2002; **324**: 776–9.

Esberger D, Jones S, Morris F. ABC of clinical electrocardiography: Junctional tachycardias. *BMJ* 2002; **324**: 662–5.

Goodacre S, Irons R. ABC of clinical electrocardiography: Atrial arrhythmias. *BMJ* 2002; **324**: 594–7.

Resuscitation Council (UK) website with more information on the peri-arrest arrhythmia algorithms.
http://www.resus.org.uk/pages/periarst.htm

Related topics of interest

Cardiac chest pain (acute coronary syndromes)

Cardiac chest pain is one of the most common reasons for emergency admission to hospital. The term acute coronary syndrome encompasses a range of acute myocardial ischaemic states from unstable angina to non-ST segment elevation myocardial infarction (MI) and ST segment elevation MI. The mortality of acute myocardial infarction can be reduced markedly with the early administration of thrombolytic drugs. Patients presenting with chest pain thus require a rapid assessment of their condition to determine whether or not urgent thrombolysis is indicated. At the same time, their symptoms need controlling and physical condition stabilising.

Angina and non-ST segment elevation myocardial infarction

Angina is defined as unstable when attacks are increasingly frequent and/or prolonged, occur at rest, or are brought on with minor provocation. The vast majority of such patients have atheromatous obstructive coronary disease. The clinical presentation of unstable angina and non-ST segment elevation MI may be indistinguishable; it is simply that the ischaemia of the latter is severe enough to cause myocardial damage and the release of detectable quantities of markers of myocyte necrosis. Cardiac troponin is a more specific and sensitive marker of myocyte necrosis than creatine kinase, which is a better indicator of infarct size.

Treatment aims
1. Pain relief.
2. Reduction of platelet activity and thus thrombus formation.
3. Prevention of progression to MI or limitation of myocardial damage in the event of infarction.
4. Restoration of blood supply to muscle distal to coronary occlusion.

Immediate actions
- *Oxygen* by facemask or nasal cannulae.
- *Intravenous access.*
- *Pain control.* Give diamorphine 2.5–5 mg i.v. by slow injection (1 mg min^{-1}) repeated as required together with an antiemetic e.g. metoclopramide 10 mg or cyclizine 25–50 mg i.v. The equivalent dose of morphine is 5–10 mg i.v. by slow injection (2 mg min^{-1}).
- *Aspirin* 75 mg orally or 300 mg chewed then swallowed. Clopidogrel can be used in those allergic to aspirin.
- *12 lead ECG* and continuous ECG monitoring (CXR later).
- *Blood tests.* FBC, U&Es, glucose, troponin, cholesterol.

The patient should then be admitted to a critical care unit for bed rest, monitoring, and continued management.

Antianginal therapy

Nitrates

Nitrates reduce the pain of unstable angina. Sublingual glyceryl trinitrate (GTN) provides rapid but transient relief. A continuous intravenous infusion of isosorbide dinitrate ($2-10\,mg\,h^{-1}$) or GTN ($10-200\,\mu g\,min^{-1}$) should be titrated against the clinical response. Headache, nausea or hypotension may limit the use of nitrates. It is not known whether the use of intravenous nitrates will prevent progression to infarction.

Beta-blockade

Treatment usually relieves symptoms and may prevent progression to infarction. Early (within 12 h) intravenous therapy followed by oral treatment reduces the risk of progressing to infarction from 32 to 28%. Intravenous therapy is associated with an increased risk of adverse events in patients with first-degree heart block or bundle branch block.

Antiplatelet therapy

Thromboxane A$_2$ promotes the aggregation of platelets. **Aspirin** inhibits its synthesis, reduces the incidence of MI and improves the survival of patients with unstable angina. Given early enough, aspirin will save 20–30 lives per 1000 infarcts. Following the initial dose, it should be continued indefinitely at 75 mg daily.

Other drugs that inhibit platelet aggregation include **clopidogrel,** which inhibits adenosine diphosphate binding to platelet receptors, and **tirofiban,** a glycoprotein IIb/IIIa receptor inhibitor.

Anticoagulants

Unfractionated heparin

When given by intravenous infusion, unfractionated heparin (UFH) reduces symptomatic and silent ischaemic episodes in patients with unstable angina. It has been difficult to see this translated into a difference in outcome, however; in a meta-analysis of studies comparing groups treated with UFH and aspirin in combination, or aspirin alone, the incidence of death or infarction was 7.9% in the combined therapy groups versus 10.4% with aspirin alone. There is probably a small but clinically significant benefit in combined therapy.

Low molecular weight heparins

The anticoagulant effect of low molecular weight heparin (LMWH) is more predictable than UFH: it can be given by s.c. injection in a fixed dose adjusted for body weight and anticoagulation monitoring is not required. The combination of LMWHs and aspirin is more effective than aspirin alone in reducing the incidence of MI or death. This combination is more effective than UFH in reducing the need for early revascularisation procedures.

Revascularisation

Revascularisation comprises either coronary artery bypass grafting (CABG) or percutaneous coronary intervention (PCI) (e.g. coronary stenting or transluminal coronary angioplasty). Acute complications, procedure-related death and MI are all more common in patients with unstable angina, regardless of the procedure, than in patients having the same procedure for stable angina. Where it is suitable on angiographic grounds, PCI will, over a 5-year period, avoid the need for CABG in most patients. Outcome following CABG performed on patients with unstable angina is as good as that performed on those with stable angina, once they survive the early complications (90% survival at 5 years, 80% at 10 years, and relief of angina).

Patients with angina resistant to medical therapy or which persists after 48 h of inpatient treatment require urgent angiography to determine suitability for revascularisation. Patients whose symptoms settle should be investigated non-invasively for severe residual ischaemia (exercise ECG, stressed myocardial perfusion imaging, stress echocardiography).

Acute ST segment elevation myocardial infarction

Acute ST segment elevation MI usually occurs when an epicardial coronary artery is completely occluded by thrombus forming on a ruptured atheromatous plaque.

Given early enough, aspirin will save 20–30 lives per 1000 infarcts. Giving thrombolytic drugs early enough will save 30 lives per 1000 infarcts. The difference between thrombolysis during the first hour following the onset of symptoms and the second to third hour is 10–12 lives saved per 1000 infarcts. There is a synergistic effect when aspirin is given with thrombolysis (further reduction in mortality than when either therapy is used alone). When experienced personnel and appropriate facilities are available, PCI reduces mortality even more than thrombolysis.

Thrombolysis

- *Indications.* Patients within 12 h of the onset of major symptoms suggestive of acute MI. Supporting ECG changes are ST elevation > 0.2 mV in more than two adjacent chest leads or > 0.1 mV in limb leads, or new left bundle branch block.
- *Absolute contraindications.* Active haemorrhage. Recent CNS infarction, haemorrhage or surgery. Trauma or malignancy.
- *Relative contraindications.* Recent non-CNS surgery (< 10 days). Recent trauma (< 10 days). Recent gastrointestinal haemorrhage. Coagulation disorders. Pregnancy or < 10 days post partum. Severe hypertension (diastolic > 130 mmHg).

Thrombolytic drugs
DO NOT WAIT FOR CONFIRMATORY LAB RESULTS OF MI

1. Streptokinase (for almost all patients). Streptokinase is a fibrin non-specific plasminogen activator. It causes widespread activation of circulating plasminogen resulting in a systemic lytic state. It is antigenic. It should be given within 12 h of maximal symptoms.
Dose: 1.5 million units in 0.9% sodium chloride given over 60 min.

2. t-PA (tissue plasminogen activator) with intravenous heparin. t-PA is a fibrin specific plasminogen activator which produces direct activation at the site of the fibrin clot occluding the coronary artery. It is indicated if:

- Streptokinase given between 5 days to 12 months previously.
- Patient aged <75 years, with a large anterior MI, and within 6h of onset of symptoms (large infarcts are defined by ST segment elevation in more than six of the 12 ECG leads).
- Severe persistent hypotension, especially if aggravated by streptokinase.

Dose: 15 mg bolus i.v., then infusion of $0.75\,mg\,kg^{-1}$ over 30 min (max 50 mg), then $0.5\,mg\,kg^{-1}$ over 60 min (max 35 mg).

The dose of i.v. heparin is 5000 units bolus, then 1000 units h^{-1} for 48 h. Heparin is commenced simultaneously with tPA.

3. Tenecteplase. Tenecteplase is the most recent thrombolytic drug. It is given as a single intravenous bolus (0.5–$0.6\,mg\,kg^{-1}$ up to maximum of 50 mg) over 5 s, which makes it ideal for pre-hospital use. For the same reason, it is the thrombolytic of choice during resuscitation of a patient in cardiac arrest from a suspected pulmonary embolus. It is very expensive.

Alternatives to thrombolysis
Emergency coronary angiography with angioplasty, placement of intraluminal stents, intracoronary thrombolysis and emergency CABG are the subject of current investigation and should be considered if available. At present, emergency angiography is not widely available in many countries.

Other drugs
1. Beta-blockade. This should be started as soon as possible by either the oral or intravenous route unless contraindicated (e.g. asthma, bradycardia, first-degree or left bundle branch block). Drugs in common use include metoprolol and atenolol. Beta-blockade probably reduces mortality, arrhythmias (including VF), cardiac rupture and reinfarction rate.

2. ACE inhibitor. After 48 h an ACE inhibitor should be started. Captopril 12.5 mg bd increasing to 50 mg has been shown to be effective. Captopril given in this way will save an extra five lives per 1000 patients with MI. The benefit continues for at least 1 year. Evidence from the SAVE study suggests that patients with poor left ventricular function following an MI treated with captopril 50 mg tds had a reduced mortality (over 40 lives per 1000 patients), fewer recurrent MIs and reduced need for hospitalisation for heart failure over a 3.5-year period. Longer-acting ACE inhibitors (e.g. ramipril, perindopril, trandolapril) have been developed and shown to be effective. They are usually better tolerated than captopril.

3. Aspirin. Aspirin should be continued after thrombolysis because it reduces the chances of reocclusion.

4. Insulin. An intravenous sliding scale infusion should be commenced in all patients with an admission blood sugar $>11\,mmol\,l^{-1}$.

Consider:

5. Heparin. Intravenous heparin is started in conjunction with t-PA and continued for at least 24 h. While there is no convincing evidence that heparin infusions are beneficial after streptokinase they are often initiated within 6–12 h of thrombolysis. After intravenous heparin has been stopped, s.c. heparin (5000 units bd) should be continued for all patients at risk from DVT. Compression stockings should be worn.

6. Warfarin. Oral anticoagulation is given to patients with large anterior myocardial infarctions and continued for 3 months.

7. Spironolactone in addition to ACE inhibitors and diuretics for those patients with New York Heart Association (NYHA) grade 3 or 4 heart failure.

Rehabilitation

Survivors should start a cardiac rehabilitation programme and be given advice about their risk factors (family history, smoking, hyperlipidaemias, hypertension and diabetes mellitus).

Cholesterol-lowering drugs: three recent large clinical trials have all confirmed that cholesterol lowering is a safe and effective means of preventing initial or recurrent coronary events in at-risk patients. In the CARE trial, pravastatin (a competitive inhibitor of cholesterol biosynthesis) saved 150 fatal and non-fatal CVS events per 1000 patients treated for 5 years when it was given to post-MI patients with average cholesterol levels. Patients aged >60 years and women showed the greatest benefit. Pravastatin does not interact with warfarin.

Further reading

Antman EM. Decision making with cardiac troponin tests. *N Engl J Med* 2002; **346**: 2079–82.
Grech ED, Ramsdale DR. Acute coronary syndrome: unstable angina and non-ST segment elevation myocardial infarction. *BMJ* 2003; **326**: 1259–61.
www.escardio.org
NICE guidance on the use of drugs for early thrombolysis in the treatment of acute myocardial infarction.
http://www.nice.org.uk/cat.asp?c=38399
Owen A. Intravenous β-blockade in acute myocardial infarction. *BMJ* 1998; **317**: 226–7
Task Force on the Management of Acute Coronary Syndromes of the European Society of Cardiology. Management of acute coronary syndromes in patients without persistent ST-segment elevation. *Eur Heart J* 2002; **23**: 1809–40.

Related topics of interest

Cardiac failure

Cardiac failure occurs when the heart fails to maintain an adequate circulation despite adequate filling pressures. This results in failure to meet tissue oxygen and metabolic requirements. Cardiogenic shock is severe acute cardiac failure and is defined by a systolic BP < 90 mmHg with evidence of impaired tissue perfusion. This condition has a poor prognosis.

Factors affecting cardiac output

Cardiac output is the product of stroke volume and heart rate. Stroke volume is determined by preload, contractility and afterload. Cardiac output is optimised by manipulation of these factors.

Preload

This refers to the diastolic myocardial tension or left ventricular (LV) end-diastolic volume. Increasing preload increases cardiac output by the Frank–Starling mechanism when LV function is normal. In patients with poor LV function, decreasing preload may improve cardiac output if left atrial pressures are high. Preload may be increased by volume loading and decreased by diuresis and venodilatation.

In cardiac failure with abnormal LV systolic function, reducing preload may be deleterious.

Contractility

This is the force of LV contraction independent of preload and afterload. Contractility is increased by inotropic drugs and by treatment of ischaemia and hypoxia. It is decreased by ischaemia, hypoxia and negatively inotropic drugs.

Afterload

This refers to the systolic myocardial wall tension. It is increased with high intraventricular pressures, increased aortic impedance/systemic vascular resistance (SVR), increased ventricular radius and negative intrathoracic pressure. Afterload is decreased by reduced aortic impedance/SVR, reduced intraventricular pressure, positive intrathoracic pressure and increased ventricular wall thickness.

The failing heart is generally more afterload dependent (compared with the heart with normal LV function, which is preload dependent).

Heart rate

Heart rate is increased in most patients with cardiac failure as an acute compensatory mechanism. However, increased heart rate results in reduced diastolic filling time, reduced time for coronary perfusion (which occurs during diastole) and increased cardiac work.

Rhythm

Arrhythmias with loss of coordinated atrial activity (atrial fibrillation, atrial flutter and heart block) can impair ventricular filling, resulting in lowered stroke volumes which may trigger cardiac failure in susceptible patients.

Manipulation of these factors to improve cardiac output must be performed without increasing myocardial work or oxygen demand.

Clinical features

The main symptoms of cardiac failure are dyspnoea, orthopnoea, paroxysmal nocturnal dyspnoea (PND) due to pulmonary congestion, and fatigue (due to low cardiac output). The main signs are due to:

- Sympathetic stimulation: tachycardia, sweating, peripheral vasoconstriction.
- Myocardial dysfunction: cardiomegaly, added heart sounds (gallop rhythm), functional tricuspid and mitral regurgitation.
- Sodium and water retention: elevated venous pressure, pulmonary and peripheral oedema, pleural effusions, hepatomegaly and ascites.

Similar symptoms may be caused by non-cardiogenic pulmonary oedema, pulmonary pathology and non-pulmonary causes (e.g. obesity, psychogenic). Gallop rhythms may occur normally in the aged and in pregnancy. Oedema may be caused by renal and liver disease and venous insufficiency. Patients in cardiac failure with normal LV systolic function often have normal-sized hearts.

Sudden deterioration in well-compensated chronic cardiac failure may be caused by ischaemia/infarct, arrhythmias, pulmonary embolism, hypertension or increased cardiac work, e.g. due to asthma, infection or poor compliance with medical therapy.

Consider occult cardiac failure in patients difficult to wean from ventilation.

Investigations

- Investigations for coexisting and precipitating conditions.
- Full blood count, urea, electrolytes, creatinine, cardiac enzymes and thyroid function tests.
- ECG for diagnosis of myocardial ischaemia/infarct and arrhythmias.
- CXR for assessment of cardiac size and shape and pulmonary oedema.
- Arterial blood gas and lactate for assessment of severity of decompensation.
- Echocardiogram for confirmation of diagnosis, assessment of cause and severity.
- Other investigations:
  - Stress testing and coronary angiography for coronary artery disease.
  - Electrophysiological studies and radiofrequency ablation for arrhythmias.
  - Endomyocardial biopsy for diagnosis of infiltrative diseases.

Management

Aims
- To reduce cardiac work and optimise coronary O_2 supply.

- To improve cardiac output to meet tissue needs.
- To treat precipitating event and underlying cause.

General treatment

- Rest will reduce metabolic requirements.
- O_2 by mask or nasal prongs. In acute pulmonary oedema, mask CPAP is useful. It improves oxygenation by re-expanding flooded alveoli. The increased functional residual capacity positions the lung on a more favourable part of its compliance curve and reduces work of breathing. CPAP increases pericardial pressure, which reduces LV afterload by reducing transmural pressure, thus enhancing cardiac performance. Intubation and ventilation may be required in fulminant pulmonary oedema and ventilatory compromise.
- Drugs:
  - Nitrates cause venodilatation and reduce preload. In comparison with high-dose furosemide, first-line therapy with nitrates will improve outcome from heart failure.
  - Diuretics: in acute heart failure, furosemide produces rapid venodilatation followed by diuresis. However, in chronic congestive heart failure (CHF), furosemide stimulates the renin–angiotensin aldosterone system and causes an initial increase of afterload with reduction of stroke volume and cardiac output and increased pulmonary capillary pressure. In chronic CHF, if large doses of diuretic are needed, thiazides or metalozone may be considered. Spironolactone improves long-term survival in patients with severe, chronic heart failure.
  - Vasodilators: in acute heart failure with evidence of increased afterload, a short acting vasodilator such as GTN or sodium nitroprusside can be given, the dose being titrated against effect. Both systolic and diastolic function may be improved. Angiotensin-converting enzyme (ACE) inhibitors improve exercise tolerance and signs and symptoms of heart failure and reduce mortality. To prevent hypotension they should be introduced cautiously in severe heart failure.
  - Calcium channel blockers reduce afterload. However, they make heart failure worse and may increase the risk of death.
- Inotropes: improve cardiac output and tissue perfusion (see p. 186).
  - Dobutamine is an inotrope and a vasodilator and may be the drug of choice in heart failure. However, it often causes tachycardia and may occasionally cause severe hypotension.
  - Adrenaline (epinephrine) increases cardiac output but often at the cost of tachycardia and increased cardiac work.
  - Noradrenaline (norepinephrine) causes less tachycardia but is not ideal in vasoconstricted states.
  - Phosphodiesterase inhibitors have independent lusitropic effects in addition to inotropic effects. They are useful in diastolic failure. Because of their different site of action, they may also be useful in down-regulated states.
  - Digoxin: in the critically ill, its role is restricted to the treatment of atrial fibrillation. Digoxin has a narrow therapeutic index with increased risk of toxicity in renal failure. It is a poor inotrope, especially in the presence of high sympathetic activity, and may reduce cardiac output in cardiogenic shock by increasing SVR.

- Beta-blockers counteract the harmful effects of the sympathetic nervous system that are activated during heart failure. They improve survival in severe heart failure after acute myocardial infarction (AMI).

Mechanical support devices

The introduction of ciclosporin in the 1980s established heart transplantation as the most effective therapy for end-stage heart disease, with 10-year survival rates after transplantation approaching 50%. Increasing numbers of patients require continuous intravenous inotropic support until a suitable donor heart becomes available – and up to 30% die before that occurs. Efforts aimed at increasing the supply of donor organs have failed, emphasising the need for alternatives to cardiac transplantation. The most promising alternative is mechanical support with ventricular assist devices, which decrease the work of the heart while improving coronary perfusion. Although mechanical assist devices may not be appropriate in the management of all critically ill patients with cardiac failure, their use is becoming more widespread.

Intra-aortic balloon counterpulsation

The intra-aortic balloon pump (IABP) uses counterpulsation timed to the cardiac cycle. Counterpulsation provides both an augmented diastolic arterial pressure and a decreased end-diastolic pressure (afterload). The IABP increases coronary artery perfusion, increases myocardial oxygen supply, decreases myocardial oxygen demand, decreases myocardial work by reducing afterload, increases blood pressure and decreases pulmonary artery pressure.

Indications for an IABP include acute LV failure after cardiac surgery, severe unstable angina, cardiogenic shock after MI and as a bridge to cardiac transplantation.

The IABP is contraindicated in severe aortic insufficiency, aortic aneurysm and severe peripheral vascular disease. The balloon catheter is inserted either percutaneously or surgically by cutdown into the femoral artery. The catheter tip is positioned in the descending thoracic aorta, distal to the subclavian artery and proximal to renal arteries.

The balloon is connected to a console that regulates the inflation or deflation of the balloon with helium. Complications of the IABP include limb ischaemia, bleeding from insertion site, infection, vessel dissection, embolism and thrombosis, inappropriate timing causing increased afterload, haemolysis, arterial obstruction (renal/subclavian) due to improper positioning, balloon rupture and gas loss, and aortic valve rupture.

Ventricular assist devices

Ventricular assist devices (VADs) were used initially as a means of supporting a patient while a suitable donor heart was found for transplant. However, with improved reliability and miniaturisation of the pumps, VADs are being used as a bridge to recovery. In this setting, the function of the heart is virtually taken over by the device, enabling the heart to recover from a potentially reversible insult (e.g. viral myocarditis) before removal. Despite substantial cost, VADs are also being used to treat end-stage cardiac failure. Their use is limited to specialist cardiac centres.

Specific treatment
- Treatment of arrhythmias: anti-arrhythmic drugs, radiofrequency ablation, pacemakers, implantable cardioverter-defibrillators.
- Treatment of coronary artery disease: coronary angioplasty +/− stent, CABG.
- Other surgical treatment: cardiomyoplasty, cardiomyomectomy, cardiac transplantation.

Outcome
Cardiac failure has a high mortality. More than 30% of patients will die within a year of diagnosis. Cardiogenic shock is associated with an initial mortality of >50%.

Further reading

Cowie MR, Zaphiriou A. Management of chronic heart failure. *BMJ* 2002; **325**: 422–5.
Davies MK, Gibbs CR, Lip GYH. *ABC of Heart Failure*. London: BMJ Books, 2000.
Jessup M, Brozena S. Heart failure. *N Engl J Med* 2003; **348**: 2007–18.
McMurray J, Pfeffer MA. New therapeutic options in congestive heart failure: Part I. *Circulation* 2002; **105**: 2099–106.
McMurray J. Pfeffer MA. New therapeutic options in congestive heart failure: Part II. *Circulation* 2002; **105**: 2223–8.
Suttner SW, Piper SN, Boldt J. The heart in the elderly critically ill patient. *Curr Opin Crit Care* 2002; **8**: 389–94.

Related topics of interest

Inotropes and vasopressors (p. 186)

Cardiac output – measurement

Martin Schuster-Bruce

The maintenance of adequate tissue perfusion is one of the primary goals in the management of the critically ill. Cardiac output is the major determinant of oxygen delivery and the variable that can be most effectively manipulated therapeutically. Preload, afterload, cardiac contractility and compliance affect cardiac output. The monitoring and manipulation of cardiac filling and cardiac output form the basis of much of critical care practice.

Clinical

Clinical assessment, vital signs, urine output and core/peripheral temperature gradients can provide valuable information about the cardiac output and circulation. In all forms of shock there is evidence of poor end-organ perfusion (oliguria, altered mental state, lactic acidosis). In low cardiac output states the peripheries are cool and the pulse volume low, whereas in septic shock the peripheries are warm and the pulse volume high. However, in critically ill patients with multisystem failure, clinical assessment alone may be inadequate and the accuracy of estimation of volume status compared with invasive techniques may be as low as 30%.

Pulmonary artery flotation catheter

The pulmonary artery flotation catheter (PAFC) enables catheterisation of the right heart and pulmonary artery without the need for X-ray, through a percutaneous sheath placed in a central vein. The waveform and pressure are monitored continually. The balloon is inflated and the catheter 'floated' through the tricuspid valve into the right ventricle and finally 'wedged' in the pulmonary artery. It enables direct measurement of central venous pressure, pulmonary artery pressure (PAP) and pulmonary artery occlusion pressure (PAOP).

Preload
Inflation of the balloon isolates a pulmonary vascular segment, and flow in that segment ceases. The PAOP reflects left ventricular end-diastolic volume and is used as an indicator of the preload of the left ventricle. PAOP is measured at end-expiration to minimise the effect of intrathoracic pressure.

Cardiac output
The addition of a thermistor near the tip allows determination of cardiac output by the thermodilution technique. A known volume of liquid at a known temperature is injected as a bolus into the atrium. This mixes with and cools the blood, causing a

drop in temperature at the thermistor in the pulmonary artery. The dilution curve is analysed by computer to calculate the cardiac output. The mean of three consecutive measurements, taken randomly through the respiratory cycle, is calculated. The precision of the measurements is at best 4–9%. The results will be inaccurate in the presence of intracardiac shunts or pulmonary/tricuspid regurgitation.

Complications of PAFC include all those of central venous catheterisation plus trauma to the atria, ventricles and valves, arrhythmias, pulmonary infarction and haemorrhage, catheter knotting and infection (particularly after 72 h).

Derived variables

Measurement of cardiac output, intravascular pressures and heart rate allows the calculation of a number of haemodynamic and oxygen transport variables. Body surface area is used to index the variables and compensate for differences in patient size (Table 4).

Pulmonary and systemic vascular resistance can be useful in diagnosis of the type of shock and estimate the afterload of the right and left ventricles, respectively.

Semi-continuous cardiac output and mixed venous oxygen saturation

Intermittent cold bolus injections are replaced by pulses of heat emitted from a thermal filament attached to the catheter. The cardiac output is updated every 30 s and the average over the last 5 min displayed. It is as accurate and reproducible as intermittent thermodilution in routine practice. However, the response time is too slow for immediate detection of acute changes in cardiac output and rapid infusion of cold solutions can interfere with measurements. The addition of a fibreoptic oximeter at the tip provides continuous mixed venous oxygen saturation. Based on the Fick principle, when oxygen consumption is constant, changes in mixed venous oxygen saturation are directly proportional to cardiac output.

There are no unambiguous data showing that the use of a PAFC reduces mortality and the frequency of use is reducing dramatically. Indications for considering a PAFC include:

1. Assessment of intravascular volume, cardiac output, SvO_2, DO_2 and VO_2.

Table 4 Normal values of cardiac output parameters

Variable	Calculation	Normal range
Cardiac index	CO/BSA	2.8–4.2 l min^{-1} m^{-2}
Stroke volume	CO/HR	80 ml
Left ventricular stroke work index	$CI \times (MAP - PAOP) \times 0.0136$	44–64 g m^{-1} m^{-2}
Right ventricular stroke work index	$CI \times (MPAP - CVP) \times 0.0136$	7–12 g m^{-1} m^{-2}
Systemic vascular resistance	$(MAP - CVP) \times 80/CO$	1000–1200 dyn s cm^{-5} m^{-2}
Pulmonary vascular resistance	$(MPAP - PAOP) \times 80/CO$	60–120 dyn s cm^{-5} m^{-2}
Oxygen delivery	$CO \times CaO_2$	850–1050 ml min^{-1}
Oxygen consumption	$CO \times (CaO_2 - CvO_2)$	180–300 ml min^{-1}

2. Rational use of volume, inotropes and vasoactive drugs.
3. Manipulation of PAOP and PAP in acute respiratory distress syndrome.

Many still consider the PAFC to be the gold standard device for measuring cardiac output; however, several new devices are available that are less invasive and they are gradually replacing the PAFC.

Lithium indicator dilution (LiDCO™)

In small doses lithium is non-toxic and it can be measured easily *in vivo* using a lithium-sensitive electrode ion. A small dose of lithium is injected into a central vein as an intravenous bolus, and the cardiac output is derived from the dilution curve generated by a sensor attached to a standard radial arterial line.

Transpulmonary cold indicator dilution (PiCCO™)

An injection of cold solution is made into a central vein, in exactly the same fashion as with the PAFC. Instead of sensing a temperature change in the pulmonary artery, a special femoral arterial line incorporating a thermistor generates a dilution curve from the temperature change in the aorta. Further analysis of the dilution curve allows determination of intrathoracic blood volume (ITBV) and extravascular lung water (EVLW). ITBV is a global preload indicator, while EVLW is a measure of pulmonary oedema and can be used as a brake on further fluid resuscitation.

Pulse contour (PulseCO™, PiCCO™)

Nominal beat-to-beat stroke volume is calculated by analysis of the arterial waveform. This is then converted to actual stroke volume by calibration of the algorithms by either lithium or transpulmonary indicator dilution cardiac output. The devices provide true beat-by-beat cardiac output measurement but require recalibration every 4–6 h or after significant changes in vascular resistance.

Fick partial rebreathing method (NICO™)

This device consists of a rebreathing loop incorporated into the breathing circuit and measures end-tidal and volumetric breath-by-breath CO_2 elimination. The technique is based on the CO_2 Fick equation for cardiac output (CO):

$$CO = \frac{\dot{V}CO_2}{CvCO_2 - CaCO_2}$$

where $\dot{V}CO_2$ = CO_2 elimination rate
$CvCO_2$ = mixed venous CO_2 content
$CaCO_2$ = arterial CO_2 content

The arterial CO_2 content can be estimated from the end-tidal CO_2, while the volumetric sensor measures the CO_2 elimination rate. Comparing baseline CO_2 excretion with that during a short period of CO_2 rebreathing, mixed venous CO_2 remains constant and can be mathematically removed from the equation. Hence, the cardiac output is equal to the change in elimination of CO_2 divided by a change in the end-tidal CO_2 between the two periods.

Clearly the use of this device is restricted to intubated patients and errors arise if the end-tidal CO_2 does not approximate arterial CO_2 or there are leaks in the breathing circuit.

Aortic Doppler flow probes

When a sound wave is reflected off a moving object the frequency is shifted by an amount proportional to the relative velocity of the object. This is the Doppler principle. Reflected signals from a probe placed in the oesophagus are analysed to produce a velocity–time curve for blood flow in the aorta. From analysis of the area under the curve, cardiac output and SV can be calculated. The shape of the curve gives an indication of the volume status, inotropic state and vascular resistance.

The accuracy of the measurements depends on the assumption that the cross-sectional area of the aorta is constant throughout the cardiac cycle, that the angle of the probe to the direction of blood flow is constant and that there is laminar flow within the aorta. Additionally, since flow is measured in the descending aorta, which represents only 70% of the total cardiac output, the displayed cardiac output has to be adjusted accordingly.

There is reasonable correlation between Doppler and thermodilution estimates of cardiac output, though relative rather than absolute values are obtained and some operator dependence has been noted. The major advantage of this technique is that the probes are relatively non-invasive and easy to place, although in some patients signal strength can be poor.

Echocardiography

Echocardiography utilises an ultrasound beam to generate intermittent real-time images of the heart. It has been performed traditionally via the transthoracic approach, but up to 30% of mechanically ventilated patients have poor transthoracic windows, particularly those who have undergone cardiothoracic surgery. Transoesophageal echocardiography (TOE) uses a transducer mounted on the tip of an endoscope. The image obtained is more refined since the transducer within the oesphagus is juxtaposed against the heart and it is easier to maintain a stable transducer position. TOE can be used to assess preload either qualitatively (signs of hypovolaemia include left ventricular outflow tract turbulence and systolic cavity obliteration) or by measurement of the volume of the ventricle. Cardiac performance can be estimated by the calculation of ejection fractions and from Doppler velocity traces of aortic flow. However, echocardiography is a poor indicator of cardiac filling and its chief advantage is its ability to detect other cardiac pathologies. TOE is sensitive enough to detect ischaemia by regional wall motion abnormalities prior to any ECG changes. Other diagnostic uses include the detection of aortic dissection or trauma, cardiac tamponade, valvular lesions and intracardiac thrombus.

Further reading

Allsager CM, Swanevelder J. Measuring cardiac output. *BJA CEPD Rev* 2003; **3**: 15–19.

Hudson E, Beale R. Lung water and blood volume measurements in the critically ill. *Curr Opin Crit Care* 2000; **6**: 222–6.

Jonas MM, Tanser SJ. Lithium dilution measurements of cardiac output and arterial pulse waveform analysis: an indicator dilution calibrated beat-to-beat system for continuous estimation of cardiac output. *Curr Opin Crit Care* 2002; **8**: 257–61.

Cardiac pacing

Jas Soar

Cardiac pacing is necessary when normal impulse formation fails (bradyarrhythmias) or conduction fails (heart block) and there is a decrease in cardiac output with associated hypotension or syncope. Pacing can also be used to override tachyarrhythmias. Antiarrhythmia devices also enable cardioversion and defibrillation.

Permanent pacemakers

Assessment of a patient with a permanent pacemaker should include the following key points:

1. Why was the patient's heart paced? Indications include symptomatic heart block, sinus node disease, carotid sinus or malignant vasovagal syndromes. The underlying cause may be idiopathic or include congenital abnormalities, ischaemic heart disease, valve disorders, connective tissue diseases and problems associated with antiarrhythmic drug therapy. An ECG rhythm strip will indicate the underlying rhythm or if the patient is pacemaker dependent.

2. What type of pacemaker is fitted? Pacemakers are classified using the North American Society of Pacing and Electrophysiology/British Pacing and Electrophysiology Group (NASPE/BPEG) five-letter code (NBG code). The first letter refers to the paced chamber and the second to the sensed chamber. The chamber codes are A (atrium), V (ventricle), D (dual), O (none) or S (single – atrium or ventricle). The third letter refers to the sensing mode and may be T (triggering), I (inhibition), D (dual, inhibition and triggering) or O (none, pacemaker in asynchronous mode). The fourth letter indicates rate response to activity (e.g. mechanical vibration, acceleration or changes in minute ventilation) and may be O (none) or R (rate modulation). The fifth letter refers to multi-site pacing (i.e. more than one stimulation site in any single cardiac chamber or a combination) and may be A (atrium), V (ventricle), D (dual) or O (none). There is a separate NASPE/BPEG coding system (NBD code) for implantable cardioverter-defibrillators (ICDs).

Temporary pacemakers

1. Indications include:
- Life-threatening bradyarrhythmia until a permanent pacemaker is implanted.
- Temporary bradyarrhythmia. Transient atrioventricular block may occur after MI, cardiac surgery, especially valve surgery, or with drug therapy, e.g. amiodarone toxicity.

- Pacemaker-dependent patients who develop pacemaker malfunction. Temporary pacing allows the permanent pacemaker to be changed.
- Patients undergoing surgical procedures at risk of life-threatening bradyarrhythmia.
- Temporary overdrive pacing may be used to control tachyarrhythmias.

2. Several methods of temporary pacing are available. They may enable pacing at a fixed rate (asynchronous or non-demand) or on demand. Fixed rate systems produce electrical stimuli at the selected rate regardless of any intrinsic cardiac activity. If the pacing stimulus falls on the apex of a T wave, ventricular tachycardia or ventricular fibrillation can occur. Demand pacing is preferable as it senses intrinsic QRS complexes and only delivers electrical stimuli when needed.

- *Transvenous pacing* is the commonest temporary mode. A single bipolar right ventricular lead is placed with fluoroscopy. Temporary dual chamber pacing is also possible. The lead is connected to a pacing box. The commonest modes are VOO or VVI. Leads can stay in place for 1–2 weeks although puncture site infection and septicaemia is a risk.
- *Transcutaneous pacing* is rapid, safe and easy to initiate. Adhesive electrodes with a large surface area are used. The negative electrode is placed anteriorly (cardiac apex) and the second electrode posteriorly (below the tip of the scapula). Multifunction electrodes (pacing and defibrillation) are placed in the usual positions for defibrillation. The electrical stimulus causes skeletal muscle contraction. Patients often require analgesia and sedation to tolerate transcutaneous pacing. In an emergency, transcutaneous pacing buys time for transvenous pacing to be initiated.
- *Epicardial pacing* is common after cardiac surgery. Wires are positioned on the atrial and ventricular surfaces at the end of surgery and passed out through the chest wall.
- *Transoesophageal pacing.* The posterior left atrium comes into close proximity with the oesophagus. Ventricular capture is difficult to achieve and use of this method is limited.
- *Percussion pacing* by gentle blows over the precordium lateral to the lower sternal edge may produce a cardiac output in patients with ventricular standstill where P waves are seen. This temporising manoeuvre may buy time to institute other therapies and avoid the need for CPR.

Pacemaker problems

It is important to ensure that a palpable pulse accompanies electrical activity on the ECG. A CXR will show position of leads and may indicate misplacement, dislodgement or damage.

1. Failure to capture. The ECG shows pacing spikes with no following P or QRS waves. Myocardial ischaemia at the site of electrode attachment or of conducting pathways can cause loss of capture of the pacemaker impulse by the heart. There may be scarring at the contact site. Increasing the generator output may correct this. Potassium abnormalities also cause failure to capture. These affects are amplified in critically ill patients who may have hypoxia, acidosis and other metabolic abnormalities. Antiarrhythmic drug therapy may also alter the threshold for pacing.

2. Failure to pace. There are no pacing spikes when they should occur. Battery failure, loose connections and lead damage should be excluded.

3. Failure to sense. Pacing spikes occur inappropriately. May precipitate ventricular arrhythmias.

4. Oversensing. Pacemaker is inhibited by non-cardiac stimuli. Electromagnetic interference from diathermy, MRI scanners and mobile phones (in close proximity) can interfere with pacemakers. Patient shivering can also interfere with pacemaker function.

5. Defibrillation. Paddles should be placed at least 12–15 cm from the pacing unit.

Permanent pacemakers can be converted to a VOO (asynchronous) mode by placing a magnet over the pacemaker box. It is preferable to use the programming transceiver for this adjustment as a magnet may result in an unpredictable resetting.

Implantable cardioverter-defibrillators (ICDs)

Critical care staff are increasingly likely to encounter patients with ICDs. The list of indications for which they are beneficial is growing. These include idiopathic ventricular fibrillation, hereditary long QT syndromes and hypertrophic cardiomyopathy. These devices deliver low-energy shocks (less than 30 J).

ICDs can also be classified by a four-letter (NBD) code. The first letter refers to the chamber shocked and the second to the antitachycardia pacing chamber (O = none, A = atrium, V = ventricle, D = dual). The third letter refers to the mode of tachycardia detection (E = electrical, H = haemodynamic). The fourth letter refers to the antibradycardia pacing chamber (O, A, V, D).

Early intervention can be life-saving in ICD-related emergencies. These include lack of response to ventricular tachyarrhythmias, pacing failure and multiple shocks. A magnet placed on top of all ICD models will temporarily disable the tachyarrhythmia function. The magnetic field closes a reed switch in the generator circuit. Different models of ICD will respond slightly differently. The pacing function should continue whilst the magnet is in place. If there is time, it is preferable to contact the ICD programmer to change the settings.

Diathermy during surgery can be used safely if the ICD is deactivated before the procedure and reactivated and reassessed immediately afterwards. Peripheral nerve stimulators used to assess neuromuscular blockade may interfere with pacemakers and ICDs. The 2 Hz frequency (120 beats min^{-1}) used for 'train of four' assessment is unlikely to trigger the ICD unless the detection rate is very low (in patients with slow ventricular tachycardia). Transcutaneous electrical nerve stimulation (TENS) should be avoided as it can trigger spurious shocks.

The ICD patient in cardiac arrest should receive standard cardiopulmonary resuscitation (including prompt external defibrillation). The ICD should be deactivated if resuscitative efforts are unsuccessful to avoid inadvertent shocks during postmortem examination or removal of the ICD.

Multiple ICD discharges in a short period of time constitute a serious situation. Causes include ventricular electrical storm, inefficient defibrillation, non-sustained ventricular tachycardia and inappropriate shocks caused by supraventricular tachyarrhythmias or oversensing of signals. Antiarrhythmic drugs may increase defibrillation energy requirements.

Deactivation of an ICD with the consent of the patient or relatives should be considered when withdrawing treatment or instituting a do not attempt resuscitation (DNAR) order.

Further reading

ACC/AHA 2002 guideline update for implantation of cardiac pacemakers and antiarrhythmia devices. A report of the American College of Cardiology/American Heart Association task force on practice guidelines (ACC/AHA/NASPE committee on pacemaker implantation). Executive summary available. *Circulation* 2002; **106**: 2145–61.
Full text available on line at:
http://www.americanheart.org/downloadable/heart/1032981283481CleanPacemaker FinalFT.pdf
Bernstein AD, *et al.* The revised NASPE/BPEG generic code for antibradycardia, adaptive-rate and multisite pacing. J Pacing Clin Electrophysiol 2002; **25(2)**: 260–4.
Full text available on line at:
http://www.naspe.org/pdf_files/RevisedNASPE_BPEGGeneric.pdf
Cardiac Pacing. *Resuscitation Council (UK) Advanced Life Support Course Provider Manual*, 4th edn, 2000.
Kaushik V, Leon AR, Forrester JS, Trohman RG. Bradyarrhythmias, temporary and permanent pacing. *Crit Care Med* 2000; **28(10 Suppl)**: N121–8.

Related topics of interest

Cardiac arrhythmias (p. 75)
Cardiopulmonary resuscitation (p. 104)

Cardiac valve disease

Cathal Nolan

Life expectancy of patients with valvular heart lesions has improved dramatically over the past 15 years. This coincides with a reduction in rheumatic fever in the developed world, better non-invasive monitoring of cardiac function and improved prostheses and surgical techniques. There has also been a greater understanding of valvular pathology and timing of surgical intervention.

Surgery on stenotic lesions may be deferred until symptoms appear. Regurgitant lesions, however, may cause severe left ventricular dysfunction before symptoms occur. Conservation of the native valve structure is preferable to mechanical replacement where possible.

Aortic stenosis

Aortic stenosis may be congenital (bicuspid valve) or acquired (calcification, rheumatic fever). Symptoms include dyspnoea, angina and syncope. Signs include a slow rising anacrotic pulse and an ejection-systolic murmur that is loudest at the 2nd right intercostal space and radiating to the neck. There may be an associated thrill if there is severe stenosis, when the murmur occurs late. The S_2 is soft and there may be reversed splitting of the second sound.

Investigation
- ECG findings may be those of left ventricular hypertrophy.
- CXR: the heart is of normal size unless there is left ventricular dilatation. There may be aortic calcification or post-stenotic dilatation of the aorta.
- Doppler echocardiography enables estimation of the valve area, the transvalvular gradient, ventricular hypertrophy and ejection fraction.
- Cardiac catheterisation will add to the echocardiographic findings as well as define the anatomy of the coronary arteries.

Management
The cardiac output is 'fixed'; the blood pressure is thus directly related to SVR. Tachycardia will reduce time for diastolic myocardial perfusion and should be avoided. The presence of symptoms and a documented stenotic valve should prompt immediate valve replacement. Seventy-five per cent of patients with symptomatic aortic stenosis die within 3 years of the onset of symptoms unless the valve is replaced. A gradient of $>50\,mmHg$ or a valve area $<0.8\,cm^2$ represents severe stenosis. Balloon aortic valvotomy is a palliative procedure only and is associated with serious complications (death, stroke, aortic rupture and aortic regurgitation in 10% of

cases). Mortality with this procedure is 60% at 18 months, which is similar to no treatment. Antibiotic prophylaxis against infective endocarditis is essential.

Mitral stenosis

Most cases of mitral stenosis are due to rheumatic fever but other causes include left atrial myxoma, calcification of the annulus and SLE. Symptoms include dyspnoea, recurrent bronchitis, palpitations (atrial fibrillation), haemoptysis (due to pulmonary oedema) and acute neurological events (due to embolism). Signs are mitral facies, small volume pulse (+/- atrial fibrillation), tapping apex beat (palpable S_1), parasternal heave (RVH), loud S_1 and opening snap (if non-calcified). A diastolic murmur with or without presystolic accentuation may be present if the patient is in sinus rhythm.

Investigations
- The ECG may show P mitrale, atrial fibrillation or right ventricular hypertrophy.
- CXR: there may be an enlarged left atrium, calcification of the valve and pulmonary venous congestion.
- Echocardiography enables an accurate calculation of the valve area (mitral stenosis is severe if the area is $< 1\,cm^2$).

Management
Digoxin or beta-blockers will increase diastolic filling time and reduce the heart rate. If atrial fibrillation is present, anticoagulation is needed to prevent neurological complications. Antibiotic prophylaxis is required to prevent infective endocarditis. Preload should be optimised and tachycardia avoided. Hypoxia will increase pulmonary vasoconstriction, putting further strain on the right ventricle. The high left atrial pressure associated with mitral stenosis eventually causes pulmonary hypertension. Balloon valvotomy or valve replacement should be performed before irreversible pulmonary hypertension results.

Mitral regurgitation

The causes include infective endocarditis, myxomatous degeneration of the mitral valve (including mitral valve prolapse), collagen vascular disease, rheumatic fever and spontaneous rupture of the chordae. Regurgitation may be acute or chronic. In acute mitral regurgitation there is sudden volume overload on the left atrium and pulmonary veins leading to pulmonary oedema. In chronic mitral regurgitation the volume overload is compensated for by the development of cardiac hypertrophy. Symptoms are those of left and right heart failure. There is cardiac enlargement; the apex beat is displaced and there may be a parasternal heave. The S_1 is followed by a pansystolic murmur which radiates to the axilla. A third heart sound signifies reduced compliance.

Investigations
- ECG signs include left ventricular hypertrophy, P mitrale and possibly atrial fibrillation.

- Echocardiography or cardiac catheterisation may show the enlarged cardiac chambers and permit estimation of the severity of regurgitation.

Management

The amount of blood regurgitated will depend on the gradient across the valve, the heart rate, and the SVR (a slow heart rate and raised SVR favour regurgitation). Vasodilators and a mild tachycardia will reduce regurgitation. Antibiotic prophylaxis against infective endocarditis is required.

Aortic regurgitation

Chronic aortic regurgitation is due to disease of the aortic leaflets (infective endocarditis, rheumatic fever or the seronegative arthropathies) or disease affecting the aortic root (Marfan's syndrome, aortic dissection, syphilis or idiopathic associated with ageing and hypertension). Symptoms include fatigue, dyspnoea, orthopnoea (signs of left heart failure) or angina. The increased stroke volume produces a large pulse pressure with a Waterhammer (collapsing) pulse. Corrigan's sign (visible carotid pulses) and head nodding may be apparent. Quincke's sign (nail bed capillary pulsation) and pistol-shot femoral pulses are also a feature. The apex beat is displaced. The murmur of aortic regurgitation is typically high-pitched and early in diastole. The Austin Flint murmur (due to the aortic jet impinging on the mitral valve apparatus) may contribute to a physiological mitral stenosis (due to early closure of the mitral valve).

Investigations
- The ECG may show left ventricular hypertrophy with or without strain.
- The CXR shows cardiomegaly.
- Echocardiography or cardiac catheterisation enables measurement of the aortic valve gradient and the extent of regurgitation. Left ventricular size and function may also be assessed.

Management

Vasodilators such as nifedipine or ACE inhibitors are used to reduce the afterload. If the patient is asymptomatic, these can delay the need for surgery for 2–3 years. Surgery should be performed on the valve before the LV end-systolic dimension exceeds 55 mm or the ejection fraction falls below 55%. Acute aortic regurgitation or mitral regurgitation is a surgical emergency. The left ventricle does not have time to adapt in the face of increased volume load, which causes cardiogenic shock and pulmonary oedema. The coronary blood vessels are affected both by the reduction in perfusion and the increase in left ventricular end-diastolic pressure, thus making myocardial ischaemia worse. Infective endocarditis is the usual cause. Concerns of valve replacement in infected patients are offset by the life-threatening nature of the insult; the risk of prosthetic valve infection is 10%. Antibiotic prophylaxis against infective endocarditis is required.

Further reading

Anonymous. ACC/AHA guidelines for the management of patients with valvular heart disease. A report of the American College of Cardiology/American Heart Association. Task Force on Practice Guidelines (Committee on Management of Patients with Valvular Heart Disease). *J Am Coll Cardiol* 1998; **32**: 1486–588.

Borer JS, Bonow RO. Contemporary approach to aortic and mitral regurgitation. *Circulation* 2003; **108**: 2432–8.

Goldsmith I, Turpie AG, Lip GY. ABC of antithrombotic therapy: valvular heart disease and prosthetic heart valve. *BMJ* 2002; **325**: 1228–31.

Roldan CA. Valvular disease associated with systemic illness. *Cardiol Clin* 1998; **16**: 531–50.

Starr A, Fessler CL, Grunkemeier G, He GW. Heart valve replacement surgery: past, present and future. *Clin Exp Pharmacol Physiol* 2002; **29**: 735–8.

Related topics of interest

Cardiopulmonary resuscitation

In adults the commonest arrhythmia at the onset of cardiac arrest is ventricular fibrillation (VF) or pulseless ventricular tachycardia (VT). The definitive treatment of these arrhythmias – defibrillation – must be administered promptly. Survival from out-of-hospital VF falls by 7–10% for every minute after collapse. Advanced life support (ALS) is the process that attempts to deliver the definitive treatment for the underlying rhythm. Basic life support (BLS) extends the interval between the onset of the collapse and the development of irreversible organ damage and provides the opportunity for ALS to be effective.

Basic life support

Basic life support refers to maintaining airway patency, and supporting breathing and circulation without the use of equipment. It consists of the initial assessment, airway maintenance, expired air ventilation (rescue breathing) and chest compressions. Failure of the circulation to deliver oxygenated blood to the brain for 3–4 min (less if the patient was initially hypoxic) will lead to irreversible cerebral damage. The purpose of BLS is to maintain adequate ventilation and circulation until the underlying cause of the cardiac arrest can be treated.

During two-person CPR, 15 chest compressions (rate $100\,min^{-1}$ with 4–5 cm sternal depression) are given for every two breaths (400–600 ml). In the hospital, BLS usually includes the use of simple adjuncts, such as an oral airway and pocket mask.

Advanced life support

The universal adult ALS treatment algorithm outlines the treatment of all cardiac arrest rhythms (Figure 4). After the initial assessment it divides into two pathways: arrest in VF/VT (shockable rhythms that require defibrillation) and other rhythms that are not treated with defibrillation (non-shockable). It is essential to remember that early defibrillation, adequate oxygenation and ventilation through a clear airway, and chest compressions, are always more important than giving drugs.

Above all, **treat the patient, not the monitor**.

Defibrillation

When using a monophasic defibrillator, the initial three shocks in the treatment sequence of VF/VT should be delivered at 200 J, 200 J and 360 J. Thereafter, each shock should be at 360 J. All new defibrillators deliver shocks with biphasic waveforms, which are effective at lower energy levels. Some manufacturers of biphasic defibrillators recommend delivery of fixed energy shocks (typically 150 J), whereas others recommend escalating energy levels (up to 360 J). Most of these newer defibrillators incorporate impedance compensation, which means that the shock waveform and duration is modified according to the patient's transthoracic impedance. Defibrillators should always be charged with the paddles held against the patient's chest wall.

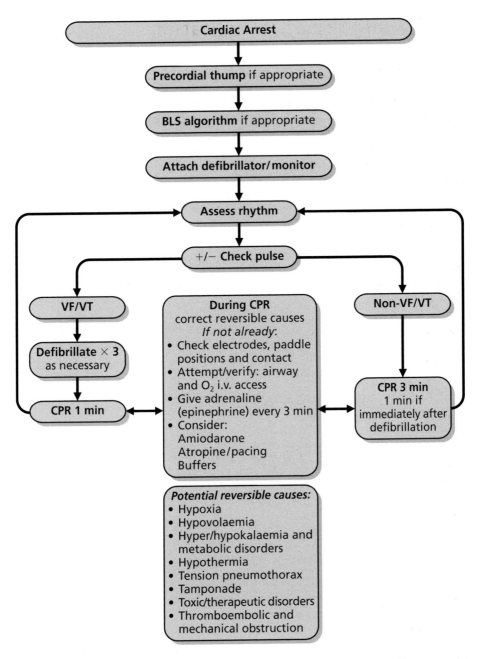

Figure 4 Advanced life support algorithm for the management of cardiac arrest in adults.

Self-adhesive defibrillator patches are preferable to paddles; they enable monitoring, defibrillation and external pacing, and are probably safer.

Vasopressor agents

Adrenaline (epinephrine) improves myocardial and cerebral blood flow and resuscitation rates in experimental animals. There is no clinical evidence that it improves neurological outcome in humans. Vasopressin also improves resuscitation rates in experimental animals, but studies in humans have failed to show a significant improvement in long-term survival. In North America, vasopressin is recommended as an alternative to adrenaline, but the lack of convincing evidence for benefit has kept it out of European resuscitation guidelines.

Antiarrhythmic drug therapy

Haemodynamically significant bradycardias should be treated with atropine, usually using aliquots of 0.5 mg up to a total dose of 3 mg i.v., which is sufficient to totally block vagal activity. In asystole or pulseless electrical activity (PEA) with rate less than 60 min^{-1}, a single dose of 3 mg should be given.

In shock refractory VF/VT (failure to defibrillate after three shocks), amiodarone 300 mg produces higher short-term (admission to hospital) survival rates than either placebo or lidocaine (lignocaine). Despite lacking data on long-term outcome, amiodarone 300 mg is recommended for those patients who remain in VF/VT after three shocks.

Buffer agents

There are no robust clinical data supporting the use of buffers in cardiac arrest; however, sodium bicarbonate is indicated in cardiac arrest associated with hyperkalaemia or following tricyclic antidepressant overdose. Despite lacking data, some continue to advocate the use of sodium bicarbonate in severe acidosis (pH < 7.1, base excess < −10).

The denervated heart

A denervated heart (as occurs following heart transplantation) is exquisitely sensitive to the actions of adenosine. Supraventricular tachyarrhythmias in a denervated heart should not be treated with adenosine. In the presence of severe bradycardia that does not respond to atropine or pacing, an adenosine antagonist (e.g. aminophylline) should be considered.

Return of spontaneous circulation (ROSC)

Patients who are successfully resuscitated should be referred immediately for post resuscitation care.

Further reading

Adult Advanced Life Support Guidelines of the ERC:
   http://www.erc.edu/uniweb/pdf/AALSguidelines.pdf
Colquhoun MC, Handley AJ, Evans TR (eds). *ABC of Resuscitation*, 5th edn. London: BMJ
   Books, 2003.
Parr MJA, Craft TM. *Resuscitation: Key Data – Third Edition*. Oxford: BIOS Scientific Publish-
   ers, 1998.

Related topics of interest

Cardiac chest pain (acute coronary syndrome) (p. 81)
Cardiac pacing (p. 96)
Post resuscitation care (p. 230)

Central venous pressure

Central venous pressure (CVP) measurement is one of the most commonly used monitors in critically ill patients. The CVP is not a measure of blood volume but enables assessment of the ability of the right heart to accept and deliver blood. CVP is influenced by several factors: venous return, right heart compliance, intrathoracic pressure and patient position. Venous blood returning to the right atrium is delivered via the superior vena cava, the inferior vena cava and the coronary veins. Right ventricular compliance is the change in end-diastolic pressure with change in ventricular volume. In a healthy heart, volume administration does not cause a dramatic rise in end-diastolic pressure; the ventricle is compliant. Certain disease states cause the ventricle to be less compliant or stiff, e.g. pericardial effusion, cardiomyopathies or cardiac failure.

The correct catheter position for valid CVP monitoring is in the superior vena cava. The patient should be supine and the zero point level with the mid-axillary line in the fourth intercostal space.

A normal CVP is said to be 0–8 mmHg, but critically ill patients frequently require a higher CVP than this to achieve an optimal cardiac output. The absolute value is not as important as the response to therapy. Serial measurements are essential to enable assessment of intravascular volume. Central venous pressure is an unreliable reflection of left atrial pressure in the seriously ill.

Catheter insertion sites

Internal jugular vein
- *Advantages.* Large vessel. Easy to locate/access. Short straight path to SVC. Low rate of complications.
- *Disadvantages.* Uncomfortable for the patient. Difficult to dress/nurse. Close to carotid artery.

Subclavian vein
- *Advantages.* Large vessel. High flow rates possible. Lowest infection rate and incidence of catheter-related thrombosis of all the sites. Easy to dress. Less restrictive for patient.
- *Disadvantages.* Risk of pneumothorax. Close to subclavian artery. Difficult to control bleeding (non-compressible vessel).

Basilic vein
- *Advantages.* Accessible during resuscitation.
- *Disadvantages.* Increased risk of phlebitis. Catheter movement with arm movement. Greater distance to superior vena cava. High rate of misplacement.

Femoral vein
- *Advantages.* Easy access. Large vessel. High flow rates possible. Accessible during resuscitation.
- *Disadvantages.* Decreased patient mobility. Increased risk of thrombosis. Risk of femoral artery puncture. Dressing problematic.

Insertion guidelines

All central venous insertion sites risk air entrainment and consequent embolism as well as infection. Thus, the patient should be positioned with head down tilt (Trendelenburg). This produces venous engorgement as well as reducing the risk of air entrainment. Femoral venous cannulation does not require the patient to be head down. Central venous catheter insertion should always be performed as a sterile procedure to reduce the risk of catheter-related infection. Consideration should also be given to the use of antimicrobial-impregnated catheters and catheters should be removed as soon as they are no longer needed. Use continuous ECG monitoring; insertion of wires or catheters into the right ventricle may trigger cardiac arrhythmias. Get a CXR after insertion of the central venous catheter to check for catheter position and exclude complications.

Ultrasound locating devices

The National Institute for Clinical Excellence (NICE) has issued guidance for the use of two-dimensional (2D) ultrasound imaging for the placement of central venous lines. It recommends 2D ultrasound imaging guidance as the preferred method for insertion of central venous catheters into the internal jugular vein in adults and children in elective situations. It also considers that although 2D ultrasound imaging guidance in central line placement may eventually become the routine method for placing such lines, the landmark method will remain important in some circumstances, such as emergencies, and when ultrasound equipment and/or expertise might not be immediately available. Consequently, it is important that clinicians maintain their ability to use the landmark method and that the method continues to be taught alongside the 2D ultrasound-guided technique.

The normal waveform

- The **a wave**. This occurs during atrial contraction. Some blood regurgitates into the vena cavae during atrial systole. In addition, venous inflow stops and the rise in venous pressure contributes to the a wave. A large a wave occurs in tricuspid stenosis, pulmonary stenosis, in complete heart block (cannon wave) and in severe pulmonary hypertension. There is no a wave in atrial fibrillation.
- The **c wave**. This is the transmitted manifestation of the rise in atrial pressure produced as the tricuspid valve bulges into the right atrium during ventricular contraction.
- The **v wave** mirrors the rise in atrial pressure during atrial filling before the tricuspid valve opens. A large v wave occurs in tricuspid incompetence and is known as a giant v wave.

Further reading

McGee DC, Gould MK. Preventing complications of central venous catheterization. *N Engl J Med* 2003; **348**: 1123–33.

NICE guidance on the use of ultrasound devices in central line insertion:
http://www.nice.org.uk/pdf/Ultrasound_49_GUIDANCE.pdf

Related topics of interest

Arterial cannulation (p. 35)
Cardiac failure (p. 86)
Cardiac output – measurement (p. 91)

Chest tube thoracostomy

Indications

The indications for insertion of a chest drain include the drainage of established or threatened collections of air, blood, fluid or pus from the pleural cavity. According to guidelines produced by the British Thoracic Society, a simple, spontaneous pneumothorax can be aspirated without the need for a chest drain. However, any patient developing a pneumothorax while receiving positive pressure ventilation should have a chest drain inserted. Without chest drainage, 50% of these will develop into a tension pneumothorax. A tension pneumothorax requires immediate decompression. For patients *in extremis* a cannula in the 2nd intercostal space in the mid-clavicular line of the affected side will reverse the life-threatening mediastinal compression while preparations are made for chest drainage. A patient with fractured ribs who requires intubation and positive pressure ventilation may need to have a chest tube inserted prophylactically. This is indicated particularly before interhospital transfer or prolonged anaesthesia for associated injuries; under these circumstances a developing tension pneumothorax is likely to be discovered late. If the patient has a few, undisplaced rib fractures, it may be reasonable to undertake short procedures requiring positive pressure ventilation without placement of a chest tube. However, the anaesthetist must be alert to any signs of a pneumothorax and must ensure easy immediate access to the chest for needle decompression and chest tube placement. Computed tomography (CT) scanning of patients with serious injuries may reveal occult pneumothoraces, which are visible on the CT scan but not on a plain chest radiograph. There is no consensus on whether these should be drained routinely.

Pleural effusions that cannot be drained by repeated thoracocentesis may require the insertion of a chest drain. Many of these may be managed more appropriately, and less traumatically, with the insertion of a narrow bore (e.g.10F) drain using a Seldinger technique.

Equipment

Drainage of blood from an adult requires at least a 32F chest drain; smaller drains will tend to become blocked. Never use sharp trocars for chest drain insertion – they may lacerate the lung or pulmonary vessels. The chest drain is usually attached to an underwater seal bottle. Some chest drainage systems will enable the re-infusion of blood collected from a massive haemothorax. A purpose-designed bag with a built-in flutter valve can be used instead of an underwater seal. This is particularly useful in the pre-hospital environment or if the patient requires interhospital transfer.

Technique

Give the patient additional oxygen to breathe. Infiltrate local anaesthesia into the skin and along the proposed incision line. Under aseptic conditions insert the drain in the 5th intercostal space just anterior to the mid-axillary line. Define the track down to parietal pleura using blunt dissection, staying close to the upper border of the rib. Puncture the pleura with the blunt tip of a clamp. Remove the clamp and use a finger to 'sweep' the pleural cavity and exclude adhesions or abdominal viscera prior to insertion of the drain.

Connect the drain to an underwater seal or flutter valve. Insert sutures across the skin incision. These can be tightened after drain removal. Traditional 'purse string' sutures produce very poor cosmetic results and are now less often used. Apply a clean dressing and obtain a CXR to confirm an acceptable position of the drain.

Seldinger chest drains

A relatively recent development is equipment that enables insertion of chest drains using a Seldinger technique. A Tuohy-type needle is used to identify the pleural space, a guidewire is inserted and a chest drain is placed over the wire. The advantages of this technique are that it requires a very small incision, is less painful and, once the drain is placed, there is minimal leakage of blood or fluid from the insertion site. However, if the collection of fluid or air is small, or if there is adherent pleura, it is possible to inadvertently place the wire and drain in the lung.

Bronchopleural fistulae

Bronchopleural fistulae cause large air leaks. A bronchoscopy will exclude the presence of a ruptured bronchus. If the lung is non-compliant or the air leak is large, and a major airway injury has been excluded, continuous, high-flow suction (20–$30\,cmH_2O$) may be applied to the drainage system. This may help to bring the visceral and parietal pleural surfaces together.

Complications

Intercostal vessels or nerves may be inadvertently damaged during chest tube insertion. It is possible to lacerate the lung or pulmonary vessels, particularly if a sharp introducer is used. A common error committed by the inexperienced is to place the tube outside the pleural cavity (extrapleural or intra-abdominal). Inadequately tied drains will fall out. A persistent air leak will occur if the proximal side-hole of the chest tube is outside the pleural cavity. Empyema occurs in about 2% of patients having chest tubes inserted. It is particularly likely after blunt trauma.

Removal of chest drains

While the indications for chest drain insertion are relatively clear, explicit guidance on removal of chest drains is hard to find. Chest tubes inserted to drain a pneumothorax are removed on resolution of the pneumothorax. Assuming there is no air leak or excessive drainage of fluid ($>100\,ml\;day^{-1}$), chest tubes inserted prophylactically into patients with rib fractures can probably be removed after the patient has been stabilised and any early, prolonged surgery has been completed.

Further reading

Feliciano DV. Tube thoracostomy. In: Benumoff JL (ed.), *Clinical Procedures in Anesthesia and Intensive Care*. Philadelphia: JB Lippincott, 1992.

Laws D, Neveille E, Duffy J, on behalf of the British Thoracic Society Pleural Disease Group, a subgroup of the British Thoracic Society Standards of Care Committee. BTS guidelines for the insertion of a chest drain. *Thorax* 2003; **58(Suppl II)**: ii53–9.

Related topics of interest

Trauma – primary survey (p. 315)
Trauma – secondary survey (p. 318)
Trauma – anaesthesia and critical care (p. 322)

Chronic obstructive pulmonary disease

Chronic obstructive pulmonary disease (COPD) is a slowly progressive disorder and is the fourth leading cause of death worldwide. Up to 20% of cigarette smokers develop clinically significant COPD, which is a disease almost entirely confined to smokers. Other less common causes include occupational exposure to pulmonary toxins and hereditary α1-antitrypsin deficiency.

There is no agreed definition of COPD. The main feature of the disease is slowly progressive chronic airflow limitation with a reduced FEV_1 and FEV_1/VC ratio. There is usually underlying chronic bronchitis and emphysema. Wall fibrosis follows airway inflammatory processes. There may be an element of reversibility to the airflow obstruction but most of the obstruction is fixed. There is mucosal hypertrophy, increased mucous secretion, increased bronchial reactivity and reduced pulmonary compliance. Emphysema is a histological diagnosis, although the CXR is often suggestive. Elastic tissue destruction results in dilatation of the terminal airways and reduced elasticity.

Diagnosis of COPD

This requires both:

1. A history of chronic progressive symptoms (cough and/or wheeze with or without breathlessness).
2. Objective evidence of airway obstruction (spirometry) that does not return to normal with treatment.

Severe COPD is associated with marked reductions in forced inspiratory and expiratory flows. This causes early airway closure and air trapping with patients breathing at abnormally high lung volumes. This, in turn, results in smaller tidal volumes and a more rapid respiratory rate to maintain a normal minute ventilation, especially during an acute exacerbation. The efficiency of respiratory muscles is impaired at these high volumes and rapid rates, and eventually fatigue will precipitate further respiratory failure.

Exacerbation of COPD

A recent consensus definition of an exacerbation of COPD is a sustained worsening of the patient's condition from the stable state and beyond normal day-to-day variation, which is acute in onset and necessitates a change in regular medication. Previous viral infection accounts for 30% of exacerbations and bacterial infection is present in 30–50% of cases.

Differential diagnosis of an exacerbation of COPD

This includes:

- Pneumonia.
- Segmental pulmonary collapse due to secretions (particularly associated with

surgery, chest trauma and depressed level of consciousness which cause hypoventilation and ineffective cough).
- Pneumothorax (a lung bulla may be misdiagnosed as a pneumothorax).
- Heart failure.
- Pulmonary embolus.
- Lung cancer.
- Airway obstruction.

Clinical features

1. Symptoms. Cough, sputum production and dyspnoea.

2. Signs. Pyrexia, hyperinflation, respiratory distress, use of accessory muscles, decreased breath sounds, wheeze, cyanosis and signs of cor pulmonale.

Investigations

1. CXR. Hyperinflation with flat diaphragms, more than six anterior ribs visible, bullae, areas of consolidation due to infection. Malignancy may be present. Pulmonary oedema may be difficult to diagnose because of the abnormal pulmonary pathology. Pulmonary hypertension results in large proximal pulmonary artery shadows with peripheral attenuation of vessel markings.

2. Lung function tests. Demonstrate an obstructive pattern with $FEV_1/FVC < 70\%$, high residual volume and total lung capacity, transfer factor for CO is low. The pattern is mainly irreversible.

3. Arterial blood gas analysis. Patients with an exacerbation of COPD are often severely hypoxaemic. Increased resistance and hyperinflation increases ventilation–perfusion (V/Q) mismatch, which often causes significant hypercarbia.

4. Blood count. To assess polycythaemia and neutrophilia.

5. ECG. Is often normal but may show signs of right atrial and ventricular enlargement associated with pulmonary hypertension.

Treatment

1. Controlled oxygen therapy. COPD patients with acute respiratory failure are often profoundly hypoxaemic and restoration of an adequate PaO_2 is a priority. Those patients who are chronically hypoxaemic will have developed compensatory mechanisms such as an increased haematocrit and a high oxygen extraction ratio. The aim of oxygen therapy should be to increase the PaO_2 to approximately 8 kPa. This marks the end of the steep portion of the oxygen dissociation curve and will provide acceptable arterial oxygen saturation. Increased airway resistance reduces ventilation in some zones of the lungs (low V/Q) and hyperinflation reduces blood flow in distended alveoli (high V/Q). These alterations in V/Q mismatch are the main reason for an increase in $PaCO_2$ despite maintenance of minute ventilation. The degree of V/Q mismatch is limited by hypoxic vasoconstriction. Administration of high-concentration oxygen will abolish the hypoxic vasoconstriction reflex and exacerbate the V/Q mismatch. This may cause a profound rise in $PaCO_2$ with the onset of CO_2 narcosis and respiratory arrest. It is this mechanism and not the elimination of 'hypoxic drive' that necessitates carefully titrated oxygen therapy. Oxygen is provided using a Venturi mask and the FIO_2 is increased in increments of 0.04 starting at 0.24 or 0.28. Arterial blood gases should be checked every 30 min. If the PaO_2 remains <8.0 kPa and the $PaCO_2$ has not increased by more than 2 kPa, the FIO_2 can be increased to the next level. If it is not possible to achieve adequate arterial oxygenation without a steep increase in $PaCO_2$, ventilatory assistance will be required.

2. Bronchodilators. β_2 agonists (salbutamol or terbutaline) are best given by nebuliser (salbutamol is also available as an intravenous preparation). They act as bronchodilators and enhance mucociliary clearance. They may cause hypokalaemia, tachycardia and tremor.

The anticholinergic ipratropium is used in conjunction with β_2 agonists for its bronchodilator action. It has a slower onset of action, with a peak effect at 60–90 min. Dry mouth and urinary retention are side effects.

Aminophylline by continuous infusion is used as an adjunct to β_2 agonists but is of unproven efficacy. Loading doses should be avoided in patients already taking theophylline preparations. Levels must be monitored because of narrow therapeutic limits.

3. Antibiotics. Most exacerbations are treated as infections, although it is common that no particular organism is identified as the cause. The most common organisms responsible for infective exacerbations are *Haemophilus influenzae*, *Streptococcus pneumoniae* and *Moraxella catarrhalis*. In patients with very severe COPD ($FEV_1 < 30\%$ predicted) Gram-negative organisms, particularly Enterobacteriaceae and *Pseudomonas*, are also important. Antibiotic prescribing should follow local protocols that are governed by organism sensitivities. Amoxicillin and tetracycline are common first-line treatments for out-of-hospital exacerbations. In-hospital acquired and life-threatening infection should be managed with more aggressive intravenous therapy.

4. Steroids. Although fewer than 25% of patients with COPD are steroid responsive, steroids are often given during an acute exacerbation. Courses of steroid should be tapered rapidly. Commonly, hydrocortisone 200 mg, 6-hourly is commenced, converted to oral prednisolone 30 mg after improvement and withdrawn over 7–14 days.

5. Secretion clearance. Sputum retention is common in COPD. Mucolytics are of unproven benefit. Physiotherapy and tracheal suction are crucial in intubated patients with extensive sputum production, though they may be detrimental in the absence of sputum production. Bronchoscopy and tracheal suction may be beneficial in the presence of large airway obstruction due to mucous plugging and may be required to aid the diagnosis of infection or malignancy. Tracheostomy aids weaning and pulmonary toilet for those with ineffective coughs.

6. Diuretics/vasodilators. Hypoxia and acidosis increase pulmonary artery pressure (which may be chronically raised) and precipitate right heart failure. In this situation oxygen, diuretics and vasodilators may improve heart function. Electrolyte abnormalities (hypokalaemia, hypomagnesaemia, hypophosphataemia) secondary to diuresis should be prevented or corrected.

7. Nutrition. Avoid excessive carbohydrate loads in those patients with CO_2 retention.

8. Ventilatory support. Non-invasive positive pressure ventilation (NPPV) can be provided with a nasal or facemask. Several randomised controlled trials have shown that NPPV reduces the need for intubation, the length of hospital stay, the risk of nosocomial pneumonia and mortality in patients with exacerbation of COPD. It is most effective when the pH is between 7.30 and 7.35.

Invasive positive pressure ventilation following intubation may be required for patients who fail to improve with a non-invasive strategy. Respiratory muscle activity will account for up to 50% of oxygen consumption in patients with severe COPD. Resting these muscles by mechanical ventilation allows correction of hypoxia, oxygen utilisation by other tissues and the correction of acidosis. Where possible, spontaneous ventilation is preserved, excessive inflation pressures avoided ($<35\,mmHg$) and a degree of respiratory acidosis is accepted. Relative hypoxia is acceptable provided sufficient oxygen is available to meet the metabolic requirements of the tissues. Patients with severe COPD may have auto-PEEP due to early airway closure and gas trapping which results in volume trauma and barotrauma. Adequate time for expiration must be allowed.

The potential difficulties in weaning patients with COPD from ventilatory support do not preclude intubation for selected cases. The decision to admit these patients to a critical care environment and the decision to intubate must be made by senior clinicians. Many patients with COPD progress to end-stage respiratory failure where aggressive intensive care management is futile. Where prolonged intubation is probable, early tracheostomy is likely to provide better conditions for weaning from ventilation.

Criteria supporting the use of intubation and mechanical ventilation include:

- A reversible reason for the current decline (e.g. pneumonia).
- A quality of life/level of activity prior to this exacerbation that is acceptable to the patient.

Criteria against intubation and mechanical ventilation include:

- Where aggressive management is likely to be futile.
- Previous severe COPD unresponsive to optimal therapy.
- Poor quality of life, with an expected outcome that would be unacceptable to the patient.
- Severe co-morbidity (e.g. heart failure, neoplasia).
- The need for continuous home oxygen.

Doxapram

Doxapram is a respiratory stimulant that acts principally on peripheral chemoreceptors. It may provide time for other therapies to take effect and avoid the need for ventilatory support. Doxapram should be considered if the pH is <7.26 and the $PaCO_2$ is $>6.5\,kPa$.

Outcome

The outcome from the management of an acute exacerbation of COPD is not related to the patient's age or the $PaCO_2$. Hospital survival of an acute exacerbation exceeds 80% but long-term survival is poor and dependent on the respiratory reserve and co-morbidity.

Prevention of exacerbations of COPD requires the following:

- Cessation of smoking.
- Weight loss if obese.
- Avoidance of sedatives (including excess alcohol).
- Prevention of infection (influenza and pneumococcal vaccination).
- Control of cardiovascular disease and fluid overload.
- Venesection for polycythaemia (decreases the risk of thrombosis and cardiac work).

Cor pulmonale

This chronic lung disease results in hypoxic pulmonary vasoconstriction and eventually leads to chronic pulmonary hypertension and right heart failure.

The features include a raised venous pressure, peripheral oedema, hepatomegaly and ascites. Tricuspid regurgitation may be present. A left parasternal heave and loud pulmonary component of the second heart sound are features. The CXR demonstrates cardiomegaly and large pulmonary arteries. The ECG shows P pulmonale, right axis deviation, right ventricular hypertrophy with strain pattern, or right bundle branch block.

Pulmonary vasodilators

- In patients whose arterial PaO_2 is always $<7.3\,kPa$, domiciliary oxygen for more than 15 h per day prolongs life.
- Systemic vasodilators (calcium antagonists).

Further reading

British Thoracic Society Guidelines for the management of chronic obstructive pulmonary disease. *Thorax* 1997; **52(Suppl 5)**: S1–32.
www.brit-thoracic.org.uk/copd/index.html
Calverley PMA, Walker P. Chronic obstructive pulmonary disease. *Lancet* 2003; **362**: 1053–61.
Lieshing T, Kwok H, Hill NS. Acute applications of noninvasive positive pressure ventilation. *Chest* 2003; **124**: 699–713.

Related topics of interest

Asthma (p. 38)
Pneumonia (p. 223 and p. 227)
Weaning from ventilation (p. 331)

Coma

Coma is the manifestation of a depressed level of consciousness. Coma is usually defined as a Glasgow Coma Scale (GCS) of 8 or less. Coma reflects pathology in the reticular activating system of the brain stem or the cerebral cortex. The principals of critical care management of coma include:

- Protecting the patient from further injury.
- Diagnosing the underlying cause.
- Managing the patient to ensure an optimal outcome.

Causes of coma

- Primary cerebral lesion: head injury, intracranial haemorrhage, meningitis/encephalitis, abscess, tumour, hydrocephalus, cerebral oedema and epilepsy.
- Secondary to systemic illness: any cause of hypoxia and hypotension (e.g. cardiac arrest and shock), liver failure, renal failure, CO_2 narcosis, hypoglycaemia, ketoacidosis, electrolyte abnormalities, hyper and hypo-osmolar states, myxoedema, hypothermia, sepsis (including tropical diseases).
- Drug induced: therapeutic drugs, drugs in overdose or non-therapeutic drugs and poisons, anaesthetic agents, benzodiazepines, opioids, antidepressants, alcohol.

Assessment

- A rapid assessment with simultaneous resuscitation following the ABC format is required.
- The history will often provide the likely diagnosis.
- Exclude hypoxia and hypotension. Assess respiration (absent in brain stem death and following overdosage of certain drugs).
- Assess external signs of head injury (if suspicious, immobilise cervical spine). NB. Blood in external auditory meatus or from the nose or over the mastoid area is a sign of base of skull fracture.
- Assess and record the GCS.
- Localising neurological signs suggest intracranial pathology.
- Examine the pupils for asymmetry, size and reactions. Bilateral unreactive pupils suggest brain stem pathology. A unilateral dilated and unreactive pupil suggests ipsilateral III nerve palsy. Meiosis suggests opioids or brain stem disease. Dysconjugate gaze suggests cranial nerve lesion (III, IV or VI) or internuclear ophthalmoplegia. Conjugate gaze deviation suggests an ipsilateral frontal lesion. Fundoscopy for retinopathy (hypertensive, diabetic) and papilloedema.
- Consider assessment of other cranial nerves.
- Meningism suggests meningitis or subarachnoid haemorrhage.
- Assess temperature. Pyrexia suggests sepsis, meningitis. Exclude hypothermia.
- Look for venepuncture marks (opioid overdose, other illicit drugs, septicaemia and intracerebral abscess).
- Examine the abdomen for signs of liver and renal disease.

Investigations

- Blood sugar on fingerprick test.
- Laboratory blood sugar, urea, creatinine, electrolytes, liver function tests and full blood count.
- Drug screen for suspected agents and hold urine for toxicology.
- Blood alcohol level.
- CT/MRI scan.
- Lumbar puncture is rarely required as an urgent procedure and should never be performed in the presence of signs of raised intracranial pressure (ICP).
- EEG is useful to demonstrate abnormal activity.

Management

- Specific therapy is directed at the underlying pathology.
- Hypoxia and hypotension must be rapidly corrected.
- GCS < 10 may require intubation to protect the airway, prevent secondary brain injury and facilitate investigation (e.g. CT scan).
- Ventilate the patient's lungs to achieve a normal PaO_2 and $PaCO_2$ if there is any ventilatory failure.
- Hypoglycaemia is corrected with 50 ml i.v. 50% glucose.
- Give thiamine 100 mg if suspicion of history of alcohol abuse.
- Correct electrolyte abnormalities and ensure adequate hydration.
- Commence early enteral nutrition.
- Commence DVT prophylaxis.
- Consider the use of anticonvulsants.
- Consider insertion of ICP monitor.
- Initiate therapy to reduce a raised ICP if present.
- Consider cerebral protective therapy (hypothermia, reduce $CMRO_2$).

Specific antagonists:

- Naloxone for opioid overdose.
- Flumazenil for benzodiazepine overdose.

Extradural haemorrhage

It usually results from a head injury. There may be an initial lucid period followed by a rapid deterioration in GCS, progressing to coma often with focal signs (lateralising weakness or pupillary signs). This is consistent with a minor brain injury with a rapid accumulation of blood from a middle meningeal artery rupture. Surgical drainage following CT scan localisation has a relatively good prognosis provided the time period to surgery was short and the initial GCS immediately after injury was high.

Subdural haemorrhage

Acute presentations following trauma are associated with severe underlying brain injury, initial low GCS post injury and a poor prognosis. In acute head injury, subdural haemorrhage is more common than extradural haemorrhage and the onset of coma is immediate.

Chronic subdural haematoma presents days to weeks after head trauma that is often described as trivial. Presentation may be vague with a fluctuating level of consciousness, agitation, confusion, seizures, localising signs or a slowly evolving stroke. Diagnosis is made by CT or MRI scan. Treatment is by surgical drainage.

Intracerebral haemorrhage

Intracerebral haemorrhage is associated with hypertension, haemorrhage into a neoplasm, haemorrhage into an infarct, AV malformations, vasculitis, coagulopathy (including post-thrombolysis) and mycotic aneurysms associated with bacterial endocarditis.

Clinical features are governed by the area of involvement. Extensive haemorrhage presents as sudden onset of coma, drowsiness and/or neurological deficit. The rate of evolution depends on the site and size of the bleed. Some are amenable to surgical drainage.

Intracerebral infarction

Cerebral infarction follows thrombosis or embolism. Few of these patients benefit from intensive care management. Those that may benefit include those with embolic strokes where the source of the embolism is amenable to therapy, those with thrombosis secondary to medical intervention (e.g. post carotid or neurosurgery) or where surgery, invasive radiology or thrombolysis may be of use. Management is largely supportive.

Brain death

(see p. 55)

Vegetative state

In this uncommon state, there is severe cortical damage but with preservation of some brain stem activity. Vegetative states usually follow severe hypoxic brain injury or severe head injury. Consciousness is impaired, although there may be eye opening, and there is no voluntary movement. It is a diagnosis that can be made only after a prolonged period of observation (months), at which stage it is usually permanent.

Locked-in syndrome

Locked-in syndrome is a state of normal consciousness but with impaired movement due to lower cranial nerve damage and brain stem/spinal cord damage that results in paralysis. Careful assessment of responsiveness is required and the EEG will demonstrate awake rhythms.

Pseudo-coma/psychogenic coma

This is a diagnosis of exclusion. Signs are usually not consistent with accepted neurological damage. Cranial nerve reflexes will remain intact and the EEG will demonstrate awake rhythms.

Global ischaemia

Global cerebral ischaemia is the usual result of a prolonged period of circulatory arrest but will also result from prolonged periods of severe hypoxia and/or hypotension of any cause. Prognosis is related to the duration of the ischaemic/hypoxic period and the presence of co-morbidity. Less than 10% of patients demonstrating severe global ischaemic injury will regain independent activity. Recovery can be delayed and prolonged, which leads to a guarded prognosis. After 6 months the potential for major improvement in patients with severe brain injury is small: patients with potential for significant recovery will have demonstrated improvements within the first 72 h. If there is improvement in cranial nerve activity and motor activity during this period, continued aggressive intensive care may be indicated. Seizures in the initial post resuscitation period do not correlate with outcome but myoclonic activity carries a poor prognosis. EEG and evoked potentials may provide some aid to judging prognosis.

Further reading

Chiappa KH, Hill RA. Evaluation and prognostication in coma. *Electroencephalogr Clin Neurophysiol* 1998; **106**: 149–55.

Giacino JT. Disorders of consciousness: differential diagnosis and neuropathological features. *Semin Neurol* 1997; **17**: 105–11.

Scheuer ML. Continuous EEG monitoring in the intensive care unit. *Epilepsia* 2002; **43(Suppl 3)**: 114–27.

Related topics of interest

Brain death and organ donation (p. 55)
Status epilepticus (p. 291)

Critical illness polyneuromyopathy

Rachel Markham

Critically ill patients may develop profound acute muscle weakness that cannot be explained by physical inactivity alone. Historically, clinicians have sought to classify the cause between myopathy, neuromuscular junction abnormalities, neuropathy and neuromyopathy. Abnormal electrophysiological tests and muscle biopsies are common. However, the management of the patient is not currently influenced by such differentiation.

Risk factors

- Duration of assisted ventilation (up to 25% of patients ventilated for >7 days may develop critical illness polyneuromyopathy).
- Duration of multiple organ failure (MOF) or sepsis.
- Exogenous steroids.
- Hyperglycaemia – there is a lower incidence in postoperative patients who have been managed with strict blood sugar control.
- Hypoalbuminaemia.
- Neuromuscular blocking drugs.
- Total parenteral nutrition.
- CNS disorders.
- Female sex.
- The elderly.

Clinical features

- Motor weakness, which can be assessed using the Medical Research Council (MRC) sum-score (Table 5).
- Failure to wean from ventilation. Respiratory muscle weakness can be assessed using simple bedside measurements such as vital capacity or maximal inspiratory pressure but is greatly influenced by the patient's cooperation, coordination and motivation.

Typically, there is a symmetrical, flaccid, tetraparesis sparing the facial muscles. There may be reduced or absent tendon reflexes with or without muscle wasting. Sensorimotor axonopathy and muscle abnormalities seen on biopsy but not related to nerve involvement are common.

Table 5 MRC sum-score

Movement tested on each side	Score for each movement
Arm abduction	**0** = no movement
Flexion at the elbow	**1** = flicker of movement
Wrist extension	**2** = movement with gravity eliminated
Hip flexion	**3** = movement against gravity
Extension at the knee	**4** = movement against resistance
Foot dorsiflexion	**5** = normal power

Each limb is scored from 0 to 15. The total score ranges from 0 (tetraplegia) to 60.

Differential diagnosis

- Spinal cord injury.
- Guillain–Barré syndrome.
- Botulism.
- Organophosphate poisoning.
- Myasthenia gravis.
- Motor neurone disease.
- Acid maltase myopathy.

Management

There is little in the way of evidence-based medicine or randomised controlled trials on this topic. Management is aimed at the treatment or avoidance of risk factors. This includes the effective prevention and treatment of sepsis and MOF, minimising the duration of sedation and assisted ventilation, and avoidance of neuromuscular blocking drugs (especially continuous infusion) and steroids wherever possible. Strict blood sugar control using insulin is the only strategy that has been shown, in a randomised controlled trial, to reduce the incidence of acute critical illness polyneuromyopathy.

Physical rehabilitation and psychological support are both important in the effective management of such patients.

Prognosis

Effectively managed patients show recovery but there is an increased mortality due to the underlying condition, especially in sepsis and MOF. Survivors usually show a complete or almost complete recovery of neuromuscular function over a period of weeks to months.

Further reading

Berghe Gvd, Wouters P, Weekers F, *et al*. Intensive insulin therapy in critically ill patients. *N Engl J Med* 2001; **345**: 1359–67.

Hund E. Myopathy in critically ill patients. *Crit Care Med* 1999; **27**: 2544–7.

Nates JL, Cooper DJ, Day B, Tuxen DV. Acute weakness syndromes in critically ill patients – a reappraisal. *Anaesth Intensive Care* 1997; **25**: 502–13.

Sharshar T, Outin MD, de Jonghe B. Neuromuscular abnormalities in critical illness. In: Vincent JL (ed.), *Yearbook of Intensive Care and Emergency Medicine*. Berlin: Springer-Verlag, 2003, pp. 776–87.

Related topics of interest

Guillain–Barré syndrome (p. 161)
Myasthenia gravis (p. 204)
Psychological aspects of critical care (p. 236)
SIRS, sepsis and multiple organ failure (p. 276)
Weaning from ventilation (p. 331)

Death certification

The medical certificates that are completed for transmission to the Registrar of Births and Deaths serve both legal and statistical purposes. A death must be registered before a funeral director can proceed with the final arrangements for the body. There are three types of death certificate:

- Stillborn certificate (after 24 weeks of pregnancy).
- Neonatal Death Certificate (any death up to 28 days of age).
- Medical Certificate of Death (any other death).

The certificate should be completed only by a medical practitioner who attended the deceased during their final illness.

Cause of death statement

The cause of death on a death certificate should refer to the state or condition directly leading to death. The mode of dying should not be stated (e.g. heart failure, cardiac arrest, renal failure, coma, old age). The addition of acute or chronic to any of these terms does not make them acceptable as a cause of death. Abbreviations or medical symbols should be avoided. Registrars of Births and Deaths are instructed to refer Medical Certificates to the Coroner for further enquiry if only a mode of death (and not a cause) has been recorded. This will almost certainly result in unnecessary delay and distress to the deceased's family.

The Coroner

A death should be referred to the Coroner if:

- The cause of death is unknown.
- The deceased was not seen by the certifying doctor either after death or within the 14 days before death.
- The death was violent or unnatural or there are suspicious circumstances.
- The death may be due to an accident (whenever it occurred).
- The death may be due to self-neglect or neglect by others.
- The death may be due to an industrial disease or may be related to the deceased's employment.
- The death may be due to an abortion.
- The death occurred during an operation or before recovery from anaesthesia was complete.
- The death may be a suicide.
- The death occurred during or shortly after detention in police or prison custody.

Death related to employment

Categories of death that may be of industrial origin are given in Table 6.

A more complete list is found on the reverse of each death certificate.

If there is any doubt whether a death should be reported the advice of the local Coroner's officer should be sought.

Table 6 Death in employment

Disease	Causes include
Malignant diseases	
Skin	Radiation and sunlight pitch or tar, mineral oils
Lung	Asbestos, nickel, radiation
Nasal	Wood or leather work, nickel
Pleura	Asbestos
Urinary tract	Benzidine, dyestuff, chemicals in rubber
Liver	PVC manufacture
Bone	Radiation
Infectious diseases	
Anthrax	Imported bone, bonemeal, hide or fur
Brucellosis	Farming or veterinary
Leptospirosis	Farming, sewer or underground workers
Rabies	Animal handling
Pneumoconiosis	Mining and quarrying, potteries, asbestos

Where the death has been reported to the Coroner, the death certificate will be issued by the Coroner and sent directly to the Registrar of Births and Deaths. This normally takes approximately 2 working days to complete. In some cases when the death has been discussed with the Coroner's officer, a doctor will be given permission to issue a death certificate without further enquiry.

What happens next?

The death certificate is taken to the Registrar's office usually by a close relative and the deceased's death recorded. The Registrar will issue two certificates. A white certificate which is for Department of Social Services purposes and will ensure that any benefits (such as a widow's pension) that are due from the state can be claimed for. The green certificate is for the funeral director and authorises burial or the application for cremation.

The Registrar is also able to issue certified copies of the death certificate, which will be required for probate or insurance purposes. Such certificates are needed to access bank accounts, pension policies or investments for instance.

Further reading

Completion of Medical Certificates of Cause of Death, May 1990. Office of Population Censuses & Surveys, St Catherine's House, 10 Kingsway, London WC2B 6JP.

Coroner's review. An independent review, commissioned by the Home Office, of the coronial service in England, Wales and Northern Ireland, including death certification, reporting in 2002. http://www.coronersreview.org.uk/

Related topics of interest

Brain death and organ donation (p. 55)

Diabetes mellitus

Patients with diabetes may require critical care due to end organ damage secondary to chronic disease or as an acute diabetic emergency.

Most cases of insulin dependent diabetes mellitus (IDDM) are associated with autoimmune destruction of pancreatic cells producing insulin deficiency, but it may also follow pancreatitis or pancreatectomy. In non-insulin dependent diabetes mellitus (NIDDM) there is insulin resistance; insulin levels are initially high but later in the disease process they are reduced and overt hyperglycaemia develops. In the critical care setting, hyperglycaemia in IDDM should be managed by infusions of a short-acting insulin and frequent blood sugar measurement. The same is often true for NIDDM patients who can usually return to non-insulin control after resolution of their acute illness. Hyperglycaemia also occurs in normal individuals secondary to administration of glucose-containing solutions, corticosteroids, catecholamines, and the stress response. In this non-diabetic group, the hyperglycaemia resolves with the clinical illness and long-term anti-diabetes treatment is rarely required.

Long-standing diabetes causes end organ damage, producing severe morbidity and increased mortality.

- Vascular disease (15–60%), coronary artery disease, cerebrovascular disease.
- Hypertension (30–60%).
- Cardiomyopathy.
- Nephropathy.
- Retinopathy.
- Autonomic neuropathy (risk of arrhythmias, cardiac arrest, respiratory arrest and hypoglycaemia).
- Infection.
- Increased respiratory disease.
- Neuropathy.

Treatment is directed at both maintaining normoglycaemia (blood glucose 6–10 mmol l^{-1}) and at associated disorders.

Specific diabetic emergencies

Diabetic ketoacidosis (DKA)

DKA accounts for the majority of diabetic emergencies admitted to critical care units. It is usually seen in patients with IDDM and evolves over several days. Lack of insulin combined with increases in glucagon, catecholamines and cortisol stimulates lipolysis, free fatty acid production and ketogenesis. Accumulation of ketoacids (β-hydroxybutyrate and acetoacetate) causes metabolic acidosis. Increased gluconeogenesis and glycolysis cause hyperglycaemia; glucose is not taken up peripherally because of the lack of insulin. The renal retention threshold for glucose is exceeded and glycosuria and ketonuria cause considerable loss of water and electrolytes. Hypovolaemia ensues and impaired tissue perfusion invokes anaerobic metabolism, which adds to the metabolic acidosis. The degree of hyperglycaemia is variable in DKA: up to 15% may have normal or only slightly elevated blood glucose.

Clinical features

These include thirst, polyuria, nausea, abdominal pain, vomiting, weight loss, confusion progressing to coma, hyperventilation (Kussmaul respiration) due to acidosis, ketone breath, dehydration and hypovolaemia.

Precipitants

These include infection, surgery, myocardial infarction and non-compliance with drug therapy.

Investigations

Blood sugar, urea, creatinine and electrolytes (potassium should be measured frequently as deficits are often large and only become obvious once treatment has been commenced). Serum bicarbonate $<16\,mmol\,l^{-1}$ signifies a severe acidosis and is an indication for arterial blood gas (ABG) analysis. Serum lactate, urinary ketones, serum osmolality and calculation of anion gap, amylase (which may be raised in the absence of pancreatitis), full blood count and ECG. Do a septic screen: blood culture, urine for microscopy and culture, CXR and sputum culture if signs of infection.

Management

- Severe DKA has a mortality rate of 5%.
- Follow the ABC principles of acute management and resuscitation.
- Intubation is required if consciousness is obtunded significantly. There is risk of aspiration from both the depressed level of consciousness and gastric dilatation. When assisted ventilation is used, the minute ventilation must take into account the large respiratory compensation of the spontaneously ventilating patient; an inadequate minute volume at this stage may precipitate profound acidosis and cardiovascular decompensation.

Fluid resuscitation

Hypovolaemia must be reversed rapidly to ensure adequate tissue perfusion; the overall fluid deficit can then be replaced over a longer period. The volumes infused must be assessed repeatedly against resuscitative end points (heart rate, blood pressure, peripheral perfusion, CVP).

Average losses are around 5–10 l of water and 400–700 mmol of sodium. Hypotension is corrected initially with 0.9% sodium chloride; a bolus of 1 l is followed typically by an infusion of approximately $200\,ml\,h^{-1}$. Once volume and serum sodium have been restored and blood sugar is approaching normal levels ($<15\,mmol\,l^{-1}$), 5% dextrose can be substituted. Some clinicians prefer to use half-normal saline at an early stage as it approximates more closely to the urinary sodium and water losses.

In general, the fluid and electrolyte deficits should be corrected over a 48–72 h period. Regular measurement of urine output and blood electrolytes enables fluid replacement to be tailored individually.

The potassium debt is typically 250–700 mmol. Potassium, magnesium and phosphate require regular measurement and replacement. Acidosis and excess potassium administration may cause hyperkalaemia, while fluid and insulin will cause hypokalaemia. Potassium requirements range from 10 to $40\,mmol\,h^{-1}$; some should be given as potassium phosphate to replace lost phosphate.

The magnesium deficit mirrors that of potassium. Initial replacement is started at

$10–20\,mmol\,h^{-1}$. Hypomagnesaemia may contribute to insulin resistance and increase the risk of arrhythmias.

During fluid and electrolyte replacement there is a risk of volume overload; hypernatraemia and hyperchloraemic acidosis from excess sodium chloride infusion; hypokalaemia, hypophosphataemia and hypomagnesaemia may result from inadequate replacement; hypoglycaemia from excess insulin; and cerebral oedema from excess fluid and too rapid replacement.

Insulin infusion
An insulin infusion $(2–5\,U\,h^{-1})$ is commenced and titrated against frequent blood glucose measurements. Insulin resistance is seen in around 10% of IDDM. The blood glucose level should be corrected over 48–72h (at a rate of $2–3\,mmol\,h^{-1}$), as rapid correction is likely to result in osmotic shifts and serious complications.

Correction of acidosis
The metabolic acidosis will improve with restoration of tissue perfusion and reduction in ketosis. There is no role for sodium bicarbonate, which is associated with numerous side effects including: adverse effects on tissue oxygenation, because of increased haemoglobin oxygen affinity; increased carbon dioxide production, which will require increased minute ventilation; paradoxical intracellular and cerebrospinal acidosis; a high osmotic and sodium load, with the risk of volume overload; hypokalaemia; and hypocalcaemia.

A nasogastric tube should be inserted, stress ulcer prophylaxis initiated and early enteral feeding commenced.

DVT prophylaxis
Deep vein thrombosis prophylaxis with compression stockings or mechanical compression devices and subcutaneous heparin should be used.

Hyperglycaemic hyperosmolar state
Hyperglycaemic hyperosmolar state (HHS), formerly known as hyperglycaemic hyperosmolar non-ketotic coma, occurs much less frequently than DKA. The new terminology reflects that an altered sensorium may be present without coma and there may be variable degrees of ketosis. The mortality associated with HHS is 15–30%. Severe hyperglycaemia and fluid depletion develops over a period of days or weeks with no or mild ketosis. It is seen usually in elderly patients with uncontrolled NIDDM, but may also be the first presentation of late-onset diabetes. Precipitants include infection, steroid and diuretic use, an excessive glucose intake and intercurrent surgery or illness. The characteristic presentation is of non-specific anorexia, malaise and weakness, which progresses to coma, severe dehydration and renal impairment. The severe dehydration and renal impairment will result in a metabolic acidosis but severe ketosis is not a feature. Coma will necessitate intubation, and the patient is likely to be obtunded for several days. The principles of fluid replacement are the same as for DKA but the dehydration is often more severe and replacement should be more gradual as the risk of cerebral oedema is higher: 0.9% sodium chloride is used to correct hypotension, and half-normal saline is used to replace the water and sodium losses. The fluid deficits should be corrected over a period of days. Despite the levels of hyperglycaemia often exceeding those seen in DKA, the insulin

requirements are lower than for DKA. Thrombotic events are more common in HHS and are a major cause of morbidity and mortality. For this reason, these patients should be fully anticoagulated with heparin.

Hypoglycaemia

Life-threatening hypoglycaemia may be seen in diabetics and non-diabetics. Coma in diabetics is most commonly due to hypoglycaemia. Hypoglycaemia (blood glucose $<2.5\,mmol\,l^{-1}$) may be precipitated by:

- Inadequate diet carbohydrate, missed meals.
- Excess glucose uptake (exercise, insulin overdose).
- Change in therapy/commencement of insulin therapy.
- Liver failure.
- Alcohol (inhibition of gluconeogenesis).
- Hypoadrenalism (including Addison's disease), hypopituitarism.

The threshold for symptoms and clinical features of hypoglycaemia varies widely:

- Nausea, vomiting.
- Sweating, tachycardia, tremor (may be absent with autonomic neuropathy).
- Altered behaviour, confusion, agitation and depressed level of consciousness.
- Seizures, coma and focal neurological signs; permanent neurological damage occurs rapidly because of the brain's dependence on glucose for metabolism and the lack of any significant brain stores of glycogen.

Management

Sufficient glucose must be given to rapidly reverse hypoglycaemia. High-concentration glucose (e.g. 50 ml 20% glucose) must be given without delay and repeated if necessary. Blood sugar levels are measured frequently and a continuous infusion of glucose may be required to maintain normoglycaemia.

Injection of glucagon 1 mg (i.m/s.c.) can be used if there is no venous access or glucose solution immediately available; glucose should be given as soon as possible.

Intensive insulin treatment in critically ill patients

Hyperglycaemia and insulin resistance are common in critically ill patients; the role of intensive insulin treatment to maintain tight control of blood glucose in these patients has been evaluated recently. In a prospective, randomised, controlled study of mechanically ventilated adults, intensive insulin therapy, targeted to a blood glucose of $4.4-6.1\,mmol\,l^{-1}$, reduced mortality to 4.6% compared with a conventional treatment group (target blood glucose $10.0 -11.1\,mmol\,l^{-1}$), which had a mortality rate of 8%. The benefit of intensive insulin therapy was attributable mainly to its effect on mortality among patients who remained in the intensive care unit for more than 5 days. The greatest reduction in mortality involved deaths due to MOF with a proven septic focus. Intensive insulin therapy also reduced overall in-hospital mortality by 34%, bloodstream infections by 46%, acute renal failure requiring dialysis or haemofiltration by 41%, the median number of red cell transfusions by 50% and critical illness polyneuropathy by 44%; in addition patients receiving intensive therapy were less likely to require prolonged mechanical ventilation and intensive care.

Controlling blood glucose this tightly requires close attention to detail if serious hypoglycaemic episodes are to be prevented. A specific protocol (e.g. Bath Insulin Protocol), which involves 1–2-hourly blood glucose measurement, is essential and needs to be agreed upon and introduced.

Further reading

Boord JB, Graber AL, Christman JW, Powers AC. Practical management of diabetes in criti-cally ill patients. *Am J Respir Crit Care Med* 2001; **164**: 1763–7.

Genuth SM. Diabetic ketoacidosis and hyperglycaemic hyperosmolar coma. *Curr Ther Endocrinol Metab* 1997; **6**: 438–47.

Lebovitz HE. Diabetic ketoacidosis. *Lancet* 1995; **346**: 767–72.

Van den Berghe G, Wouters P, Weekers F, *et al.* Intensive insulin therapy in the critically ill patients. *N Eng J Med* 2001; **345**: 1359–67.

Related topics of interest

Bath Insulin Infusion Protocol v5.1

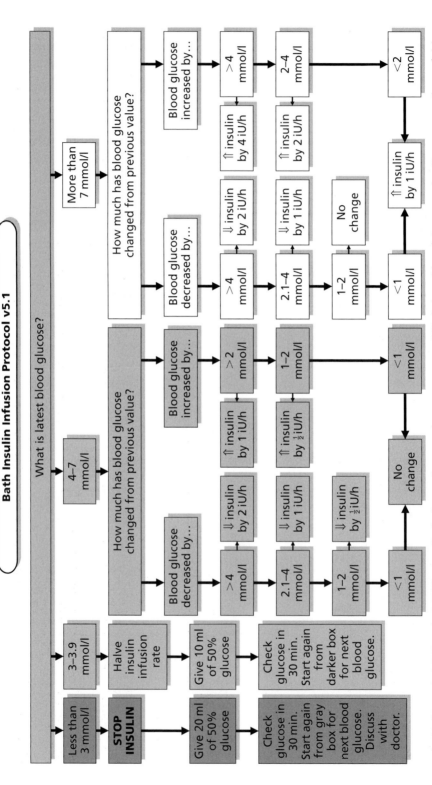

Bath Critical Care Unit 08/05/03 Version 5.1 While every effort has been made to ensure its accuracy, no responsibility for loss or injury whatsoever occasioned to any person acting or refraining from action as a result of using this protocol can be accepted by the authors or the Royal United Hospital, Bath NHS Trust.

Exclusions

This protocol is NOT suitable for patients with diabetic ketoacidosis, patients who are eating or children under the age of 16

Start protocol when blood sugar rises above 7 mmol/l

Insulin infusion

Use Insulin Actrapid 50 iU in 50 ml 0.9% NaCl running through a dedicated cannula or central line lumen.
Round insulin infusion rates to the nearest 0.5 ml/h.

Starting rate for insulin infusion

Blood glucose	Rate (ml/h)
>12	4
7.1–12	2
3–7	0
<3	give 20 ml 50% glucose, recheck glucose in 30 min, discuss with doctor

Blood glucose testing

Test blood glucose each hour if blood glucose is more than 7 mmol/l.
Use the same blood glucose testing machine each time.
If blood glucose is stable between 4 and 7 and the insulin dose has only changed by 1 ml/h or less in the last 2 h, blood glucose can be measured every 2 h.

Feeding

Continuous feeding is recommended with this protocol.
If enteral feed is stopped, halve the insulin infusion and measure blood glucose hourly. When enteral feed is restarted, measure the blood glucose hourly and simply follow the protocol (i.e. do not automatically increase insulin infusion when feed goes on).
Stop protocol when patient is taking food orally (even if NG supplements being given at night). Consider if insulin necessary by another route.

Other infusions (especially anitbiotics)

Should be made up with water or saline if possible, or if not, with the minimum volume of glucose.
Immunoglobulin infusion may cause over-reading of blood glucose with advantage II glucometer.

Ward discharge

Patients should be converted to a standard sliding scale before ward discharge. This should always run with a glucose or TPN infusion.

Figure 5 Bath insulin infusion protocol v5.1.

Drug overdose

Minh Tran

Drug overdose may be accidental or intentional as seen in suicidal or parasuicidal patients. The number of drugs available is enormous and clinical presentations vary greatly. However, basic and advanced life supportive measures remain the mainstay of treatment and the majority of patients will recover without the need for specific measures. A systematic approach to assessment and management comprises resuscitation, substance identification, drug elimination and specific treatment.

Resuscitation

Resuscitation should follow the well-established 'ABC' principles. However, there are specific problems:

- Hypothermia is common especially at the extremes of age. Core temperature should be measured (see p. 174).
- Hyperthermia is relatively uncommon but is seen with salicylates, amphetamines, cocaine and anticholinergic drugs. Neuroleptic malignant syndrome and malignant hyperthermia are rare causes. Sepsis may be the cause, particularly in obtunded patients.
- Rhabdomyolysis should be excluded in hypothermic, comatose or traumatised patients. It may also occur in narcotic and cocaine abuse without coma, or it may complicate prolonged seizures.

Substance identification

The history is often unreliable but important information includes:

- Drug: name(s), dosage, when taken, route taken.
- Circumstance: intention, witnesses, empty bottles, packets, syringes, associated trauma.
- Background: previous attempt(s), past medical history, allergy.
- Symptoms and signs: description and first aid prior to presentation. A full physical examination is essential.

Investigations

Identify the drug (blood, urine or gastric aspirate) and decide on the need for a specific treatment. It is often routine practice to check for paracetamol, aspirin and alcohol. Other helpful investigations might include:

- Blood count and coagulation.

- Urea, creatinine and electrolytes, liver function tests and CPK.
- Serum osmolality (ethanol, methanol and ethylene glycol).
- Arterial blood gas analysis.
- CXR in obtunded or intubated patients.
- 12-lead ECG.

Drug elimination

There are a number of strategies for drug elimination:

External decontamination is indicated for toxins that can be absorbed transdermally, e.g. organophosphates and hydrocarbons.

Induced emesis with syrup of ipecacuanha is not indicated when time of ingestion is more than 1 h. Less than 40% of ingested substance is usually recovered. It is contraindicated in children less than 6 months old, when there is coma or a depressed level of consciousness, following ingestion of caustic agents, alkalis and hydrocarbons. Potential complications include aspiration, Mallory–Weiss tears, protracted vomiting and gastric rupture. Its routine administration in the emergency department should be abandoned.

Gastric lavage is generally only useful within 1 h of ingestion but worthwhile recovery of some drugs (e.g. salicylate, theophylline) may occur later. It is not effective against alcohol ingestion and is potentially harmful following petroleum product and caustic ingestion. It should be performed only when the airway is protected. Complications include aspiration and inhalation of gastric contents, oropharyngeal trauma and oesophageal perforation. There is no certain evidence that its use improves clinical outcome and it may cause significant morbidity.

Activated charcoal (AC) is an effective adsorbent for many drugs. It is superior to emesis or lavage. Activated charcoal does not bind elemental metal (e.g. iron, lithium), alcohol (e.g. ethanol, methanol), cyanide or some pesticides (Malathion, DDT). Commercially available AC is an aqueous slurry with added cathartic and flavouring. AC should be considered only in life-threatening overdose of carbamazepine, dapsone, phenobarbital, quinine and theophylline. Its use in salicylate poisoning is controversial. No controlled study has yet demonstrated that AC reduces morbidity and mortality.

Cathartics cause diarrhoea and are used in combination with AC. Fluid and electrolyte losses may be excessive. Its sole use has no role in routine practice.

Endoscopy may be used for iron, alkali or acid ingestion, where gastric lavage and AC may cause further harm.

Surgical removal is rarely indicated (e.g. iron overdose, body packers).

Diuresis relies on bulk flow to decrease drug concentrations in blood. Intravenous fluid with or without a diuretic is used to produce a urine output of $2\text{--}5\,\text{ml}\,\text{kg}^{-1}\text{h}^{-1}$. Electrolyte and volume status must be closely monitored. There is a major risk of fluid overload. Alkalinisation with sodium bicarbonate may enhance barbiturate and salicylate elimination but is generally no longer recommended.

Haemodialysis is effective for low molecular weight compounds with small volume of distribution, low protein binding, low lipid solubility and low spontaneous clearance. Examples include methanol, ethanol, ethylene glycol, salicylates, lithium and chloral hydrate.

Haemoperfusion using either charcoal or resin columns may be useful for lipid-soluble drugs such as theophylline and barbiturates.

Specific treatment

Tricyclic antidepressants (TCAs)

Toxicity from TCAs remains one of the most common causes of serious drug poisoning as well as poisoning death. TCAs produce severe neurological (altered level of consciousness and seizures) and cardiovascular toxicity (atrial and ventricular arrhythmias and myocardial depression). A quinidine-like action on myocardial sodium channels is thought to be the underlying mechanism.

Drug levels are probably not helpful in predicting toxicity; however, ECG changes offer a more useful assessment. QRS width of 0.10–0.15 s correlates with an increased risk for seizures, whereas QRS >0.16 heralds tendency for both seizures and arrhythmias. A QRS width <0.10 does not rule out the possibility of significant toxicity. Also R_{aVR} of ≥3 mm is the only ECG variable that significantly predicts adverse outcomes.

There is no specific antidote, and rapid metabolism results in recovery within 24 h. Gastric elimination and AC are effective up to 24 h after ingestion. Bicarbonate therapy is an effective treatment in reducing toxicity, particularly when arrhythmias occur. It alkalinises the blood to pH of 7.5–7.55, thus increasing protein binding of the drugs, resulting in less free drug and lower toxicity. Ventricular arrhythmias usually respond to correction of acidosis and hypoxia. When arrhythmias are resistant to bicarbonate therapy, lidocaine (lignocaine) and phenytoin may help. Magnesium is useful in the presence of torsades de pointes. Beta-blockers should be used with caution. Procainamide is contraindicated as it can worsen the cardiovascular toxicity via its shared class Ia-antiarrhythmic properties.

Selective serotonin reuptake inhibitors (SSRIs)

These drugs represent a new group of 'cleaner' antidepressants. They are safer in overdose than TCAs or monoamine oxidase inhibitors (MAOIs). Neurological and cardiovascular toxicities rarely occur. Symptoms of overdose include tachycardia, drowsiness, tremor and nausea. Serious toxicity is unlikely, and if present should alert to the possibility of co-ingestants. When SSRI overdose patients present to the Emergency Department, if a careful history and examination and ECGs fail to detect co-ingestion, they should be monitored for a few hours. If no symptoms or signs appear after 1–3 h, they may be discharged from medical observation.

Serotonin syndrome is a potentially serious adverse reaction caused by excessive serotonin availability in the CNS. Drug interactions between SSRIs and other antidepressants (TCAs and MAOIs) are implicated, as well as between one of the antidepressants and other drug classes such as opioid (pethidine, tramadol), pantazocine, lithium, bromocriptine, sympathomimetics (pseudoephedrine, cocaine). Signs and symptoms of serotonin syndrome include neurobehavioural (altered mental state, agitation, confusion, seizures), autonomic (hypothermia, diaphoresis, diarrhoea, salivation, tachycardia, hypertension) and neuromuscular (myoclonus, hyper-reflexia, tremor, muscle rigidity, ataxia and nystagmus). It is important to recognise the syndrome first. Once identified, the treatment becomes simpler, with discontinuation of serotonergic drugs, support care, assisted ventilation if required, temperature control, sedation and muscle relaxation. The use of serotonin receptor antagonists, cyprohep-tadine or propranolol offers some benefits.

Paracetamol

Ingestion of $>150\,mg\,kg^{-1}$ by a child or $>7.5\,g$ by an adult is considered toxic. A single dose of 15 g carries great risk of liver damage, but it is possible to get liver toxicity from ingesting recommended doses, especially in the setting of fasting and malnutrition. Paracetamol is metabolised by the liver via glucuronidation and sulphation. Approximately 55% and 30% of paracetamol is normally excreted in urine in the form of glucuronide and sulphate metabolites, respectively. A small fraction is metabolised via the microsomal cytochrome P450 mixed-function oxidase system to reactive intermediates. N-acetyl-p-benzo-quinone (NAPQI) is the reactive metabolite responsible for the observed hepatotoxicity. At recommended doses, only trace amounts of NAPQI are formed. These are readily inactivated by the endogenous store of glutathione. When a large quantity of paracetamol is ingested, or when the hepatic glutathione store is depleted, excess NAPQI binds covalently to hepatocyte proteins, causing cell death.

In the early phase ($<20\,h$) there are relatively few symptoms apart from some abdominal pain, and nausea and vomiting. In the 2nd phase ($>20\,h$), clinical (pain and tenderness) and biochemical signs of hepatocellular necrosis are present. In the 3rd phase (days 3–4) liver damage is maximal. The recovery phase lasts for 7–8 days.

Treatment goals include inhibition of absorption of ingested drugs, removal of absorbed drugs, prevention of conversion of paracetamol into reactive metabolites (NAPQI) and, finally, treatment of hepatic failure and other complications once they occur.

Although gastric lavage, activated charcoal and ipecacuanha are all able to reduce the paracetamol absorption if used within the first 2 h after ingestion, gastric lavage plus activated charcoal does not seem to be superior to activated charcoal alone which has the best risk:benefit ratio. N-acetylcysteine (NAC) is an antidote which has demonstrated virtually total protection against hepatotoxicity if given within 8–10 h of paracetamol ingestion. It serves as a sulphur donor to replenish glutathione, and hence prevents accumulation of the toxic metabolite. Initiating NAC later than 8 h after ingestion affords less antidotal protection. Also, chronic ethanol abuse or concurrent use of enzyme-inducing medications may increase risk of hepatotoxicity. Delayed NAC therapy (more than 24 h after ingestion) and continuing past 72 h is considered beneficial in patients with hepatotoxicity. Methionine is an oral alternative. Activated charcoal binds acetylcysteine, and hence reduces its effectiveness. NAC is indicated if more than 10 g has been ingested, or if there is doubt about the amount taken or if the paracetamol level (taken at least 4 h after ingestion) is above the hepatotoxic line of the Rumack–Matthew nomogram. No N-acetylcysteine regime has been shown to be more effective than any other. NAC may cause urticaria, bronchospasm and anaphylaxis, especially with rapid administration. No evidence supports haemoperfusion or cimetidine for paracetamol overdose. Liver transplantation has the potential to be life-saving in fulminant hepatic failure.

Aspirin

Absorption may be delayed (enteric formulations) and blood concentrations within 6 h may be misleadingly low. Aspirin toxicity causes hyperventilation, tinitus, vasodilatation and an initial respiratory alkalosis that progresses to metabolic acidosis. Delirium may result in severe overdose. Metabolic acidosis, non-cardiac pulmonary oedema and altered level of consciousness are typical of chronic overdose. There is no specific antidote. Gastric emptying may be useful up to 4 h after ingestion. If the plasma salicylate concentration is >350 mg l^{-1} in children or >500 mg l^{-1} in adults, sodium bicarbonate may enhance urine excretion. Severe overdose (plasma level >700 mg l^{-1}) is an indication for haemodialysis.

Anticholinergic drugs

Atropine and other belladonna alkaloids, antihistamines, phenothiazines and tricyclic antidepressants have anticholinergic activity. This results in hyperthermia, dilated pupils, loss of sweating, delirium, visual hallucination, ataxia, dystonic reactions, seizures, coma, respiratory depression, labile blood pressure, arrhythmias, urinary retention and ileus.

Management comprises resuscitation, GI elimination and supportive care. Physostigmine, an anticholinesterase, crosses the blood–brain barrier and may be useful in severe cases but is not widely available.

Amphetamines and ecstasy (MDMA)

These drugs cause sympathomimetic effects, including arrhythmias, hypertension, seizures, coma, hyperthermia, rhabdomyolysis, renal and hepatic failure, intracerebral haemorrhage and infarction and hyponatraemia. There are no specific antidotes but beta-blockers can be used to treat arrhythmias.

Benzodiazepines

Supportive care alone will usually result in a good recovery. The antagonist flumazenil may be used but its short half-life dictates the need for an infusion and it may precipitate seizures, particularly in chronic benzodiazepine users.

Beta-blockers

Beta-blockers will cause bradyarrhythmias, atrioventricular block and hypotension. They may cause an altered mental state, delirium, coma and seizures. Sotalol may cause VT (sometimes torsades de pointes). Bradycardia is treated with atropine. Isoprenaline and cardiac pacing may also be useful in refractory cases. Intravenous glucagon, 3.5–5 mg (or 50–150 µg/kg^{-1}), is used as a beta-receptor independent inotrope and chronotrope in refractory bradycardia and hypotension. An infusion of 1–5 mg h^{-1} may be required to maintain chronotropic and inotropic effects of glucagon.

Calcium channel blockers

In overdose, calcium channel blockers will cause hyperglycaemia, nausea and vomiting, coma, seizures, bradycardia, varying degrees of AV block, hypotension and cardiac arrest. Gastric lavage may precipitate arrhythmias. Hypotension and bradycardia may respond to 10% calcium chloride. Additional calcium (bolus or infusion) is warranted in patients who responded to the initial dose of calcium chloride. Vasopressors (catecholamines) are first-line drugs for patients experiencing circulatory shock.

Digoxin

Nausea, vomiting, drowsiness and confusion are prominent. The ECG may show many types of rhythm and conduction abnormality. Management includes gastric elimination and correction of electrolytes, particularly potassium and magnesium. Digoxin-specific antibody fragments (Fab) are indicated in arrhythmias associated with haemodynamic instability. Ventricular tachyarrhythmias may respond to phenytoin, lidocaine or amiodarone. Atropine may be effective for bradycardia but temporary pacing may be required.

Ethanol

Very high doses of ethanol will cause severe cortical and brain stem depression (coma and hypoventilation) with obvious risk of aspiration of vomit. Depressed gluconeogenesis may cause hypoglycaemia and there may be a high anion gap metabolic acidosis. Management comprises supportive care with airway protection if required, intravenous thiamine and dextrose and correction of fluid, electrolyte and acid–base disturbance. Gastric lavage may be effective within 1–2 h of massive ingestion. Haemodialysisis is rarely indicated but is effective.

Methanol

The metabolites of methanol (formaldehyde and formic acid) are toxic. The lethal dose is $1-2\,ml\,kg^{-1}$ or $80\,mg\,dl^{-1}$. A latent period of 2–18 h may occur before the onset of a triad of GI symptoms (nausea, vomiting, pain, bleeding), eye signs (blurred, cloudy vision, central scotoma, yellow spots or blindness) and metabolic acidosis. There is an elevated serum osmolality and increased anion gap. Ethanol is a competitive inhibitor for metabolism and is used as an antidote to methanol. Aim to maintain a serum ethanol level at $1\,g\,l^{-1}$ or $20\,mmol\,l^{-1}$. Haemodialysis should be considered with:

- Peak methanol levels $>15\,mmol\,l^{-1}$ ($>50\,mg\,dl^{-1}$).
- Renal failure.
- Visual impairment.
- Mental disturbance.
- Acidosis not corrected with bicarbonate therapy.

Ethylene glycol

Ethylene glycol causes an odourless intoxication with high serum osmolality, severe metabolic acidosis and oxalate crystalluria. It is associated with hyperthermia, hypoglycaemia and hypocalcaemia. Toxicity is due due to hepatic metabolites (glycoaldehyde, glycolic acid, glycoxylate and oxalate). Management is as for methanol toxicity.

Opioids

An opioid overdose will cause respiratory depression, pinpoint pupils and coma. Seizures are usually due to hypoxia but can be caused by norpethidine, the neurotoxic metabolite of pethidine. Rhabdomyolysis, endocarditis and pulmonary complications are common. Naloxone is a specific antagonist that can be given i.v. and/or i.m. Its short half-life dictates the need for repeated injections or an infusion. Titration will avoid precipitating withdrawal in habitual users.

Lithium

Polyuria, thirst, vomiting, diarrhoea and agitation are common presentations of lithium overdose. Coma, seizures and nephrogenic diabetes insipidus also occur. Serum lithium levels $>1.5\,\mathrm{mmol\,l^{-1}}$ are toxic. Fluid and electrolyte disturbances should be corrected. Consider haemodialysis when concentrations reach $2\,\mathrm{mmol\,l^{-1}}$.

Organophosphates and carbonates

Toxicity is due to cholinergic overactivity and symptoms appear within 2 h of exposure. The symptoms can be memorised with the following mnemonics:

- **DUMBELS**: **d**iarrhoea, **u**rination, **m**iosis, **b**ronchospasm, **e**mesis, **l**acrimation, **s**alivation.
- **SLUDGE**: **s**alivation and **s**weating, **l**acrimation, **u**rination, **d**iarrhoea, **g**astrointestinal pain and **e**mesis.

Observe strict isolation and avoid contact exposure. Gastric elimination is appropriate. Atropine is used treat bradycardia and pulmonary secretions. Pralidoxime is a specific reactivator of cholinesterase but is effective only if given within 24 h of exposure. Plasma cholinesterase levels require monitoring until recovery.

Further reading

Barceloux D, Mcguigan M, Hartigan-Go K. Position statement: cathartics. American Academy of Clinical Toxicology; European Association of Poisons Centres and Clinical Toxicologists. *J Toxicol Clin Toxicol* 1997; **35(7)**: 743–52.

Brok J, Buckley N, Gluud C. Interventions for paracetamol (acetaminophen) overdoses (Cochrane Review). In: *The Cochrane Library*, Issue 1, 2003.

Krenzelok EP, Mcguigan M, Lheur P. Position statement: ipecac syrup. American Academy of Clinical Toxicology; European Association of Poisons Centres and Clinical Toxicologists. *J Toxicol Clin Toxicol* 1997; **35**: 699–709.

Position statement and practice guidelines on the use of multi-dose activated charcoal in the treatment of acute poisoning. American Academy of Clinical Toxicology; European Association of Poisons Centres and Clinical Toxicologists. *J Toxicol Clin Toxicol* 1999; **37**: 731–51.

Vale JA. Position statement: gastric lavage. American Academy of Clinical Toxicology; European Association of Poisons Centres and Clinical Toxicologists. *J Toxicol Clin Toxicol* 1997; **35**: 711–19.

Related topics of interest

End-of-life care

Cynthia Uy

Recent studies on end-of-life care in the intensive care unit (ICU) have identified substantial shortcomings in current practices. These include poor pain control in a significant proportion of patients, frequent aggressive treatments, late discussion and documentation of 'Do Not Attempt Resuscitation' (DNAR) orders, patient or proxy dissatisfaction with communication from intensive care staff and lack of acknowledgement of patient treatment preferences. Wide variations in the practice and patterns of end-of-life care have also been noted within different cultures.

To rectify these deficiencies, clinicians, ethics committees, hospital administrators and medical societies are attempting to establish a standard of care for the dying patient in the ICU which focuses on issues relating to treatment choices, symptom control, terminal care and family support.

Treatment choices

Witholding or withdrawing life support precedes the majority of ICU deaths, where up to 90% of patients die after a decision to limit therapy. The decision to make the transition from curative to palliative care is not always an easy one and is influenced by several factors, which are now considered.

Patient autonomy versus paternalism

Physicians are not obliged to provide or continue treatments that are futile. Historically, they have been responsible for making end-of-life decisions. Recently there has been a shift away from this paternalistic model to one of shared decision making. Conflict will arise when doctors and patients/families have opposing views on what constitutes futile treatment, but these differences may be resolved with honesty and clarity in imparting information, exploring the options and careful deliberation.

Indices of futility

Some authorities recommend a physiological definition of futility because other definitions, which usually take quality of life into account, are laden with value judgements. Others argue that, at times, value judgement is needed, especially when treatments may confer psychological benefit to the patient. The usefulness of prognostic models (which predict mortality rates for groups of ICU patients) in guiding treatment choices are of limited use in this setting.

Cultural differences

The cultural and spiritual values of patients and families may have an impact on treatment choices. Intensive care staff should also be aware of cultural differences in grieving and bereavement and consider involvement of relevant supporters or clergy.

Cost-effectiveness of palliative care

At present, there are scarce data on the cost-effectiveness of palliative care in the ICU setting, mostly due to methodological difficulties in selecting appropriate outcome indicators in this patient population and measuring these objectively and reliably. Further studies are underway.

Family support

In their definition of palliative care, the World Health Organization stresses the holistic nature of treatment and the importance of achieving the best quality of life for families as well as patients. The needs of the family have been assessed by a number of studies and include:

- Information to clarify the dying patient's condition, treatment and prognosis.
- Assurance that the patient is comfortable.
- Psychosocial support.
- Physical support – nutrition and sleep.
- Lenient visitation rights and privacy.
- Opportunity to say goodbye.
- Bereavement support.

During the terminal phase, altering the environment by reducing lighting and sound and removing restraints, unnecessary tubes and monitors might be helpful.

Symptom control

Pain

Pain can be assessed with good history taking and pain scales. In the case of the incapacitated patient, motor activity (grimacing, agitation) and haemodynamic signs (tachycardia, hypertension) in association with autonomic signs (diaphoresis, lacrimation) could be indicators of pain. Bispectral analysis has been used as a monitor in an attempt to assess pain in the unconscious patient.

Morphine is the standard opioid used in palliation. It can be given by oral, intravenous, subcutaneous, epidural, intrathecal and intracerebroventricular routes. The half-life of 2–3 h after intravenous administration will be prolonged in renal failure. Most commonly it is administered by continuous infusion. Adverse effects include nausea, vomiting, constipation, respiratory depression, asthma and urticaria due to histamine release.

Fentanyl is a potent synthetic opioid which can be given by intravenous, intramuscular, epidural, intrathecal, sublingual and transdermal routes. It has a half-life of 30–60 min after an intravenous dose. It is metabolised by the liver and is therefore potentially useful for patients with renal failure. It causes less histamine release and has a lower incidence of hypotension than morphine.

Hydromorphone is a semisynthetic opioid structurally similar to morphine. Its higher solubility enables large doses to be administered in low volumes of solution.

Delirium and terminal agitation

In up to 50% of cases no cause will be found for the delirium. When a cause is found, it is often irreversible.

Haloperidol is the neuroleptic agent of choice and has proven efficacy in managing delirium. It can be given orally, subcutaneously, intramuscularly and intravenously. Extrapyramidal side effects may occur.

Midazolam can be used in conjunction with haloperidol in agitated delirium and can be given as a continuous intravenous or subcutaneous infusion. Other indications for its use are myoclonus, seizures, to provide sedation and adjunctive treatment of intractable vomiting where sedation is not an issue. Transient apnoea and hypotension may occur after intravenous administration.

Propofol has a comparable effect to midazolam but is expensive, occasionally painful on administration and requires a separate intravenous line.

For the rare patient who does not settle with high doses of the medications listed above, other options to consider include *barbiturates*, *chlomethiazole* (suspected alcohol withdrawal), *thioridazine* and *chlorpromazine*.

Dyspnoea

Non-pharmacological measures used to ease shortness of breath include positioning, using a cold fan to direct air to the face, relaxation training and psychotherapy. These measures have not been systematically studied.

Oxygen may relieve dyspnoea by relieving hypoxaemia. Its efficacy in dyspnoeic non-hypoxaemic cancer patients is currently being evaluated.

Opioids have been shown to relieve breathlessness by reducing respiratory rate and altering the perception of dyspnoea.

Death rattles

Swallowing difficulties, infection and general debility cause secretions to accumulate in the oropharynx and airways. In the terminal setting, noisy breathing can be very distressing for the family and staff. Anticholinergic agents are used to dry secretions.

Hyoscine hydrobromide, given subcutaneously, is the preferred drug as it also has sedative effects. Other options include *hyoscine butylbromide* and *glycopyrrolate.*

Atropine is useful but can produce an agitated delirium and should be combined with midazolam if delirium is observed.

Nausea and vomiting

These symptoms occur commonly and usually respond to a combination of antiemetics. Intractable vomiting from a bowel obstruction may be eased by the use of a nasogastric tube and continuous subcutaneous infusion of the somatostatin analogue *octreotide.*

Hydration

In the terminal phase of illness, the current palliative care view on dehydration is that it is a normal part of the dying process and, hence, most patients in a hospice setting do not receive forced nutrition or hydration. 'Starvation euphoria', which may be related to endogenous opioid production or ketosis, may actually contribute to patient comfort. A review of the literature gives conflicting reports of what symptoms may be attributed to dehydration. Thirst and dry mouth are perceived to be the main troublesome symptoms of dehydration. There is no data comparing the efficacy of palliative management for thirst and dry mouth (good mouth care, sips of water) with rehydration. There is also no evidence to date that proves rehydration generally makes patients more comfortable.

Withdrawing life support
The approaches to withdrawing ventilatory support vary. Terminal extubation with administration of analgesic agents and sedatives allows the dying process to proceed naturally.

Further reading

Prendergast TJ, Claessens MT, Luce JM. A national survey of end-of-life care for critically ill patients. *Am J Respir Crit Care Med* 1998; **158**: 1163–7.

The SUPPORT Principal Investigators. A controlled trial to improve care for seriously ill hospitalized patients. The study to understand prognoses and preferences for outcomes and risks of treatments (SUPPORT). *JAMA* 1995; **274**: 1592–8.

Truog RD, Cist AFM, Brackett SE, *et al*. Recommendations for end-of-life care in the intensive care unit: the Ethics Committee of the Society of Critical Care Medicine. *Crit Care Med* 2001; **29**: 2332–48.

Related topics of interest

Analgesia in critical care – basic (p. 17)
Analgesia in critical care – advanced (p. 22)
Sedation (p. 270)

Endocarditis

Antony Stewart

Infective endocarditis results in the formation of infective vegetations on the endocardium. The cardiac valves are most commonly involved but other areas of endocardium may also be affected, e.g. ventricular septal defect (VSD), atrial septal defect (ASD), patent ductus arteriosus (PDA) and coarctation. Endocarditis occurs in one of three groups of patients: native valve endocarditis, prosthetic valve endocarditis and endocarditis in intravenous drug users.

Causative organisms

Staphylococcus aureus is the most common organism overall.

Native valve endocarditis
The frequency of causative organisms by age group is given in Table 7.

Table 7 Frequency of causative organisms by age group

Organism	Neonate	2 months to 15 years	16–60 years	>60 years
Streptococcus spp.	20%	45%	50%	35%
Staphyloccus aureus	45%	22%	35%	25%
Coagulase-negative *Staphylococcus*	10%	5%	6%	4%
Enterococcus	<1%	5%	6%	15%
Gram-negative bacilli	10%	2%	2%	2%

- *Streptococcus bovis* is frequently associated with colonic polyps or malignancy.
- HACEK organisms (*Haemophilus parainfluenza*, *Haemophilus aphrophilus*, *Actinobacillus actinomycetemcomitans*, *Cardiobacterium hominis*, *Eikenella corrodens* and *Kingella kingae*) account for 5–10% of all native valve endocarditis patients not using intravenous (i.v.) drugs.
- Very rare: *Rickettsia* (Q fever), *brucella*, *mycoplasma*, *legionella* and *histoplasma*.

Organisms in i.v. injecting drug users
- Staphylococci (60%).
- Gram-negative organisms (10%).
- Streptococci and fungi (6–12%).

5% of patients will have more than one organism.

Prosthetic valve endocarditis

Early (within 60 days):

- *Staphylococcus aureus* (20–24%).
- Coagulase-negative staphylococci (30–35%).
- Enterocci (5–10%).
- Gram-negative organisms (10–15%).
- Fungi (5–10%).

Late onset (after 60 days):

- *Staphylococcus aureus* (10–15%).
- Coagulase-negative staphylococci (30–35%).
- Streptococci (7–10%).
- Enterococci (10–15%).
- Gram-negative organisms (2–4%).

Pathogenesis

Endocarditis most commonly involves the left side of the heart, with the mitral valve most commonly affected. Drug addicts often have right-sided involvement, most commonly of the tricuspid valve. Vegetations consisting of fibrin, platelets and infecting organisms form in areas with high velocity and abnormal blood flow, flow from high to low pressure chambers, and flow through a narrow orifice.

The risk of endocarditis is increased in patients with structural heart disease, rheumatic valve disease, and mitral valve prolapse with regurgitation or thickened mitral valve leaflets. Other risk factors include poor dental hygiene, long-term haemodialysis and diabetic patients. Patients with HIV are also at risk, most likely as a result of long-term i.v. access and i.v. drug use. However, 40–50% of cases occur in patients with no abnormalities and are usually caused by virulent organisms such as *Staphylococcus aureus*.

Prosthetic valve endocarditis accounts for 7–25% of all cases. There is no difference in incidence between mechanical and bioprosthetic valves, although mechanical valves have a greater risk of early infection.

Nosocomial infective endocarditis accounts for 7–29% of all cases of endocarditis in tertiary hospitals. At least 50% are a result of infected intravascular devices.

Clinical features

Low-virulence organisms such as *Streptococcus viridans* tend to have insidious clinical courses. Virulent organisms such as *Staphylococcus aureus* and fungi cause more dramatic presentations. Fever is present in up to 90% of patients, as are new murmurs or changing murmurs (may not be detected in tricuspid involvement). Myalgia, arthralgia, fatigue, anorexia and anaemia are common presenting features. In patients with a prosthetic valve, an unexplained fever should lead to a search for endocarditis. Embolic phenomena are common, especially if vegetations are larger than 10 mm. Splenomegaly (40%) and clubbing are both late signs. Neurological signs occur in 20–40% due to embolism, encephalopathy and haemorrhage from mycotic aneurysms. Heart failure due to fulminant valvular regurgitation and cardiac conduction abnormalities also occurs.

Immune complex deposition causes vasculitis, splinter haemorrhages, Osler's nodes in the finger pulp, Roth spots in the retina and microscopic haematuria (due to either proliferative glomerulonephritis or focal embolic glomerulonephritis). In severe cases shock and multi-organ failure are features.

Nosocomial endocarditis has an acute onset and classic signs are often absent. A persistent bacteraemia before treatment, or for >72h after removal of an infected i.v. device, should raise suspicion of endocarditis.

Diagnosis

1. Definite infective endocarditis
(a) Pathological criteria
- Microorganisms on culture or histology in a vegetation (local or embolic) or in an intracardiac abscess.
- Pathological lesions on histology confirming endocarditis.

(b) Clinical diagnosis based on major and minor criteria
- 2 major criteria, or
- 1 major and 3 minor criteria, or
- 5 minor criteria.

2. Possible infective endocarditis. Clinical findings fall short of a definite diagnosis, but endocarditis is not rejected.

3. Rejected. Firm alternative diagnosis, or resolution of clinical manifestations with 4 days or less of antibiotics, or no evidence of endocarditis at autopsy or surgery.

4. Definitions
(a)   Major criteria
Positive blood culture with typical microorganism for infective endocarditis from:
- Blood cultures more than 12h apart, or
- all three or a majority of four or more blood cultures with first and last at least 1h apart, or
- microorganisms consistent with endocarditis isolated from persistently positive blood cultures, or
- single positive blood culture for *Coxiella burnetii*.

Evidence of endocardial involvement – positive echocardiogram for endocarditis (a transoesophageal echocardiography (TOE) is recommended for patients with a prosthetic valve):
- Oscillating intracardiac mass on a valve or supporting structures, in the path of regurgitant jets or on implanted material in the absence of an alternative explanation.
- Abscess.
- New partial dehiscence of prosthetic valve or new valvular regurgitation.

(b)   Minor criteria
- Predisposing heart lesion or i.v. drug use.

- Fever $> 38.0°C$.
- Vascular phenomena.
- Immunological phenomena, e.g. glomerulonephritis, Osler's nodes, rheumatoid factor, Roth spots.
- Microbiological evidence: positive blood cultures not meeting major criteria or serological evidence of active infection with organisms consistent with infective endocarditis.
- Echocardiogram consistent with endocarditis but not meeting major criteria.

Investigations

- Blood count may show neutrophilia and anaemia.
- Urinalysis for haematuria and casts.
- Blood cultures – at least three from different sites 1 h apart and before antibiotics are given. Cultures are positive in up to 90% of patients. Culture may be negative because of prior antibiotic exposure, fastidious organisms, e.g. *Coxiella burnetii* (Q fever), fungi, anaerobes, right-sided endocarditis or non-infective endocarditis, e.g. Libman–Sacks disease in SLE or marantic endocarditis (non-thrombotic endocarditis usually seen in patients with terminal malignant disease). In patients with confirmed endocarditis or a high probability of endocarditis with negative cultures, consider further tests such as lysis centrifugation and special enriched growth mediums.
- Transthoracic echocardiography detects vegetations larger than 2–3 mm and in appropriate patients is the first-line technique. Transoesophageal echocardiography is more sensitive. Most experts would use a TOE in patients with prosthetic heart valves or if the probability of endocarditis is high. Patients should all have Doppler studies.

Management

- General resuscitative management following the ABC priorities.
- Aggressive antimicrobial therapy.
- Repeated assessment for worsening valvular function, heart failure, abscess formation, embolic phenomena (especially cerebral) and multi-organ failure.
- Cardiac surgery may be required for acute valvular regurgitation, especially aortic regurgitation which is poorly tolerated by patients, acute aortic regurgitation with early closure of the mitral valve, myocardial abscess, fungal endocarditis, valve dysfunction and persistent infection despite 7–10 days of appropriate therapy, high risk of emboli (vegetations > 10 mm), and persistent positive blood cultures despite treatment.

  Surgery for prosthetic valve endocarditis may be needed for early infection, heart failure with prosthetic valve dysfunction, fungal infection, staphylococcal infection not responding to antibiotics, perivalvular leak or abscess formation, infection with Gram-negative organisms and persistent bacteraemia after 7–10 days of appropriate antibiotics.
- There is no role for routine anticoagulation. If anticoagulation is required it should be carefully monitored as the risk of bleeding is increased.

Principles of antimicrobial therapy:

- Empirical therapy (e.g. benzylpenicillin, flucloxacillin and gentamicin) is commenced in fulminant endocarditis and then modified depending on organisms isolated from blood cultures. Rifampicin may be added if prosthetic valve endocarditis is suspected.
- Prolonged treatment is required (4–6 weeks) because the high density of microorganisms protected in vegetations is associated with a high relapse rate.
- If treatment is effective the fever should decrease in 3–7 days. A persistent fever may reflect ineffective treatment, abscess formation, septic emboli or antibiotic fever.

Prognosis

Streptococcal and tricuspid endocarditis carry a 10% mortality. The prognosis is poor (>20% mortality) in non-streptococcal disease, severe heart failure, aortic and prosthetic valve involvement, age >65, valve ring or myocardial abscess and large vegetations. Death is usually due to heart failure and embolic events. Prognosis is worst (60% mortality) in early prosthetic valve endocarditis. Recurrent or second episodes are seen in 6% of patients.

Prophylaxis

Although there is little evidence of the efficacy of antibiotic prophylaxis, it is common practice to give antibiotics to high-risk patients who are having procedures associated with the risk of bacteraemia.

The recommendations for prophylaxis vary depending on the procedure, from country to country and depending on local factors. Expert microbiologist advice should be sought.

Further reading

Dajani AS, Taubert KA, Wilson W, *et al*. Prevention of bacterial endocarditis. Recommendations by the American Heart Association. *Circulation* 1997; **96**: 358–66.

Durack DT, Lukes AS, Bright DK. New criteria for diagnosis of infective endocarditis: utilization of specific echocardiographic findings. Duke Endocarditis Service. *Am J Med* 1994; **96**: 200–9.

Mylonakis E, Calderwood SB. Infective endocarditis in adults. *N Engl J Med* 2001; **345**: 1318–30.

Related topics of interest

Epiglottitis

Acute epiglottitis is an uncommon but dangerous bacterial infection of the throat. It is usually seen in children aged less than 8 years with a peak incidence between 2 and 5 years. It may also occur in adults. The usual causative organism is *Haemophilus influenzae* type B but this is not invariable and β-haemolytic streptococci, staphylococci or pneumococci may also be isolated, especially in adult cases. The differential diagnosis in children is acute laryngotracheobronchitis (croup), which is a viral infection occurring principally in those under 3 years of age. The mortality in adults is quoted to be as high as 6–7% but this is usually due to misdiagnosis and inappropriate treatment.

Problems

1. Upper airway obstruction.
2. Lethargy and exhaustion.
3. Potential difficulty with intubation.

Diagnosis

The provisional diagnosis is made on the history and examination. Typically, the history is short with a rapid deterioration. The patient presents with a sore throat, fever, muffled voice and dysphagia. Pain may exceed that expected from the brevity of the history. Inspiratory stridor develops rapidly and progression to complete respiratory obstruction may occur within 12 h.

Children prefer to sit up and drool saliva from the mouth. Swallowing is avoided because of the extremely sore throat.

Indirect laryngoscopy should not be undertaken to confirm the diagnosis as this frequently precipitates airway obstruction, especially in children. Lateral neck X-rays may confirm a swollen epiglottis but are not essential. A sick child should not be sent to the X-ray department without the continual presence of someone skilled in paediatric intubation. A child with suspected epiglottitis will invariably require an examination of their upper airway under anaesthesia and X-rays are frequently unnecessary. The airway can then be secured with a tracheal tube.

Management

Children

The child is moved to a quiet induction area where all the necessary aids to a difficult paediatric intubation are readily to hand. The child is allowed to remain in an upright posture as sudden changes in position, especially lying down, may result in complete airway obstruction.

An inhalational induction of anaesthesia is usually preferred. Venous access can be obtained once the child is unconscious. Atropine may then be given if required. In the presence of airway obstruction it may take more than 15 min before anaesthesia is deep enough to permit safe laryngoscopy.

Laryngoscopy will show a swollen 'cherry red' epiglottis. There is often associated swelling of the aryepiglottic folds. In severe cases the only clue to the glottic opening may be bubbles issuing from behind the epiglottis during expiration.

Once intubated the child should then be transferred to a critical care area. Blood cultures and throat swabs are taken for microbiological examination. Therapy is continued with intravenous rehydration, humidified inspired gases, airway toilet and antibiotics.

Adults

The management of adult cases follows a similar course, although observation of the unintubated patient in a critical care environment has been recommended by some. The risk in this strategy is the possibility of death from sudden complete respiratory obstruction.

Antibiotics

Cefuroxime is the usual 'best bet' antibiotic until the organism's sensitivities are known. Cefotaxime is an alternative, especially in adults if broader cover for Gram-negative organisms is required.

Progress

Epiglottic oedema settles rapidly following commencement of the antibiotics and an increasing leak around the tracheal tube is expected. Once the patient is afebrile and appears well, extubation may be considered. This is usually within 24–48 hours. It is not necessary to re-examine the larynx prior to extubation.

Related topics of interest

Infection acquired in critical care (nosocomial) (p. 182)

Fibreoptic bronchoscopy

Martin Schuster-Bruce

Diagnostic uses

Fibreoptic bronchoscopy (FOB) enables direct inspection and instrumentation of the upper and lower airway. Aspiration, bronchoalveolar lavage, bronchial brushings, transbronchial biopsy and protected specimen brushings can obtain diagnostic material. Its indications comprise:

1. Investigation of atelectasis: areas of atelectasis may require bronchoscopy to exclude an obstruction.
2. Evaluation of haemoptysis.
3. Evaluation of radiological abnormalities: lesions can be biopsied but the incidence of complications, particularly pneumothorax, is highest with this technique, especially in those mechanically ventilated (as high as 20%).
4. Diagnosis of pneumonia: indicated particularly in those immunocompromised and in those with suspected nosocomial pneumonia. Protected specimen brushes or bronchoalveolar lavage affords better correlation with the infective cause of infection by reducing contamination from a colonised upper airway (see Pneumonia – hospital acquired (p. 227)).
5. Localisation of the tracheal tube tip.
6. Determination of the site of barotrauma.
7. Evaluation of major airway trauma and thermal injury.

Therapeutic uses

1. Aspiration of mucous plugs. Chest physiotherapy and suctioning are normally successful in treating mucous plugs and resultant atelectasis. If these techniques fail, bronchoscopy with bronchoalveolar lavage can be used to remove the plugs and re-expand the atelectatic lung. The relatively narrow suction channel in the FOB will limit its efficacy in the presence of very thick mucus.
2. Local treatment of haemoptysis. The FOB can be used to instil adrenaline (epinephrine) solution onto a bleeding endobronchial site or assist the placement of a Fogarty catheter into that segment to tamponade the bleeding focus.
3. Removal of aspirated foreign bodies. Although the rigid bronchoscope is traditionally the preferred instrument for the removal of foreign bodies, the FOB used with a variety of forceps and baskets has been shown to be safe and effective.
4. Treatment of bronchopulmonary fistula. Proximally located fistulas may be visualised directly, whereas more distal fistulas may be localised by systematically passing an occluding balloon into each bronchial segment. When the correct segment is located, inflation of the balloon will result in reduction of the air leak.

Airway management

Indications for bronchoscopic airway management include:

1. Tracheal intubation: especially in the setting of difficult intubation, anatomical deformity, head and neck immobility and upper airway obstruction.
2. Percutaneous tracheostomy: the FOB is used to confirm correct position of the Seldinger wire within the lumen of the trachea.
3. Bronchial intubation (double lumen tube).
4. Changing tracheal tube.
5. Placement of a nasogastric tube.

Complications

Fibreoptic bronchoscopy is a safe procedure when performed in the ICU on critically ill patients. The most common complications are oxygen desaturation, hypotension, frequent premature ventricular beats, fever and pulmonary haemorrhage. These are generally transient and rarely life threatening. Relative contraindications include difficult ventilation or oxygenation; severe coagulopathy; acute myocardial infarction or ischaemia; and status asthmaticus.

Recently, there has been interest in the use of non-invasive ventilation during FOB in non-intubated patients in which bronchoscopy would traditionally have been contraindicated due to the significant risk of oxygen desaturation.

Further reading

Ovassapian A, Randel GI. The role of the fibrescope in the critically ill. *Resp Proc Monitoring* 1995; **11(1)**: 29–50.

Silver MR, Balk RA. Bronchoscopic procedures in the intensive care unit. *Resp Proc Monitoring* 1995; **11(1)**: 97–109.

Fluid replacement therapy

Caleb McKinstry

Total body water (TBW) represents about 60% of the body weight of a young adult male. The distribution of this fluid across the primary fluid spaces is depicted in Figure 6.

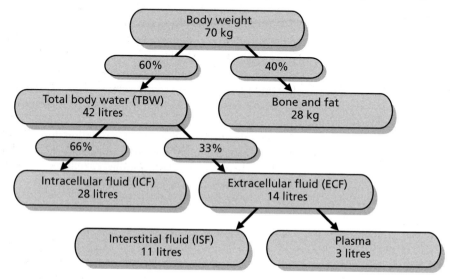

Figure 6 Distribution of fluid in the body.

Physiology

Intracellular fluid (ICF) is separated from extracellular fluid (ECF) by a cell membrane that is highly permeable to water but not to most electrolytes. Intracellular volume is maintained by the membrane sodium–potassium pump, which moves sodium out of the cell (carrying water with it) in exchange for potassium. Thus, there are significant differences in the electrolytic composition of intracellular and extracellular fluid.

The intravascular space and the interstitial fluid (ISF) are separated by the endothelial cells of the capillary wall (the capillary membrane). This wall is permeable to water and small molecules, including ions. It is impermeable to larger molecules such as proteins.

The higher hydrostatic pressure inside capillaries (compared with that in the ISF) tends to force fluid out of the vessel into the ISF.

The osmotic pressure of a solution is related directly to the number of osmotically active particles it contains. The total osmolarity of each of the fluid compartments is approximately 280 mOsml^{-1}. Oncotic pressure is that component of osmotic pressure provided by large molecules. The higher osmotic pressure inside capillaries tends to pull fluid back in to the vessels.

Electrolyte concentrations differ markedly between fluid compartments. Notably, sodium and chloride are chiefly extracellular while the majority of total body potassium is within the intracellular compartment. There is also a relatively low content of protein anions in ISF compared with ICF and plasma.

Crystalloids

The composition of some of the commonly prescribed crystalloids is given in Table 8.

A crystalloid is a solution of small non-ionic or ionic particles (e.g. sodium chloride). After intravenous administration, the distribution of a crystalloid is determined chiefly by its sodium concentration. Since sodium is confined mainly to the ECF, fluids with high sodium concentrations (e.g. 0.9% sodium chloride) will be distributed mainly through the ECF. Solutions with lower sodium concentrations (e.g. 5% glucose) will be distributed throughout both ECF and the intracellular compartment. In comparison with Hartmann's solution, the higher sodium content of normal saline will result in slightly better intravascular volume expansion. However, large quantities of normal saline will cause hyperchloraemic acidosis; the impact of this on clinical outcome is uncertain. After head injury, normal saline is the preferred resuscitation fluid because Hartmann's solution is slightly hypotonic relative to plasma and may worsen cerebral oedema.

Colloids

Colloidal solutions are fluids containing large molecules that exert an oncotic pressure at the capillary membrane. Natural colloids include blood and albumin. Artificial colloids contain large molecules such as gelatin, dextran, starch and haemoglobin. Intravenous colloids will initially expand mainly the intravascular compartment. Intravascular persistence depends on molecular size, shape, ionic charge and capillary permeability. Inflammatory conditions (e.g. sepsis) are associated with leaky capillary

Table 8 Composition of commonly prescribed crystalloids

Crystalloid	Osmolality (mosmolkg^{-1})	pH	Na^+ (mmoll^{-1})	K^+ (mmoll^{-1})	HCO_3^- (mmoll^{-1})	Cl^- (mmoll^{-1})	Ca^{2+} (mmoll^{-1})
0.9% saline	308	5.0	154	0	0	154	0
Hartmann's solution	280	6.5	131	5.0	29[a]	111	2
PlamaLyte 148	299	5.5	140	5	50[b]	98	0
5% dextrose	278	4.0	0	0	0	0	0
4% Dextrose in 0.18% saline	286	4.5	31	0	0	31	0

[a] HCO_3^- is provided as lactate.
[b] 27 mmoll^{-1} as acetate and 23 mmoll^{-1} as gluconate.

states, and under these circumstances it seems rational to limit the development of peripheral oedema by using predominantly colloids instead of crystalloids.

Blood

Blood is an appropriate replacement fluid following severe haemorrhage. It will increase the haemoglobin concentration in the circulating compartment and thus improve oxygen carriage. Blood transfusion expansion the intravascular compartment with little or no increase in interstitial fluid (see Blood and blood products, p. 41).

Albumin

Human albumin is a single polypeptide with a molecular weight of around 68 kDa. It is a negatively charged substance and is repelled by the negatively charged endothelial glycocalyx, thus extending its intravascular duration. Albumin has transport functions, is able to scavenge free radicals and has anticoagulant properties. In health, it contributes about 80% of oncotic pressure but, in the critically ill, serum albumin correlates poorly with colloid oncotic pressure. Albumin is prepared in two concentrations (4.5 and 20%) from many thousands of pooled donors. Although albumin supplied in the United Kingdom (UK) is now sourced from the United States, there remains a theoretical risk of transmission of the prion causing variant Creutzfeldt–Jakob disease. The half-life of exogenous albumin in the circulating compartment is 5–10 days assuming an intact capillary wall membrane. It is expensive to prepare but has a long shelf life. In the critically ill patient, capillary leak limits its effectiveness. The treatment of hypoalbuminaemia with albumin does not alter outcome in the critically ill. Despite the lack of robust outcome data, albumin remains a mainstay of colloid therapy in paediatric intensive care. A randomised controlled trial of saline versus albumin in 7000 critically ill patients demonstrated no difference in 28-day mortality.

Gelatins

Gelatins comprise modified bovine collagens suspended in ionic solutions. The collagen is sourced from outside the UK. Gelatin solutions have long shelf lives and, based on current knowledge, do not transmit infection. Gelatin solutions contain molecules of widely varying molecular weight. Despite a quoted average molecular weight of approximately 35 kDa, most of the molecules are considerably smaller than this and are excreted rapidly by the kidney. Thus, gelatin solutions remain in the circulating compartment for a short period. They maintain their maximal volume effect for only 1.5 h, and only 15% remains in the intravascular space 24 h after administration. Although anaphylaxis to colloids is rare, recent data indicate that gelatins are the most common to be implicated.

Dextrans

Dextrans are polysaccharide products of sucrose. Dextran 70 (average molecular weight 70 000) has an intravascular half-life of about 12 h. Dextrans cause a mild alteration in platelet stickiness and function and thus have an antithrombotic effect. They have been shown to reduce the incidence of fatal pulmonary embolism in susceptible patients. Dextran in combination with hypertonic saline (hypertonic saline dextran, HSD) has undergone extensive investigation, particularly in trauma patients. There are no robust data demonstrating improved outcome with HSD.

Hydroxyethyl starch

Hydroxyethyl starch (HES) is manufactured by polymerising cornstarch. Several HES solutions are available, each with a different average molecular weight. Most HES solutions have a longer intravascular half-life than other synthetic colloids, with a significant volume effect for at least 6 h. The higher molecular weight starch solutions (450 kDa), particularly when combined with high substitution ratios (e.g. 0.7 or 7 hydroxyethyl groups for every 10 glucose rings), prolong clotting time by impairing factor VIII and von Willebrand factor. The medium weight starches (200 kDa) used commonly in the UK have considerably less effect on coagulation. There is a theoretical concern about accumulation of higher molecular weight HES in the reticuloendothelial system. Skin deposition causing long-term itching may be a problem. There has been some concern about impairment of renal function with HES solutions. This might be related to relative dehydration, which can occur if these colloids are not given with adequate volumes of maintenance crystalloid. Newer low molecular weight starches (140 kDa with a substitution ratio of 0.4) are less likely to cause any of these complications.

Artificial oxygen carriers

Haemoglobin-based oxygen carriers (HBOCs)

Blood is the only fluid in routine use that has significant oxygen-carrying capability. While this property makes it indispensable during resuscitation of haemorrhagic shock, it is expensive, in short supply, antigenic, requires cross-matching, has a limited shelf life, requires a storage facility and carries a risk of disease transmission. Free haemoglobin causes severe renal injury. Polymerisation of the haemoglobin overcomes this problem and improves intravascular persistence. Haemoglobin solutions under development are derived from one of three sources: bovine blood, out-of-date human blood (5–13% of blood donated in the United States is discarded) and recombinant haemoglobin. The products currently under investigation do not require cross-matching, have similar oxygen dissociation curves to blood and are apparently free from risk of transmitting viral or bacterial infections. They have an intravascular half-life of up to 24 h. Some haemoglobin solutions have a significant vasopressor effect which is thought to result from scavenging endothelial nitric oxide. Polymerised bovine haemoglobin (HBOC-201) has been well tolerated in clinical trials and is licensed for clinical use in South Africa. There are now several reports involving cases in which use of this solution has been life-saving (e.g. Jehovah's Witnesses).

Perfluorocarbon emulsions

Perfluorocarbons (PFCs) are inert chemicals consisting mainly of carbon and fluorine atoms. PFCs are excreted unchanged via the lungs following plasma clearance by the reticuloendothelial system. Oxygen can dissolve 20 times more effectively in PFCs than plasma. The linear oxygen dissociation curves of these compounds means that significant oxygen carriage occurs only at an FIO_2 approaching 1.0. The emulsions consist of microdroplets of $<0.2\,\mu m$ that can pass through very small capillaries non-traversable by red cells. This may increase oxygen carriage to critically ischaemic tissues. Modest efficacy and a high incidence of flu-like symptoms are holding up the introduction of these solutions to clinical practice.

Crystalloids versus colloids

There are no robust data showing that the use of colloids in preference to crystalloids reduces the mortality of critically ill patients. Nevertheless, colloids are often prescribed by critical care physicians eager to limit the development of oedema in the patient with leaky capillaries.

Further reading

Chang TMS. Future generations of red blood cell substitutes. *J Intern Med* 2003; **253**: 527–35.
Constable P. Hyperchloremic acidosis: the classic example of strong ion acidosis. *Anesth Analg* 2003; **96**: 919–22.
McIlroy D, Kharasch ED. Acute intravascular volume expansion with rapidly administered crystalloid or colloid in the setting of moderate hypovolemia. *Anesth Analg* 2003; **96**: 1572–7.

Related topics of interest

Guillain–Barré syndrome

Guillain–Barré syndrome (GBS) is an acute inflammatory demyelinating polyradiculo-neuropathy. It is the commonest cause of acute generalised flaccid paralysis and has an incidence of 1–2 per 100000 population per annum. Around 70% of cases occur after an infection, usually viral, that often comprises a short-lived flu-like illness. It may occur following recently acquired HIV, after infection with CMV, Epstein–Barr virus, hepatitis or infectious mononucleosis. It may also occur after *Campylobacter jejuni* enteritis, a feature that carries a worse prognosis. It is likely that immune responses directed towards the infecting organisms cross-react with ganglioside surface components of peripheral nerves.

Occasionally, it occurs as a complication of an underlying systemic condition such as systemic lupus erythematosus (SLE), or Hodgkin's lymphoma. GBS should be differentiated from neuropathy of the critically ill and that associated with porphyria. It may also be confused with poisoning by neurotoxic fish or following exposure to certain heavy metals.

Approximately one-third of patients with GBS require admission to a critical care unit and subsequent ventilatory support.

Clinical features

Typically, the first symptoms of GBS may be paraesthesiae in the toes or fingers. This may progress over a few days to the major clinical manifestations: weakness of the legs, arms, face and oropharynx.

Examination may show bilateral, symmetrical, flaccid tetraparesis. There may also be facial weakness, reduced deep tendon reflexes, but only minimal sensory signs. In more severe cases progression is more rapid. There may also be respiratory muscle weakness and involvement of the extraocular muscles and dysphagia.

Two clinical variants have been described:

- The axonal form, which has a more rapid onset, anti-GM$_1$ ganglioside antibodies as a frequent finding and a generally worse prognosis.
- The Miller Fisher syndrome is, strictly, a separate condition but shares some overlap features with GBS, especially those involving the eye muscles. It comprises an acute ophthalmoparesis, areflexia without weakness and ataxia.

Autonomic dysfunction is common in severe cases. This may manifest as cardiovascular signs with both brady- and tachyarrhythmias. There may also be constipation, especially if the patient is profoundly weak.

Some patients with GBS suffer considerable pain and acutely inflamed nerves may be unusually prone to pressure palsies.

Investigation

1. Electrophysiology. Nerve conduction studies show evidence of demyelination. This may manifest as a slowed motor nerve conduction velocity or a conduction block.

Normal or only mildly abnormal results in the first week of the illness do not rule out the diagnosis.

2. Lumbar puncture. A normal CSF opening pressure and white cell count, but raised protein concentration ($>0.45\,g\,l^{-1}$) after the first week of the illness are typical.

3. Immunology. This may show antibodies to *C. jejuni*, especially in patients with the axonal form. Some patients have antibodies to myelin protein.

Management

General measures

- Careful assessment and monitoring of patients with GBS will determine those that need admission to a critical care unit. Frequent measurement of the vital capacity will enable semi-elective ventilation to be established in those becoming progressively weaker.
- Continuous ECG and direct arterial blood pressure monitoring are advised to detect those with autonomic involvement. An adequate circulating volume will minimise autonomic disturbances. Sedation may be required, especially during tracheal suction of the intubated patient. Beta-blockade may be required to control episodes of hypertension and/or tachycardia. Since hypotension and bradycardia are also likely in those with autonomic involvement, esmolol, a drug with a short half-life, given by continuous infusion, may be the best beta-blocker to use. Significant bradycardia may necessitate the insertion of a pacemaker.
- Active measures to prevent DVT should be taken.
- Attention to nutrition is important and those with dysphagia may require nasogastric or percutaneous enterostomy feeding.
- Limb pains are common, especially during passive physiotherapy. Non-steroidal anti-inflammatory drugs may control the pain but opioids are frequently required.

Specific measures

Both plasma exchange and intravenous immunoglobulin have been shown to be equally effective treatments for GBS in controlled randomised trials. Since the latter is simpler to give and less invasive, it is the treatment of choice. Immunoglobulin is given for 5 days at $0.4\,g\,kg^{-1}\,day^{-1}$.

Prognosis

The prognosis for complete recovery is good, though 10% are left with a long-term disability and 10% die from complications in the acute illness. A poor prognosis is associated with older age, preceding *C. jejuni* infection, evidence of axonal damage and a rapid onset of weakness.

Some suggest avoiding vaccinations in the future unless essential.

Further reading

Hahn AF. Guillain–Barré Syndrome. *Lancet* 1998; **352**: 635–41.

Plasma Exchange/Sandoglobulin Guillain–Barré Syndrome Trial Group. Randomised trial of plasma exchange, intravenous immunoglobulin, and combined treatments in Guillain–Barré syndrome. *Lancet* 1997; **349**: 225–30.

Related topics of interest

Head injury

Head injury accounts for approximately a third of all trauma deaths and is the leading cause of death and disability in young adults. However, severe head injury may still be compatible with a good outcome. Only preventative measures will help to address the primary brain injury. The role of critical care is to assess and resuscitate, identify intracranial pathology that can be improved by surgery, prevent secondary brain injury through monitoring and intervention and prevent other complications that will reduce the chances of the best possible recovery.

Causes of secondary brain injury and therapeutic aims

These are given in Table 9.

Table 9 Causes of secondary brain injury and therapeutic aims

Cause	Aim
Hypotension	Systolic blood pressure (SBP) $>120\,mmHg$ (maintain cerebral perfusion pressure >60–$70\,mmHg$)
Hypoxia	$SpO_2 > 95\%$
Hypo/hypercapnia	$PaCO_2 = 4.5\,kPa$
Raised intracranial pressure (ICP)	$ICP < 20$–$25\,mmHg$
Seizures	Treat convulsions with lorazepam and phenytoin
Hyperthermia	Core temperature 35–37°C (avoid hyperthermia)
Hyperglycaemia	Blood sugar 4–$7\,mmol\,l^{-1}$

Assessment and resuscitation

Initial resuscitation of patients with severe head injury should follow the ABCDE format. Hypoxia ($SpO_2 < 95\%$) and hypotension ($SBP < 90\,mmHg$) independently increase mortality after severe head injury and must be treated aggressively. A rapid neurological assessment, including response to commands and any focal signs, should be made before any sedative/paralysing drugs are given.

Management of intubation

Patients with head injuries should be sedated, paralysed, intubated and ventilated if there is airway compromise, ventilatory failure, a Glasgow Coma Score (GCS) ≤ 8 or if warranted because of another injury. The airway should also be secured if there is any doubt that there may be airway compromise, or agitation requiring sedation for a computed tomography (CT) scan. It is appropriate to sedate and intubate patients with GCS scores >8 to ensure optimal conditions for CT scanning and prevention of secondary brain injury. No head-injured adult or child should be sedated for a CT scan without control of the airway, even if this is to be reversed immediately afterwards.

Assume an unstable cervical spine injury until it is positively excluded. Oral tracheal intubation should follow a rapid sequence induction of anaesthesia and neuromuscular blockade with in-line stabilisation of the cervical spine and cricoid pressure. Try to avoid hypotension during induction of anaesthesia – all intravenous anaesthetics are cardiovascular depressants.

Once intubated, maintain sedation (+/− paralysis) and insert an orogastric tube. The oral route is preferred because of the risk of intracranial passage of a nasogastric tube in the presence of a base of skull fracture.

Breathing

All head-injured patients requiring intubation will need ventilatory support. Monitor ventilation by arterial blood gas analysis and capnography. In most cases, the patient should be ventilated to normocapnia. In the early stages after head injury the patient should not be hyperventilated excessively because it induces vasoconstriction, which results in a reduced cerebral blood flow (CBF). Long-term outcome has been shown to be worse following prolonged hyperventilation ($PaCO_2 < 3.4\,kPa$) in adults with severe head injuries. If used, hyperventilation should be titrated against the ICP and jugular bulb oxygen saturation (SjO_2).

Circulation

Control haemorrhage by whatever means is required. Large-bore intravenous cannulae are inserted and the blood pressure maintained with intravenous fluid. Avoid hypotonic solutions. In the adult, keep the blood pressure above 120 mmHg systolic (children > 90 mmHg systolic). Once hypovolaemia has been excluded, a vasopressor may be needed to counteract the vasodilatory effects of anaesthetic drugs. In the multi-trauma patient, persistent hypotension and tachycardia implies blood loss from extracranial injuries. Keep the haemoglobin concentration $>10\,g\,dl^{-1}$ to ensure adequate cerebral oxygen delivery. Circulatory monitoring should include ECG, pulse oximetry, invasive blood pressure measurement and urinary output. Severely head-injured patients should not be moved or transferred until life-threatening injuries are stable and an adequate mean arterial pressure has been achieved.

Disability

Undertake a rapid assessment of the GCS *before* anaesthesia is induced. An accurate assessment of the GCS and pupil abnormalities takes a few seconds and has therapeutic and prognostic implications (see Scoring systems (p. 266)).

Exposure

All patients should be fully exposed. Head injuries are often associated with other injuries. This exposure should include a log-roll. Assess and treat fully any life-threatening extracranial injuries. Obtain X-rays of the chest and pelvis and insert a urinary catheter. Obtain spinal X-rays during the secondary survey.

Management of critically raised ICP

Critically raised ICP secondary to a CT-proven or clinically suspected intracranial haematoma should be treated with sedation +/− neuromuscular blockade and a mannitol bolus (0.25–$0.5\,g\,kg^{-1}$). Mannitol is effective in lowering an acute rise in ICP, but the hyperosmolality and dehydration may cause hypotension. Give mannitol as a bolus and not as an infusion. The use of mannitol before ICP monitoring or CT scanning must be based on evidence of intracranial hypertension (pupil dilation, motor posturing or progressive neurological deficit). Adequate sedation is essential. Serum osmolality may be used as a guide to mannitol therapy. The osmolality should not be allowed to rise above $310\,mosmol\,kg^{-1}$. Furosemide (frusemide) may be given instead of or in conjunction with mannitol.

Patients with severe head injury should be nursed approximately 30° head-up. This enables adequate venous drainage and also reduces the risk of nosocomial pneumonia. A semi-rigid collar (if in place) should not be allowed to impede venous return and increase ICP.

Emergency craniectomy and evacuation of haematoma with insertion of an external ventricular drain to enable CSF drainage are the most appropriate surgical procedures in this setting. There may be a role for decompressive craniectomy in cases of severe brain injury with refractory intracranial hypertension. However, the true role of this procedure is still to be determined.

Steroids

Steroids have several side effects and their use outside of a randomised trial is not recommended. A large-scale randomised controlled trial of steroids (CRASH study) in head injury is underway.

Management of seizures

Seizures should be treated aggressively as they increase the cerebral metabolic rate and may lead to a critically raised ICP. Recheck the ABC sequence and then give a bolus of diazepam (0.1–$0.2\,mg\,kg^{-1}$) or lorazepam, thiopental or propofol. This is usually followed by a loading dose of phenytoin (15–$18\,mg\,kg^{-1}$).

Identifying head-injured patients who require immediate life-saving neurosurgery

Patients who have an expanding intracranial haematoma and a critically rising ICP, as shown by a deteriorating level of consciousness and/or progressive focal signs, require immediate neurosurgery. If it is necessary to transfer the patient to another centre for neurosurgery, do not delay the transfer for a CT scan if it can be performed more rapidly at the neurosurgical centre. Surgery may also be required for hydrocephalus and elevation of a depressed skull fracture.

Reducing cerebral metabolic requirements

If conventional therapy fails to control ICP adequately, an infusion of thiopental or propofol will reduce cerebral oxygen requirement ($CMRO_2$). Thiopental is given by infusion while monitoring the EEG to produce burst suppression. Increased temperature causes increased metabolic requirements and increased cerebral blood flow. Therapeutic hypothermia to temperatures of around 33°C has been used and there is some evidence from small studies that suggests an improved outcome following severe head injury. However, a recent multicentre trial involving nearly 400 head-injured patients found no significant differences in neurological outcomes between those who were treated with 48 h of therapeutic moderate hypothermia and those kept at normal temperature. Rapid rewarming of patients with head injuries is probably harmful and hyperthermia must be avoided. A subgroup of young patients (less than 45 years of age) who were kept normovolaemic showed a trend towards improved outcomes when treated with hypothermia. Temperatures of less than 34°C can be associated with coagulopathy and may have a negative effect on outcome, particularly in those patients with multitrauma. A further study of mild therapeutic hypothermia after head injury, using a refined protocol, is underway.

Investigations

- Blood glucose, urea, creatinine, electrolytes and osmolality.
- Blood alcohol level.
- Arterial blood gases.

Computed tomography

CT scanning is the most informative radiological investigation in the evaluation of head injury. CT scanning is needed to exclude lesions that require surgical intervention; the scans obtained have therapeutic and prognostic significance. The opportunity should also be used to scan the first and second cervical vertebrae and other areas of the cervical spine that are abnormal or inadequately seen on plain films. With the advent of multi-slice helical CT scanners, it is becoming common practice to scan the whole cervical spine of head-injured patients and use 3D reconstruction to screen for cervical injury. Adequate access to the patient, monitoring and sedation must be ensured during CT scanning.

Monitoring

1. ICP monitoring. This procedure should be undertaken in all patients with severe head injury who are being managed actively. The gold standard remains a surgically placed intraventricular catheter which also allows the removal of CSF to reduce ICP. Prolonged periods with ICP > 25 mmHg are associated with a poor outcome. Monitoring ICP enables cerebral perfusion pressure (CPP) to be measured (CPP = MAP − ICP). A CPP < 60–70 mmHg is associated with a poor outcome. Therefore, CPP is maintained at > 60–70 mmHg and this often necessitates a vasopressor such as noradrenaline (norepinephrine).

2. SjO_2. This pressure is measured by a fibreoptic catheter placed retrograde in the internal jugular vein at the level of the C_1 vertebral body. Saturation measurements enable assessment of global cerebral ischaemia or hyperaemia. Monitoring enables targeted hyperventilation, CPP management and osmotherapy. Saturations <55% are associated with a poor outcome.

3. Transcranial Doppler. This technique enables assessment of CBF velocity. A pulsatility index can be derived, which, with SjO_2, can be used to define the optimum CPP.

4. Evoked potentials and the electroencephalogram (EEG). In selected patients, these are used to assess activity and gauge the level of sedation in thiopental coma. Regular assessment of GCS is mandatory. Deterioration in the GCS and/or the onset of lateralising signs necessitates urgent investigation.

5. Intraparenchymal cerebral monitors. Microdialysis techniques and improved catheter technology make it possible to take multiple intracerebral measurements, including PaO_2, pH and lactate. The precise role of these monitors remains to be defined.

Adjunctive therapy

- Fluid balance should be carefully adjusted. Avoid large osmolar shifts, hyponatraemia and fluid overload.
- Electrolyte disturbances are common in severe head injury patients and are caused by inappropriate fluid therapy, the stress response, osmotic and loop diuretics and diabetes insipidus.
- Physiotherapy is important in preventing chest infection and limb contractures but adequate sedation is required to prevent increases in ICP.
- Prophylactic antibiotics are required only for invasive procedures.
- Prophylactic anticonvulsants are often commenced in severe head injury. However, there is little evidence that anticonvulsant therapy has an impact on the development of late seizures. The relationship of early seizures to outcome is unclear.
- Early enteral nutrition reduces the incidence of gastric erosions and nosocomial chest infection and reduces the negative nitrogen balance that accompanies severe head injury.
- DVT prophylaxis should be initiated early. Compression stockings and calf compression devices may be used shortly after admission. Heparin therapy is often delayed because of the presence of intracerebral blood and the risk of further bleeding.

Outcome

Outcome is determined largely by the initial mechanism of injury. The post-injury GCS provides a prognostic guide. Roughly a third of patients that survive a head injury with an initial GCS of less than 9 will never regain independent activity.

The remaining survivors can be expected to be independent or requiring some assistance.

Further reading

Biros MH, Heegaard W. Prehospital and resuscitative care of the head-injured patient. *Curr Opin Crit Care* 2002; **7**: 444–9.

Brain Trauma Foundation (BTF), a not-for-profit organization dedicated to improving the outcome of brain trauma patients. Provides access to BTF education and clinical research programmes and evidence-based guidelines. Links to other web sites on traumatic brain injury:

http://www.braintrauma.org/

Bullock R, Chesnut RM, Clifton G, *et al.*Guidelines for the management of severe head injury. Brain Trauma Foundation. *Eur J Emerg Med* 1996; **3**: 109–27.

Chesnut RM. Guidelines for the management of severe head injury. In: Vincent JL (ed.), *Yearbook of Intensive Care and Emergency Medicine*. Berlin: Springer, 1997, pp. 749–65.

European Brain Injury Consortium:

http://homepages.ed.ac.uk/gdm/EBIC/

Lee LA, Sharar SR, Lam AM. Perioperative head injury management in the multiply injured trauma patient. *Int Anesthesiol Clin* 2002; **40**: 31–52.

Marion DW. Moderate hypothermia in severe head injuries: the present and the future. *Curr Opin Crit Care* 2002; **8**: 111–14.

Marshall LF. Head injury: recent past, present, and future. *Neurosurgery* 2000; **47**: 546–61.

Roberts I. CRASH trial: the first large-scale randomized controlled trial in head injury. *ANZ J Surg* 2002; **72**: 600.

Related topics of interest

Brain death and organ donation (p. 55)
Coma (p. 120)
Status epilepticus (p. 291)
Trauma – primary survey (p. 315)
Trauma – secondary survey (p. 318)
Trauma – anaesthesia and critical care (p. 322)

Hyperthermia

Richard Protheroe

Hyperthermia is a core temperature $>37.5°C$. Severe hyperthermia is defined as a core temperature $>40°C$ or an increase in body temperature at a rate greater than $2°C$ per hour. Hyperthermia increases metabolic rate and oxygen consumption, which precipitates an increase in cardiac output and minute ventilation to meet demand. The increased carbon dioxide production is initially compensated for by tachypnoea, but the patient soon starts to develop a respiratory acidosis. This is compounded by the metabolic acidosis, which is caused by an increasing oxygen debt and lactic acidosis. Sweating and vasodilatation cause hypovolaemia, which exacerbates the metabolic derangement if left untreated. Central nervous system (CNS) dysfunction (delirium, seizures, coma and permanent damage), rhabdomyolysis, acute renal failure, myocardial ischaemia and dysfunction may all follow.

Aetiology

The aetiology of hyperthermia falls into two categories: increased heat production or decreased heat loss.

Increased heat production
1. Pyrogens/toxins. For example, in sepsis, following burns, or blood transfusion reactions.
2. Drug reactions. As a consequence of excessive dosage of the drug or as an abnormal reaction to normal doses. Potential triggers include 3,4-methylenedioxymethamphetamine (MDMA, 'ecstasy'), thyroxine, monoamine oxidase inhibitors (MAOIs), tricyclic antidepressants, amphetamines and cocaine. Hyperthermia following a drug reaction may manifest as the neuroleptic malignant syndrome (NMS) or serotonin syndrome.
3. Endocrine. Associated with hyperthyroidism or phaeochromocytoma.
4. Hypothalamic injury. Following cerebral hypoxia, oedema, or head injury/trauma.
5. Malignant hyperthermia (MH).

Decreased heat loss
1. Excessive conservation. Especially in neonates and children.
2. Heat stroke. Results from thermoregulatory failure coupled with an exaggerated acute-phase response and possibly with altered expression of heatshock proteins. Defined clinically as core body temperature $>40°C$, accompanied by hot, dry skin and CNS abnormality (delirium, convulsions or coma). Heat stoke is caused by exposure to a high environmental temperature (classic, or non-exertional, heat stroke) or from strenuous exercise (exertional heat stroke).
3. Drug effects. For example, as a predicted effect of anticholinergic administration.

Management

1. General cooling measures. Decrease ambient temperature, exposure of the patient and skin wetting in combination with cold air fans to provide efficient cooling. Application of ice packs to extremities may be used but is less efficient. Other measures include cold fluid given intravenously or intraperitoneally, cardiac bypass and cooling of blood volume.

2. Definitive treatment. The underlying condition is treated using dantrolene (e.g. in MH, NMS, MDMA poisoning) and mannitol (rhabdomyolysis, acute renal failure).

3. General critical care. Invasive monitoring to optimise fluid balance, sedation and ventilation if required.

MDMA (ecstasy)

MDMA is an amphetamine derivative that was first used as an appetite suppressant, but is now a recreational substance of abuse. There is a range of adverse effects unrelated to dose or frequency of use. Psychosis, sudden cardiac death, seizures, tachycardia, hepatitis, subarachnoid haemorrhage and acute renal failure may all occur. An acute syndrome comprising hyperthermia disseminated intravascular coagulation (DIC), rhabdomyolysis, acute renal failure and death may present in patients with a pre-existing metabolic myopathy or a genetic predisposition. Hyperpyrexia and myoglobinuria are triggered by a combination of sympathetic overactivity, vigorous muscular activity as well as disturbance of central control. The aetiology is an augmentation of central serotonin function by stimulation of neuronal serotonin release.

The peak temperature and duration of hyperthermia are important prognostic factors and any temperature $>40°C$ must be treated aggressively. Due to the similarity between this condition and MH, intravenous dantrolene has been accepted as part of the treatment. Serotonin antagonists or inhibitors of serotonin synthesis have been suggested as alternative therapies.

Serotonin syndrome

A potentially severe adverse drug reaction, this syndrome is characterised by a triad of altered mental state, autonomic dysfunction (including hyperthermia) and neuromuscular abnormalities. The syndrome may follow the administration of selective serotonin re-uptake inhibitors (SSRIs) such as sertraline, fluoxetine, paroxetine and fluvoxamine. It occurs either in overdosage, in interaction with excess serotonin precursors or agonists (tryptophan, LSD, lithium, L-dopa), in interaction with agents enhancing serotonin (MDMA) or in drug interactions with non-SSRIs such as clomipramine or impramine or with MAOIs.

The cause of the syndrome appears to be excessive stimulation of serotonin receptors and, as such, the syndrome shows a similarity to both MDMA poisoning and the neuroleptic malignant syndrome. Treatment involves withdrawal of the precipitating agents and general supportive measures, although in severe cases serotonin antagonists such as chlorpromazine, cyproheptadine and methysergide as well as dantrolene may be used.

Neuroleptic malignant syndrome

This is an idiosyncratic complication of treatment with neuroleptic drugs such as the butyrophenones and phenothiazines. Patients are usually catatonic with extrapyramidal and autonomic effects, including hyperthermia. The aetiology of NMS is unknown but appears to be related to antidopaminergic activity of the precipitating drug on dopamine receptors in the striatum and the hypothalamus, suggesting a possible imbalance between noradrenaline (norepinephrine) and dopamine. There is no evidence of an association with malignant hyperthermia.

Clinical features include hyperthermia, muscle rigidity and sympathetic overactivity. Treatment involves withdrawal of the agent and general supportive and cooling measures.

Malignant hyperthermia

This is a rare pharmacogenetic syndrome with an incidence of between 1:10000 and 1:200000. Most recent estimates of the population prevalence of the genetic susceptibility are between 1:5000 and 1:10000. It shows autosomal dominant inheritance with variable penetrance. The associated gene is on the long arm of chromosome 19. Other gene sites have been proposed and there may be considerable genetic heterogeneity. MH presents either during or immediately following general anaesthesia. The cardinal signs are hyperthermia, and a combined respiratory and metabolic acidosis often with associated muscle rigidity. Dysfunction of the sarcoplasmic reticulum increases intracellular ionic calcium, and results in depletion of high-energy muscle phosphate stores, increased metabolic rate, hypercapnia and heat production, increased oxygen consumption and a metabolic acidosis. It results from exposure to the trigger agents, namely succinylcholine and volatile anaesthetic agents.

On suspicion of MH, all trigger agents must be stopped immediately. The temperature, ECG, BP and end-tidal CO_2 levels should all be monitored and arterial blood gas analysis performed. Venous blood should be sampled intermittently for potassium, creatine kinase and myoglobin, as well as FBC and a clotting screen. The urine output should be monitored and urine tested for myoglobin.

Dantrolene is given in bolus doses of $1\,mg\,kg^{-1}$ at 10 min intervals until the patient responds, up to a maximum dose of $10\,mg\,kg^{-1}$. The average dose is about $3\,mg\,kg^{-1}$. Dantrolene uncouples the excitation–contraction mechanism by acting at the interface between the t-tubular system and sarcoplasmic reticulum. It is a yellow/orange powder stored in a vial of 20 mg with 3 g of mannitol and sodium hydroxide. It is stored below 30°C and protected from light. Reconstitution is with 60 ml of sterile water (it takes some time to dissolve) and forms an alkaline solution of pH 9.5.

General cooling measures should be undertaken and any hyperkalaemia treated with insulin and dextrose, calcium chloride and hyperventilation. Rehydration with intravenous fluids and promotion of a diuresis with furosemide (frusemide) or mannitol will help to prevent myoglobin-induced renal damage. DIC may develop. After successful treatment of a suspected MH reaction, the patient must be referred to a specialist centre for confirmation of the diagnosis and counselling.

Further reading

Bouchama A, Knochel JP. Heat stroke. *N Engl J Med* 2002; **346**: 1978–88.
Halsall PJ, Hopkins PM. Malignant hyperthermia. *Br J Anaesth CEPD Rev* 2003; **3**: 5–9.
Hopkins PM. Malignant hyperthermia: advances in clinical management and diagnosis. *Br J Anaesth* 2000; **85**: 118–28.
Martin T. Serotonin syndrome. *Ann Emerg Med* 1996; **28**: 520–6.

Related topics of interest

Drug overdose (p. 136)
Hypothermia (p. 174)

Hypothermia

Tim Murphy

Normal body temperature is maintained between 36 and 37.5°C. Hypothermia is defined as a core temperature of less than 35°C and can be divided into mild (35–32°C), moderate (32–28°C) or severe (28°C or less). It may be induced or accidental. Induced hypothermia has been used for cerebral protection in neurosurgery, cardiac surgery and critical care to reduce the cerebral metabolic oxygen requirement, and in the post resuscitation management of cardiac arrest. In the UK 0.7% of all hospital admissions and 3% of elderly patients admitted suffer from accidental hypothermia. Internationally, death rates attributable to hypothermia vary widely and do not seem to depend only on the ambient temperature.

Aetiology

Accidental hypothermia can occur in individuals with normal thermoregulation exposed to severe cold. When thermoregulation is impaired, it may occur following only a mild cold insult. Common causes include environmental exposure and water immersion. Patients with trauma, burns and neurological impairment (strokes, head injuries, diabetic coma and spinal cord injury) are at high risk. Patients with impaired thermoregulation include the elderly, babies, those with debilitation from any cause and those taking depressant drugs, especially alcohol and some recreational drugs.

Clinical signs

Most organ systems exhibit a progressive depression of function with decreasing temperature.

1. Cardiovascular effects. Mild hypothermia causes sympathetic stimulation, leading to vasoconstriction, tachycardia and increased cardiac output. As the temperature drops further, there is progressive cardiovascular depression. ECG changes are common. Progressive bradycardia and prolonged PR and QT intervals occur. Widening of the QRS complex is a late finding. The 'J' wave at the junction of the QRS and T wave is a relatively constant finding below a core temperature of 33°C. It is not, however, specific to hypothermia. Atrial fibrillation is common in hypothermia. Below 28°C, ventricular fibrillation (VF) may occur spontaneously and asystole usually occurs below 20°C. Arrhythmias are more likely at low temperatures because conducting tissues lose their conduction advantage over surrounding tissues.

2. Respiratory effects. Mild hypothermia causes respiratory stimulation; then progressive depression occurs. Both respiratory rate and tidal volume decrease.

Respiratory drive ceases at 24°C. There is also early depression of the cough reflex, which makes aspiration more likely.

3. Central nervous system effects. Mild hypothermia causes confusion. Loss of consciousness often occurs at around 28–30°C. Cerebral blood flow decreases by 7% per °C but there is a corresponding decrease in cerebral metabolic rate. In severe hypothermia, electroencephalographic activity ceases (below 20°C) and muscle rigidity occurs.

4. Metabolic effects. Shivering occurs between core temperatures of 35 and 30°C. This involves intense energy production and large increases in oxygen consumption and basal metabolic rate. Shivering can be limited by fatigue and glycogen depletion. Below 30°C, shivering ceases and thermoregulation fails. Basal metabolic rate decreases by approximately 6% per °C drop in temperature. Oxygen consumption drops accordingly. Blood gas analysers measure blood gas values at 37°C. Blood gas values that are corrected for temperature tend to be lower as gases are more soluble in blood at lower temperatures. To interpret corrected values, results would have to be compared with the normal value for that patient temperature. It is therefore easier to interpret uncorrected arterial blood gas measurements, as it is then only necessary to compare them with the well-known normal values for 37°C. This also simplifies comparison of results from serial blood gas samples during rewarming. A mixed respiratory (decreased ventilation) and metabolic (decreased tissue perfusion) acidosis is usual. The oxyhaemoglobin dissociation curve is shifted to the left by decreased temperature, with a consequent decrease in oxygen delivery. This effect may be offset by the right shift secondary to acidosis.

5. Renal effects. Hypothermia impairs the release of antidiuretic hormone (ADH), which causes a diuresis and haemoconcentration. This hypovolaemia will become apparent during rewarming. Electrolyte changes are variable and often reflect underlying co-morbidity. Hyperkalaemia is a common finding, reflecting metabolic acidosis, failure of the kidney to excrete H^+ and failure of membrane Sodium–potassium pumps.

6. Haematological effects. At 35°C, clotting factor and platelet function is compromised. Clotting is increasingly impaired at lower temperatures and in severe cases there may be disseminated intravascular coagulation. Splenic sequestration may cause neutropenia and thrombocytopenia.

7. Endocrine effects. Hypothermia is a cause of pancreatitis. There is both reduced insulin secretion and peripheral insulin resistance. Early hyperglycaemia may proceed to hypoglycaemia in prolonged hypothermia. Plasma cortisol levels are usually high. Hypopituitarism, hypoadrenalism and hypothyroidism predispose to hypothermia.

8. Infection. Hypothermia impairs the immune responses; chest infections are particularly common.

9. Gastrointestinal. Hepatic blood flow is reduced, with implications for drug metabolism. GI motility is reduced.

Drowning

Hypothermia caused by immersion in cold water has some specific features. When an individual is immersed in cold water in outdoor clothing, his core temperature falls slowly (1 h to fall 2°C in water temperature of 5°C in laboratory conditions). When core temperature falls to 33–35°C muscles are usually considerably colder. This means that neuromuscular performance is poor and there is significant risk of aspiration and hypoxia long before any temperature-related cerebral protection, which only occurs at much lower temperatures. Head immersion speeds cooling and children cool more quickly because of their large surface area to mass ratio and lack of subcutaneous fat. Even so, the cerebral protection sometimes seen in immersed children cannot be explained by cerebral hypothermia alone. The primitive mammalian diving reflex, where sudden cooling of the face causes intense vasoconstriction, bradycardia and decreased metabolic rate, may play a part in these rare cases.

Diagnosis

A high index of suspicion and a low thermometer reading aids diagnosis. Investigations to detect the cause of unexplained hypothermia should include blood glucose, amylase, drug and toxin screen and thyroid function tests. The difference between death and hypothermia can be hard to distinguish. Many units operate a 'not dead until warm and dead' policy where patients are resuscitated until a core temperature of 34°C is achieved. Without extracorporeal rewarming this may be impossible. Patients should not be resuscitated if obviously lethal injuries are present or if chest wall rigidity prevents effective chest compressions.

Management

The underlying cause must be treated. General measures include removal from the cold environment and prevention of further heat loss. Rough handling may precipitate cardiac arrhythmias and tracheal intubation may rarely cause ventricular fibrillation. Compromised patients should be intubated carefully and their lungs ventilated with high concentrations of warmed oxygen. Cardiac massage, though less effective in hypothermia should be carried out in the normal way. Defibrillation is often ineffective below 30°C. Three shocks should be delivered and further shocks delayed until core temperature is increased. Drugs often have decreased effects in hypothermia, and may have delayed and occasionally toxic effects on rewarming. Vascular access is difficult in patients with intense peripheral vasoconstriction and may be preferable by a central venous route, particularly if vasoactive drugs are needed during resuscitation.

Rewarming

The aim of rewarming is to restore body temperature without fatal side effects. Rewarming may be passive external, active external or active internal (core rewarming). Passive external rewarming consists of placing the patient in a warm environment under insulating covers. This will not rewarm a patient in cardiac arrest. The most effective active external technique is forced air warming. Internal or core rewarming is used to rewarm patients with severe hypothermia and those in cardiac arrest. Many techniques have been described including the use of warmed humidified gases, and irrigation of the stomach, colon, bladder or pleural cavity with warmed fluid. Peritoneal dialysis or haemodialysis (combined with a warmer on the return line) are effective and may also be used to dialyse drugs or toxins if present. Cardiopulmonary bypass is the most rapid rewarming technique. It is the method of choice in patients in cardiac arrest, because it supports the circulation while rewarming. In trauma patients, systemic anticoagulation should be avoided. A significant coagulopathy is usually present and heparin-bonded systems are available to enable cardiac bypass in these circumstances. There have been no clinical trials of outcome to determine the best technique of rewarming.

Therapeutic hypothermia for out-of-hospital cardiac arrest

There is now evidence that unconscious adult patients who have suffered an out-of-hospital VF cardiac arrest in whom spontaneous circulation has been restored benefit from being cooled to 32–34°C for 12–24h. Cooling is initiated as soon as possible. Rewarming should be gradual to avoid rebound hyperthermia. Patients resuscitated from cardiac arrest caused by non-shockable rhythms may also benefit from therapeutic hypothermia.

Therapeutic hypothermia for severe head injury

There has been a great deal of interest in mild therapeutic hypothermia to improve outcome in head injury. Current evidence does not support this treatment, but another large randomised trial is underway.

Outcome

Widely different mortality rates are published for severe hypothermia. Patient populations are diverse. Low core temperature and the presence of significant co-morbidity are predictors of poor outcome.

Further reading

Clifton GL, Miller ER, Choi SC, *et al*. Lack of effect of induction of hypothermia after acute brain injury. *N Eng J Med* 2001; **344**: 556–63.

Danzl DF, Pozos RS. Accidental hypothermia. *N Engl J Med* 1994; **331**: 1756–60.

Larach MG. Accidental hypothermia. *Lancet* 1995; **345**: 493–8.

Nolan JP, Morley PT, Vanden Hoek TL, Hickey RW. Therapeutic hypothermia after cardiac arrest. An advisory statement by the Advanced Life Support Task Force of the International Liaison Committee on Resuscitation. *Resuscitation* 2003; **57**: 231–5.

Polderman KH. Application of therapeutic hypothermia in the ICU: opportunities and pitfalls of a promising treatment modality. Part 1: Indications and evidence. *Intensive Care Med* 2004; **30**: 556–75.

Related topics of interest

Hyperthermia (p. 170)

Infection control

S. Kim Jacobson

Infection control is an essential and integral part of any health care service. For infection control to be effective, it must be interdisciplinary and interdepartmental. There is mounting evidence that controlling nosocomial infection not only improves morbidity and mortality but also helps in the cost containment of medical procedures. Organisms resistant to antibiotics such as methicillin-resistant *Staphylococcus aureus* (MRSA), vancomycin-resistant enterococci (VRE), multi-resistant *Mycobacterium tuberculosis* (MRTB) and extended spectrum beta-lactamase-producing Enterobacteriaceae (ESBLs) are an increasing problem.

Alert organisms

Infection with these organisms alerts the infection control team to potential hazards in the ward. Other organisms, if a particular problem in an individual unit, can be added to the list as appropriate:

- MRSA.
- Group A beta-haemolytic streptococci (*Streptococcus pyogenes*).
- VRE.
- Multi-resistant Gram-negative organisms (e.g. ESBLs).
- *Clostridium difficile.*
- *Salmonella* spp., *Shigella* spp., *Escherichia coli* 0157.
- *Mycobacterium tuberculosis.*
- Influenza A.
- Varicella zoster (chickenpox).
- Creutzfeldt–Jakob disease, and other prion diseases.

Risk factors for acquiring an infection

- Critical care unit admission for more than 48 h.
- Trauma.
- Assisted ventilation.
- Urinary catheterisation.
- Vascular cannulae.
- Stress ulcer prophylaxis (where gastric pH is raised).
- Poor general condition of patient, e.g. malnutrition, organ failure.
- Contaminated surgical procedure.

The antibiotics given to the patient will drive the selection of resistant organisms, but the likelihood of the patient becoming infected is dependent on the above risk factors and the infection control practices adhered to in the unit.

Policies and procedures

Effective infection control in the critical care unit requires the following policies and procedures to be in place and adhered to:

- Antibiotic policies tailored to individual units.
- Asepsis and antisepsis policies tailored to individual procedures.
- Isolation procedures and indications.
- Disinfection and sterilisation policies.
- Disposal of waste policies.
- Major outbreak procedures.

Hygiene

Environmental

The patient and the medical staff are the most likely source of surgical site infection. However, the quality of the environment has some part to play. The air quality of a critical care unit must be of a high standard and the air in most units is filtered. Some critical care units utilise high-efficiency particulate air filtration (HEPA) which filters out matter down to 0.5 μm (most bacteria are larger than this).

The cleanliness of the environment is as important as the quality of the air. Obvious dirt and dust are highly likely to be contaminated and are linked strongly with outbreaks of MRSA and *Clostridium difficile*.

Hand washing

The choice of hand preparation (hand wash, antiseptic hand preparation or surgical scrub) is dependent on the degree of hand contamination and whether or not it is important to merely remove dirt and transient flora, or whether it is also important to reduce residual flora to minimum counts. This decision is ultimately dependent on the procedure about to 30 undertaken. Fundamentally, however, all clinical staff should perform hand washing before and after contact with a patient. Hand washing is defined as the removal of soil and transient organisms from the hands. For simple hand washing, plain soap and water should be used. There is no evidence that antibacterial soaps are of superior benefit. Soap does not kill the resident flora but does reduce transient flora; hence the importance of hand washing to reduce the transfer of pathogenic transient flora. The duration of hand washing is also important, as the antimicrobial agents must be allowed enough time to be effective. All soap must then be rinsed off and the hands dried thoroughly with paper towels. Cloth towels harbour organisms. The tap should be turned off using either elbows or a paper towel, which is then discarded.

When even greater reduction of transient organisms is required, hand antisepsis is necessary. This is achieved at the same time as hand washing by using soaps or detergents that contain antiseptics. It can also be achieved by using alcohol hand rub after removal of dirt, i.e. when hands are clean after initial hand washing. Large amounts of organic matter reduce the efficacy of alcohol. When dealing with more than one patient, hands can be cleansed between patients with alcohol alone provided all dirt is removed initially. The application of 70% ethanol to hands will reduce viable organism counts by 99.7%. Preparations that contain emollients bind to the stratum corneum, prolonging the duration of action, and prevent excessive drying and damage of the skin.

Surgical hand scrub is the process used to remove or destroy transient microorganisms and reduce resident flora for the duration of the procedure. The optimal duration of surgical scrub is unclear and may be agent dependent, but approximately 5 min is usually appropriate. The agents used should be those that have demonstrated persistence. The moist and warm atmosphere inside latex surgical gloves is ideal for the proliferation of microorganisms. This risk is reduced by agents that have a prolonged duration of action. Alcohol-based lotions are preferred in Europe and chlorhexidine or iodophors are more popular in the United States.

Poor compliance with these basic procedures is the most serious obstacle to adequate hand hygiene. Many studies have shown that health care workers do not wash their hands as thoroughly or as frequently as they should and audits indicate that doctors and nurses overestimate the efficacy of their hand washing.

Gloves

Gloves are not a substitute for careful hand hygiene and inappropriate use of gloves is a hazard. The appropriate use of gloves is during invasive procedures when they provide a barrier against microbial transmission to and from the patient. When gloves are used they should be discarded after contamination and after each patient. Transmission of organisms has been reported even when gloves are used. Thus, hands should be washed after removal of gloves, particularly after examining patients at risk of carrying hazardous organisms.

Selective decontamination of the digestive tract

Nosocomial infections acquired on the critical care unit are often preceded by oropharyngeal and intestinal colonisation with pathogenic organisms. Selective decontamination of the digestive tract (SDD) is a strategy that aims to eradicate colonisation of aerobic potentially pathogenic organisms from the oropharynx, stomach and gut, while leaving the normal anaerobic flora undisturbed. SDD regimens comprise topical application (oral paste and through nasogastric tube) of non-absorbed antimicrobials (usually polymyxin B, tobramycin and amphotericin B) that are active against most Gram-negative bacteria and fungi, combined, for the first 4 days, with a systemic broad-spectrum antibiotic such as cefotaxime. Several studies have demonstrated that SDD reduces the incidence of nosocomial infection but most of these have failed to show any impact on mortality. However, a few meta-analyses and a recent randomised controlled trial have shown reduced mortality rates with SDD. Despite these favourable data, concerns about the development of resistant staphylococci and enterococci, and the cost of the antimicrobial therapy, have prevented most critical care units from introducing SDD.

Further reading

De Jonge E, Schultz MJ, Spanjaard L, *et al*. Effects of selective decontamination of the digestive tract on mortality and acquisition of resistant bacteria in intensive care: a randomised controlled trial. *Lancet* 2003; **362**: 1011–16.

Pittet D, Mourouga P, Perneger TV. Compliance with hand washing in a teaching hospital. *Ann Intern Med* 1999; **130**: 126–30.

Related topics of interest

Infection acquired in critical care (nosocomial) (p. 182)

Infection acquired in hospital (nosocomial)

Susan Murray

Community-acquired infections are more likely to be caused by relatively antibiotic-sensitive organisms. Hospital-acquired infections may be due to antibiotic-resistant nosocomial bacteria or the patient's endogenous resistant flora selected by previous antibiotic therapy. Infection diagnosed 48–72 h after admission to hospital is generally considered to indicate nosocomial, rather than community-acquired, infection.

Patients in critical care units are at particularly high risk of nosocomial infection because of:

- Susceptibility to infection due an to underlying condition, e.g. burns, trauma, surgery.
- Invasive procedures, e.g. assisted ventilation, intravascular and urinary catheterisation.
- Underlying disease or drugs that depress natural barriers to bacterial colonisation e.g. diabetes mellitus, steroids, chemotherapy.
- Damage to the gut mucosa enabling bacteria and their products (e.g. endotoxins) to enter the bloodstream.

Results from the European Prevalence of Infection in Intensive Care (EPIC) study showed that 21% of patients had at least one infection acquired in a critical care unit. The major types of infection were pneumonia (47%), other lower respiratory tract infections (LRTI, 18%), urinary tract infection (UTI, 18%) and bacteraemia (12%), reflecting the difference from infection acquired on the ward where UTI predominates. This study also showed the increasing importance of Gram-positive bacteria in these infections (e.g. *Staphylococcus aureus*, coagulase-negative staphylococci and enterococci), which are often multi-resistant. The classic nosocomial pathogens such as *Pseudomonas* and *Acinetobacter* species still remain major problems on critical care units. They have a propensity to survive and transfer in this environment and have an innate resistance to antibiotics. There has been an emergence of Gram-negative bacteria which produce extended-spectrum beta-lactamase (ESBL) (e.g. Klebsielleae and *Escherichia coli*). This is of concern, because ESBL confers resistance to most beta-lactams, including the newer cephalosporins. The use of broad-spectrum antibiotics accounts also for the increasing number of fungal infections on critical care units.

Most critically ill patients will need antibiotic therapy before the microbiological diagnosis is confirmed. The choice of antibiotics will be influenced by:

- The most likely site of infection and therefore the infecting organism.
- The patient's condition, including age, allergies, previous antibiotics and renal or hepatic dysfunction.

- Local and national resistance patterns of bacteria and fungi.
- The pharmacokinetic properties of each antibiotic.

Close cooperation between microbiologists and critical care physicians to formulate and operate an antibiotic policy will help to prevent the overuse of broad-spectrum antibiotics. Whenever possible, suitable microbiological specimens (e.g. blood cultures, tissues or fluids, sputum and relevant swabs) should be taken before starting or changing antibiotics.

Respiratory tract infections

Epiglottitis (see p. 152)

Severe facial or chest trauma may lead to infection with respiratory tract flora such as *Staphylococcus aureus*, *Streptococcus pneumoniae* and *Haemophilus influenzae*. Environmental Gram-negatives and anaerobes may also be involved in the case of penetrating trauma. Initial therapy with a second- or third-generation cephalosporin with or without metronidazole is appropriate. This can be rationalised when culture results are known.

The antibiotic treatment of late-onset nosocomial pneumonia (see p. 227) needs careful consideration, taking into account local resistance patterns. In many critical care units, methicillin-resistant *Staphylococcus aureus* (MRSA) is a problem and is implicated in nosocomial pneumonia. Glycopeptides (i.e. vancomycin or teicoplanin), sometimes with additional anti-staphylococcal treatment, such as rifampicin or fusidic acid, are used for treatment. The choice depends on renal and hepatic function and the ability to monitor serum levels, which are essential for vancomycin. Alternative drugs for the treatment of resistant Gram-positive serious infections, including vancomycin-resistant bacteria, include linezolid (an oxazolidinone antibiotic) and quinupristin/dalfopristin, which is active against vancomycin-resistant enterococci.

Gram-negatives (e.g. *Pseudomonas* spp. or Enterobacteriaceae) are frequently involved and should be covered with empirical therapy (e.g. quinolones, extended-spectrum cephalosporins, carbapenems or beta-lactams + inhibitors). Aminoglycosides do not penetrate well into respiratory secretions and are not first choice for infection in this site. More intrinsically resistant flora such as *Acinetobacter* spp. and *Stenotrophomonas maltophilia* (inherently resistant to carbapenems) are now also implicated. ESBL-producing strains of Enterobacteriaceae, resistant to all beta-lactams except the carbapenems, are being found increasingly and may also be resistant to quinolones or aminoglycosides. Long courses of antibiotics and invasive therapies such as parenteral nutrition will help to select for fungal (particularly *Candida*) infections. Treatment options for *Candida* infections include the azole group of antifungals, e.g. fluconazole, and amphotericin B (standard and lipid formulations). However, non-*albicans* species of *Candida* e.g. *C. krusei* and *C. glabrata*, which are resistant to fluconazole, are beginning to appear, particularly on critical care units. Newer drugs have been developed to cover filamentous fungi including *Aspergillus* spp. e.g. itraconazole, voriconazole and caspofungin.

Viral pneumonias, e.g. chickenpox, influenza and respiratory syncytial virus (RSV), may need admission to a critical care unit and specific antiviral treatment (e.g. aciclovir, amantadine, ribavirin, respectively). Specific treatment for the recently described severe acute respiratory syndrome (SARS), which is caused by a coronavirus, has yet to be determined.

Immunocompromised patients with pneumonia should be considered on an individual patient basis as cytomegalovirus (CMV) or *Pneumocystis carinii* may be involved.

Urinary tract infection

Most patients in critical care units will have a urinary catheter *in situ*. The likelihood of the catheter becoming colonised with nosocomial bacteria increases with the duration of catheterisation. Asymptomatic bacteriuria should not be treated, but, if the patient becomes septic, UTI should be considered along with other possible sources. Empirical broad-spectrum antibiotic therapy should cover likely urinary tract pathogens (e.g. an aminoglycoside or quinolone plus ampicillin or amoxicillin). An extended-spectrum cephalosporin, carbapenem or other beta-lactam + inhibitor combination may also be used.

Nosocomial bacteraemia

Nosocomial bacteraemia may occur in association with pneumonia, UTI or localised sepsis, or it may be device related. Intravascular catheters are a significant source of bacteraemia in critically ill patients and lead to high rates of Gram-positive infections. The most frequently isolated bacteria are coagulase-negative staphylococci, which are normal skin flora but produce an extracellular slime substance which enables them to adhere to foreign materials. It also inhibits penetration by antibiotics. These staphylococci are often multiple resistant and treatment is usually with a glycopeptide. Blood cultures should be taken both through the line and peripherally. Successful treatment may not be achieved with antibiotics and often line removal is necessary. *Staphylococcus aureus*, Gram-negatives or *Candida* spp. may be the cause of line-associated sepsis, and should be treated according to sensitivity, but early removal of the line is usually necessary.

Central nervous system infection

In general, patients with CSF leak are not treated prophylactically but in the presence of a pyrexia upper respiratory tract flora, especially *Streptococcus pneumoniae*, should be covered. Cefotaxime or ceftriaxone would provide appropriate cover.

See Meningitis (p. 198)

Abdominal sepsis

In the surgical patient, treatment guidelines to cover bowel flora will depend on any antibiotics used as prophylaxis and the interval after surgery. Anaerobic cover must be included either as a broad-spectrum drug that has anaerobic activity (e.g. carbapenems, or piperacillin/tazobactam combination) or as metronidazole plus an extended-spectrum cephalosporin. A good alternative is once-daily aminoglycoside (e.g. gentamicin $4\,mg\,kg^{-1}$) combined with ampicillin or amoxicillin, and metronidazole.

Orthopaedic infection

After orthopaedic surgery, likely infecting organisms are *Staphyloccous aureus* and beta-haemolytic streptococci (groups A, C, G). If the patient has been admitted to hospital recently, the staphylococci are likely to be sensitive and would be covered by flucloxacillin. If the patient is allergic to penicillin or at risk of MRSA infection, a glycopeptide is most appropriate. If there is a likelihood of heavy environmental contamination, especially in compound fractures with exposed bone, cover should be extended to include Gram-negatives and anaerobes (e.g., with a once-daily amino-glycoside, or a quinolone, and metronidazole). Appropriate specimens, including blood cultures, tissue or bone at operation or wound swabs, should be taken.

The epidemiology of infection on critical care units must be monitored closely for increasing antibiotic resistance. Infection control measures are extremely important to help prevent the spread of multi-resistant bacteria. Antibiotic guidelines may be useful to help prevent the overuse of very broad-spectrum agents, but often therapy needs to be individualised and changed to narrow-spectrum antibiotics on the basis of culture results.

Further reading

Flanagan PG. Diagnosis of ventilator associated pneumonia. *J Hospital Infection* 1999; **41**: 87–99.

Vincent J-L. Nosocomial infections in adult intensive care units. *Lancet* 2003; **361**: 2068–77.

Vincent J-L, Bihari DJ, Suter PM, *et al*. The prevalence of nosocomial infection in intensive care units in Europe. Results of the European Prevalence of Infection in Intensive Care (EPIC) Study. *JAMA* 1995; **274**: 639–44.

Related topics of interest

Inotropes and vasopressors

Giorgia Ferro

Inotropes primarily increase the contraction of the myocardium by increasing the velocity and the force of myocardial fibre shortening. Vasopressors primarily increase peripheral vascular resistance. Many inotropes also have effects on peripheral vasculature and heart rate. After optimal volume loading, inotropes and vasopressors play a major role in the management of critically ill patients with circulatory failure.

Sympathomimetic amines

Sympathomimetic amines exert potent inotropic effects by acting on myocardial β-adrenoreceptors. Dopamine, noradrenaline (norepinephrine) and adrenaline (epinephrine) occur naturally. They are all β-agonists at low doses, with increasing α_1 effects at higher doses. The haemodynamic effects vary considerably between individuals, but all tend to increase stroke volume, cardiac output and mean arterial pressure (MAP).

Dopamine
Dopamine is the immediate biosynthetic precursor of noradrenaline. It increases cardiac contractility by direct stimulation of myocardial β_1-adrenergic receptors and indirectly through sympathetic nerve terminal release of noradrenaline. It also stimulates dopamine$_1$ receptors, causing coronary, renal, mesenteric and cerebral arterial vasodilation, as well as dopamine$_2$ receptors, resulting in vasodilation by inhibiting sympathetic nerve terminals. Although dopamine can increase renal flow and urine output, there is no evidence that an infusion of 'renal dose' low-dose dopamine confers any protection from renal dysfunction in the critically ill.

Noradrenaline (norepinephrine)
Noradrenaline is the precursor of adrenaline. It stimulates both α- and β_1-adrenergic receptors, giving it both vasopressor and inotropic properties. With small doses, cardiac output and arterial blood pressure are increased. With larger doses, vascular resistance is markedly increased and cardiac output may fall despite the positive inotropic effect. Noradrenaline is the inotrope of choice in septic shock.

Dobutamine
Dobutamine is a synthetic derivative of the sympathomimetic amine isoprenaline and is available in a racemic mixture. L-Dobutamine is primarily an α_1-adrenergic agonist with some vasoconstrictive effects, while D-dobutamine stimulates β_1- and β_2-adrenergic receptors, thus increasing myocardial contractility while producing more marked vasodilation. Use of dobutamine is popular after myocardial infarction and in cardio-

genic shock because it causes a lower increase in myocardial oxygen consumption than other inotropes. However, dobutamine-induced vasodilation can sometimes cause hypotension and arrhythmias may occur, particularly in the presence of hypovolaemia.

Adrenaline (epinephrine)

Adrenaline remains the drug of choice in cardiopulmonary resuscitation, but without proven benefit in outcome. It has both α- and β-adrenergic receptor stimulating effects. It may be used as a positive inotrope in the treatment of septic shock and cardiogenic shock, but may be associated with more lactic acidosis than other inotropes.

Isoprenaline

Isoprenaline is a synthetic catecholamine that increases both heart rate and contractility. It has been advocated for the short-term emergency treatment of heart block or severe bradycardia. However, isoprenaline causes a relatively high myocardial oxygen consumption and adrenaline will perform this task equally effectively with less myocardial oxygen demand.

Dopexamine

Dopexamine is a synthetic analogue of dopamine. It acts on β_2-receptors in cardiac muscle to produce its positive inotropic effect and on peripheral dopamine receptors to increase renal perfusion.

Administration

All catecholamines have very short biological half-lives (1–2 min) and should be given by a continuous infusion through a central venous catheter. They achieve steady state plasma concentration within about 5–10 min. Infusions should be titrated against clinical end points, such as MAP (measured from an arterial cannula), urine output, base deficit and lactate. Cardiac output can be monitored using invasive or non-invasive techniques (see p. 91).

Cardiac glycosides

Digoxin

Cardiac glycosides increase the force of myocardial contraction and slow conduction through the atrioventricular node. Digoxin is the most commonly used cardiac glycoside. The effects of digoxin are mediated largely by an increase in intracellular calcium concentration and by inhibition of the membrane sodium–potassium pump. Peripheral resistance is also increased by a direct mechanism and by increased sympathetic activity. Digoxin has a narrow therapeutic index, is highly protein-bound and is largely excreted unchanged in urine. Alteration in renal function may prolong the normal half-life of about 35 h to 5 days. It has a small inotropic effect and evaluation of efficacy in acute cardiac failure is difficult. Digoxin may reduce cardiac output in cardiogenic shock due to its effect on afterload.

The potential for toxicity in the critically ill patient is increased by hypokalaemia, hypomagnesaemia, hypercalcaemia, hypoxia and acidosis. Renal function is the most important determinant of digoxin dosage. The use of digoxin in acute congestive heart failure is limited by its delayed onset of action, except in patients with atrial fibrillation and a rapid ventricular rate, in whom it may help to control the ventricular response.

Phosphodiesterase inhibitors

These drugs cause an increase in cyclic adenosine monophosphate (cAMP) by inhibiting phosphodiesterase III, the enzyme responsible for the breakdown of cAMP. Increasing intracellular cAMP produces cardiac effects characterised by positive inotropy and lusitropy (improved diastolic relaxation). The latter effect may be beneficial in patients with reduced ventricular compliance or predominant diastolic failure.

Amrinone, milrinone, enoximone and piroximone

Amrinone, milrinone, enoximone and piroximone are phosphodiesterase inhibitors that cause a dose-dependent increase in cardiac output and reduction in right- and left-sided filling pressures and systemic vascular resistance. Their effects are additive to those of the digitalis glycosides and are synergistic with sympathomimetic amines. They might be used as an alternative or an adjunct to dobutamine. Amrinone facilitates atrioventricular conduction, causing an acceleration of ventricular rate in patients with atrial fibrillation. Enoximone has more inotropic effects than vasodilation. It is more rapidly metabolised, but the metabolite is active and its activity persists for some hours. There is evidence that prolonged use of these drugs increases mortality in patients with severe heart failure.

New drugs

Levosimendan

Levosimendan is a new inodilator. The mechanism of its actions includes calcium sensitisation of contractile proteins and opening of ATP-dependent potassium channels. The combination of positive inotropy with anti-ischaemic effects produced by potassium-channel opening offers potential benefits in comparison to currently available intravenous inotropes, which may be harmful in patients with myocardial ischaemia. In patients with heart failure, levosimendan produces dose-dependent increases in cardiac output and reduced pulmonary artery occlusion pressure. At higher doses, it can induce tachycardia and hypotension. Recent trials in patients with heart failure have suggested that short-term intravenous treatment with levosimendan might improve the long-term survival of these patients.

Toborinone

Toborinone is a novel phosphodiesterase inhibitor. Unlike other drugs that increase cAMP, it has no inotropic effects. It exhibits marked venous and arterial vasodilating properties. The absence of tachycardia reduces myocardial oxygen consumption compared with conventional inotropes. Data on safety and arrhythmias from large clinical trials are awaited.

Vasopressors

Vasopressors raise blood pressure by acting on α-adrenergic receptors to constrict peripheral vessels. This mechanism may cause adverse effects on splanchnic and peripheral perfusion. By increasing cardiac afterload, they may greatly increase myocardial oxygen consumption. These drugs are used, for instance, to counter the hypotension caused by sympathetic blockade during regional anaesthesia and include ephedrine, metaraminol and phenylephrine.

Vasopressin

Vasopressin release from the posterior pituitary is mediated by high serum osmolality or baroreflex. Vasopressin acts through V1 receptors in the blood vessels (vasoconstriction) and through V2 receptors in the kidney (antidiuretic). Under normal conditions it regulates the water balance of the body and has little influence on haemodynamics. However, in shock, it is also an important regulator of blood pressure. In septic shock, vasopressin stores may be depleted. Under these circumstances, a continuous infusion of low-dose vasopressin (0.04 units min^{-1}) will increase blood pressure significantly and enable a reduction in the dose of alternative vasopressors such as noradrenaline. Vasopressin has been advocated as an alternative to adrenaline in the treatment of cardiac arrest because of improved coronary and cerebral perfusion in animal studies. It may also be beneficial in patients with refractory hypotension after cardiopulmonary bypass.

Further reading

Bellomo R, Chapman M, Finfer S, *et al*. Low-dose dopamine in patients with early renal dysfunction: a placebo-controlled randomised trial. Australian and New Zealand Intensive Care Society (ANZICS) Clinical Trials Group. *Lancet* 2000; **356**: 2139–43.

Dellinger RP. Cardiovascular management of septic shock. *Crit Care Med* 2003; **31**: 946–55.

Felker GM, O'Connor CM. Rational use of inotropic therapy in heart failure. *Curr Cardiol Rep* 2001; **3**: 108–13.

Gibbs CR, Davies MK, Lip GY. ABC of heart failure. Management: digoxin and other inotropes, beta blockers and antiarrhythmic and antithrombotic treatment. *BMJ* 2000; **320**: 495–8

Holmes CL, Patel BM, Russell JA, *et al*. Physiology of vasopressin relevant to management of septic shock. *Chest* 2002; **121**: 1723–4.

Liver dysfunction

James Low

Although liver dysfunction associated with critical illness is common, liver failure is rarely the primary reason for admission to a critical care unit. Severe liver dysfunction is characterized by the failure of the synthetic, metabolic and excretory functions of the liver. Any or all of the functions of the liver may be impaired, depending on the aetiology and duration of the disease process. The principles behind the treatment of acute liver failure (ALF) and acute on chronic liver failure are broadly similar. Liver enzymes and plasma bilirubin are markers of liver disease. Characteristic responses of these markers are shown in Table 10.

Table 10 Patterns of liver function tests associated with liver disease

	AST/ALT	GGT	ALP	Bilirubin
Cholestasis				
Intrahepatic	++	++	++	+++
Extrahepatic	+	++++	++++	++++
Cirrhosis				
Alcoholic	N/+	++++	N/+	N/+
Primary biliary cirrhosis	+	+++	++	++
Hepatitis				
Chronic active hepatitis	++	++	+	+
Acute viral hepatitis	++++	++	N/+	++
Drug-induced hepatitis	++	++	N/+	++
ICU Jaundice	N/+	N/+	N/+	++

AST, aspartate aminotransferase; ALT, alanine aminotransferase; GGT, gamma-glutamyltransferase; ALP, alkaline phosphatase.

Acute liver failure

Definition

Acute liver failure is the onset of hepatic encephalopathy within 8 weeks of presentation and in the absence of pre-existing liver disease. The definition is further refined by the terms 'hyperacute' (encephalopathy within 8 days from the onset of jaundice), 'acute' (jaundice to encephalopathy 8–28 days) and 'subacute' (jaundice to encephalopathy 4–26 weeks). Hepatic encephalopathy is classified clinically into four grades:

1. Altered mood; impaired intellect, concentration and psychomotor function, but rousable and coherent.

2. Inappropriate behaviour; increased drowsiness and confusion, but rousable and conversant.
3. Stuporous but rousable, often agitated and aggressive.
4. Coma; unresponsive to painful stimuli.

Aetiology
In the UK, paracetamol overdose is the most common cause of ALF, followed by viral hepatitis and drug-induced hepatotoxicity.

Prognosis of ALF

Mortality is as high as 80%. The main causes of death are cerebral oedema and multiple organ failure. The incidence of raised intracranial pressure (ICP) rises with the encephalopathy grade. The ICP is often very unstable and a rapid rise leading to herniation can occur despite initial clinical improvement. Bad prognostic features are:

- Age <10 or >40 years.
- Aetiology   Cryptogenic.
- Degree of encephalopathy   Grade 3 or 4.
- Prothrombin time (PT) >50 s.
- Plasma factor V $<20\%$.
- Serum bilirubin $>300\,\mu mol\,l^{-1}$.
- Serum creatinine $>350\,\mu mol\,l^{-1}$.
- Alpha fetoprotein   low.
- Arterial pH <7.3.
- Arterial ketone body ratio <0.6.

Chronic liver failure

The commonest cause of chronic liver disease is alcohol abuse. Other causes include infections (hepatitis B and C), drugs (methotrexate), autoimmunity (primary biliary cirrhosis), and hereditary conditions such as Wilson's disease. Common causes of acute decompensation of a patient with chronic liver disease include occult or overt GI bleeding, infection (commonly spontaneous bacterial peritonitis), hypokalaemia, constipation, systemic alkalosis, excess dietary protein, use of psychoactive drugs or benzodiazepines, portosystemic shunts, and progressive hepatic parenchymal damage.

Common to all these causes is increased production of ammonia or increased diffusion of ammonia across the blood–brain barrier. Many of these events are reversible with good recovery of liver function.

Clinical presentation and investigations
Most patients with severe chronic liver disease have subclinical hepatic encephalopathy and present commonly with mental deterioration. They are also immune suppressed and will not demonstrate the usual signs and symptoms of sepsis. Features of encephalopathy include asterexis and confusion. Other variable findings are those of underlying chronic liver disease, worsening ascites, hypoalbuminaemia and signs of thrombocytopenia or coagulopathy (prolonged PT). Investigations are aimed at

excluding common causes of acute decompensation (listed above), establishing the cause of the chronic liver disease and excluding other non-hepatic causes of acute deterioration (e.g. CVA, meningitis, alcohol intoxication, hypoglycaemia).

Variceal bleeding

Portal hypertension in excess of 12 mmHg may cause varices. The first episode of variceal haemorrhage is associated with a mortality rate of 21–50% and the risk of rebleeding is 50–70%. Two-thirds of these patients die within 1 year. Most patients with varices have cirrhosis and 40% die of associated medical problems. Treatment of variceal bleeding is with fluid resuscitation followed by urgent endoscopy. An anaesthetist should be present at endoscopy; the obtunded patient has a high risk of aspiration. Variceal band ligation is more effective than sclerotherapy; it reduces rebleeding and improves survival. Terlipressin constricts the splanchnic circulation, which reduces portal pressure. A bolus of terlipressin 2 mg i.v., followed by 1–2 mg every 4–6 h for 3 days or until bleeding stops, reduces the frequency and severity of rebleeding and improves survival rates.

These patients should be given prophylactic antibiotics. Failure of medical and endoscopic therapy is an indication for balloon tamponade. A Sengstaken–Blakemore tube is inserted, the gastric balloon inflated and traction applied gently. Do not inflate the oesophageal balloon. The gastric balloon is left inflated for a maximum of 24 h. The risk of rebleeding after deflation of the gastric balloon is 30–50%. If the facilities are available, this can be treated with by placement of a transjugular intrahepatic portosystemic shunt (TIPS).

Management of acute and chronic liver failure (Table 11)

General considerations

Patients with liver failure are critically ill and have a predictably high mortality. They should be managed in a specialist unit with access to appropriate facilities for managing the complications and to provide transplantation if required. They will usually require tracheal intubation and ventilation to protect the airway and optimise oxygenation. Invasive cardiovascular monitoring with fluid resuscitation and inotropic support should be instituted. Hypokalaemia and alkalosis are common in both conditions, often secondary to diuretics or vomiting. All electrolyte and acid–base abnormalities must be corrected aggressively. Diagnostic procedures such as CT scans, endoscopy and paracentesis should be carried out urgently to establish the aetiology and any possible complications.

Table 11 Management of acute and chronic liver failure

Acute liver failure (ALF)	Chronic liver failure (CLF)
Cardiovascular Hypovolaemia secondary to vomiting is common Stability may improve with *N*-acetylcysteine infusions $(150\,mg\,kg^{-1}\,day^{-1})$, even if the ALF is not due to paracetamol	Hypovolaemia is very common Occult gastrointestinal tract (GIT) bleeding should be excluded Central venous pressures (CVPs) may be very high secondary to high portal and intra abdominal-pressures
Renal Acute renal failure (ARF) secondary to fluid depletion is common The combination of ALF and ARF carries a very poor prognosis and early renal support should be considered	ARF secondary to sepsis and multiple organ failure (MOF) may occur but generally occurs later Hepatorenal syndrome is common. It is a functional renal failure characterised by oliguria, high urinary osmolality and low urinary sodium. The hepatorenal syndrome must be distinguished from dehydration and invasive monitoring is essential. The prognosis is related to the severity of the liver disease. By reducing portal pressure, terlipressin (0.5–2 mg, 4-hourly) can increase renal blood flow and may improve renal function
Bleeding A severe coagulopathy usually occurs due to decreased synthesis and increased consumption of clotting factors. Coagulopathy is an important prognostic factor. Transfuse clotting factors only after consultation with the local transplant centre	Patients often have a long-standing coagulopathy because of pre-existing liver disease and poor synthetic function. This may be exacerbated by hypersplenism due to portal hypertension and the consumption of clotting factors due to sepsis. Give clotting factors as required
Encephalopathy Cerebral oedema is a significant factor in the pathogenesis. Avoid hyperventilation, which will aggravate cerebral ischaemia. Give mannitol as required. Raised intracranial pressure (ICP) may develop suddenly and without clinical signs; ICP monitoring may improve the outcome	Cerebral oedema is not a common feature. There is increased production of ammonia and/or increased diffusion across the blood–brain barrier (BBB). Oral lactulose, neomycin or metronidazole may decrease ammonia production while correction of electrolyte and acid–base abnormalities will reduce diffusion across the BBB. Eradication of *H. pylori* will reduce ammonia production and may help
Infection Sepsis commonly complicates ALF but is rarely the initiating event	Systemic infection is a common cause of acute deterioration in CLF. In patients with ascites, spontaneous bacterial peritonitis is a common source. A diagnostic tap should be performed, as clinical signs of peritonitis may be absent
Nutrition Enteral feeding can be used. The use of feeds with branched-chain amino acids is controversial and has not been shown to improve outcome	High-calorie, low-protein enteral nutrition is indicated. Restrict dietary protein to 20 g a day and slowly increase until tolerance is established

Indications for liver transplantation in ALF

The 5-year survival rates for liver transplantation are now 50–85%. Criteria defining those patients with a poor prognosis who are most likely to benefit from transplantation are:

- PT > 100 s.

or

- Any three of the following:
  - Age less than 10 or greater than 40 years.
  - PT > 50 s.
  - Serum bilirubin > 300 μmol l^{-1}.
  - Non-A, non-B hepatitis, halothane or other drug aetiology.
  - Duration of jaundice before onset of encephalopathy > 2 days.

If ALF is induced by paracetamol:

- pH < 7.30.

or

- Grade 3 or 4 hepatic encephalopathy and creatinine > 300 μmol l^{-1} with PT > 100 s.

Hepatic dysfunction in acute illness

Hepatic dysfunction and jaundice are common in critically ill patients. This 'ICU jaundice' is precipitated typically by sepsis, trauma or major surgery and develops 1–2 weeks later. Plasma bilirubin rises to 150–300 μmol l^{-1} and is 70–80% conjugated. Plasma ALP may be normal or moderately elevated. Concurrent hepatic ischaemia may elevate plasma aminotransferase concentrations. Other causes of jaundice, such as extrahepatic biliary obstruction, must be excluded. The use of total parenteral nutrition (TPN) may contribute to liver dysfunction in critically ill patients; typically, plasma concentrations of ALT and ALP are doubled and the plasma bilirubin is variable. Histologically, there is fatty infiltration of the liver.

Drug-induced liver dysfunction can present with a variety of patterns: acute hepatitis (paracetamol, halothane), acute cholestatic hepatitis (flucloxacillin, erythromycin) and cholestasis without hepatitis (oral contraceptives).

The management of hepatic dysfunction in acute illness is largely supportive and aimed at treating the initiating event. Hepatic failure in association with multiple organ failure carries a very poor prognosis.

Artificial liver support

MARS (molecular absorbent recirculating system) is the only widely available therapy at present. Many toxins and metabolites that are produced in ALF cannot be removed with conventional dialysis or filtration, as they are highly protein-bound. This system enables protein-bound toxins to be removed. It does not affect synthetic liver function and is usually used with renal support. At present, it is being used for certain overdoses, as a bridge to transplant and in chronic liver failure with encephalopathy.

Further reading

Bernal W, Wendon J. Acute liver failure. *Curr Opin Anaesthesiol* 2000; **12**: 113–18.

Marrero J, Martinez FJ, Hyzy R. Advances in critical care hepatology. *Am J Resp Crit Care Med* 2003; **168**: 1421–6.

Mitzner SR, Stange J, Peszynski P, Klammt S. Extracorporeal support of the failing liver. *Curr Opin Crit Care* 2002; **8**: 171–7.

Riordan SM, Williams R. Treatment of hepatic encephalopathy. *N Engl J Med* 1997; **337**: 473–9.

Related topics of interest

Drug overdose (p. 136)
SIRS, sepsis and multiple organ failure (p. 276)

Medical emergency team (outreach critical care)

It has been stated that 'The most sophisticated intensive care often becomes unnecessarily expensive terminal care when the pre-ICU system fails.' The mortality rate following in-hospital cardiac arrests is high, with only 15% survival at 1 year. Adverse events such as cardiac arrest, unexpected death and unanticipated critical care admission are common and seen in anything from 4 to 17% of admissions. Analyses of such events show that many of them are predictable and preventable. Up to 80% of patients with in-hospital cardiac arrest have changes in vital signs within 8 h before arrest and up to 41% of admissions to critical care units are potentially avoidable. Intensive care medicine has been largely practised within the four walls of the critical care unit.

Outcome following critical care is determined by the level of care delivered before and after admission to the unit. The establishment of a hospital-wide system that rapidly detects and responds to the seriously ill and which monitors and audits quality should result in improved patient care. Such a system redefines critical care by recognising it as a process not a location. One such system is based around the medical emergency team. The MET system was introduced at Liverpool Hospital in Sydney, Australia in 1990. The MET consists of medical and nursing staff trained in the principles of advanced resuscitation and with the skills to manage in-hospital emergencies. The MET at Liverpool Hospital includes an ICU registrar, a medical registrar and a senior ICU nurse. Other systems such as the patient at risk team (PART) and modified early warning system (MEWS) and critical care liaison service have subsequently been developed elsewhere.

The MET system comprises:

- Identification of at-risk patients based on simple criteria.
- An emergency response by the MET which replaces the hospital cardiac arrest team.
- An advanced resuscitation training programme with hospital education and awareness.
- Evaluating system effectiveness by generating outcome indicators which allow:
  - Measurement of hospital quality.
  - Assessment of what is potentially preventable.
  - Assessment of end-of-life decisions.
- Feedback on effectiveness to allow quality improvement.

The MET is called according to the criteria given in Table 12.
The MET outcome indicators are:

- **Unexpected deaths** = Total deaths − deaths with a Do Not Attempt Resuscitation (DNAR) order.
- **Unexpected cardiorespiratory arrests** = Total cardiorespiratory arrests − cardiorespiratory arrests with DNAR order.
- **Unexpected admissions to ICU** = All admissions to ICU − ICU admissions from ED or OR (i.e. other critical care areas).

Table 12 Criteria for calling the MET

Acute change in:	Physiology
AIRWAY	Threatened
BREATHING	All respiratory arrests
	Respiratory rate <5
	Respiratory rate >36
CIRCULATION	All cardiac arrests
	Pulse rate <40
	Pulse rate >140
	Systolic blood pressure <90
NEUROLOGY	Sudden fall in level of consciousness
	Fall in GCS of >2 points
	Repeated or prolonged seizures
Other	Any patient you are seriously worried about that does not fit the above criteria

Clinical studies suggest the MET is associated with fewer unanticipated ICU admissions, better documentation of DNAR decisions and a reduced incidence of and mortality from unexpected cardiac arrest in hospital.

A multi-hospital, prospective, cluster randomised trial (Medical Early Response Intervention Therapy (MERIT) Study) is taking place in Australia to test the hypothesis that the implementation of the hospital-wide MET system will reduce the aggregate incidence of unanticipated ICU admissions, cardiac arrests and deaths without DNAR orders.

Further reading

Bristow PJ, Hillman KM, Chey T, *et al*. Rates of in-hospital arrests, deaths and intensive care admissions: the effect of a medical emergency team. *MJA* 2000; **173**: 236–40.

Buist MD, Moore GE, Bernard SA, *et al*. Effects of a medical emergency team on reduction of incidence of and mortality from unexpected cardiac arrests in hospital: preliminary study. *BMJ* 2002; **324**: 1–6.

Hillman K, Parr M, Flabouris A, Bishop G, Stewart A. Redefining in-hospital resuscitation: the concept of the medical emergency team. *Resuscitation* 2001; **48**: 105–10.

Hourihan F, Bishop G, Hillman KM, *et al*. The medical emergency team: a new strategy to identify and intervene in high risk patients. *Clin Intensive Care* 1995; **6**: 269–72

Related topics of interest

Admission and discharge criteria (p. 1)

Meningitis

Jeff Handel

Bacterial infection is the usual cause of meningitis in patients admitted to critical care units. A variety of viruses (particularly herpes simplex) may cause meningoencephalitis and opportunistic organisms including protozoa and fungi may cause meningitis in immunocompromised patients. Non-infective processes, such as connective tissue disorders and malignant infiltration, may also cause meningitis.

Epidemiology

Bacterial meningitis is more common in childhood. The peak incidence of about 1:1000 occurs in children under 1 year of age. The likely causative organism depends upon the age group. Group B streptococci (*Streptococcus agalactiae*), K1 capsulate *Escherichia coli* and *Listeria monocytogenes* are the commonest organisms in neonates. In older children bacterial meningitis is usually caused by *Neisseria meningitidis* (meningococcus) and *Streptococcus pneumoniae* (pneumococcus). The incidence of *Haemophilus influenzae* meningitis has declined by more than 99% in countries that have adopted universal immunisation using an effective conjugated vaccine against this organism.

In adults, the most common infecting organisms are meningococci and pneumococci, the latter being more common in elderly patients. A few cases are caused by Gram-negative bacilli and *L. monocytogenes* following ingestion of contaminated food such as unpasteurised soft cheeses. Infection with *Listeria* is more common at the extremes of age, and in pregnant women and immunocompromised patients. Post-traumatic meningitis is usually caused by pneumococcus, whereas device (CSF drains and shunts)-associated meningitis is usually caused by coagulase-negative staphylococci or *Staphylococcus aureus*. Tuberculous meningitis is more common in children, the elderly, the immunocompromised and the immigrant population.

Pathology

An intense inflammatory process in the meninges extending into the brain is caused by the presence of bacteria and their fragments in the CSF. The inflammatory reaction causes cell damage and death from oedema, the generation of cytotoxic free radicals and the release of excitatory neurotransmitters in the presence of tissue hypoxia. These effects are compounded by intracranial hypertension, which impairs cerebral perfusion and ultimately may cause brain stem herniation.

Clinical features

The classical features of meningism – headache, neck stiffness, fever, reduced conscious level, Kernig's and Brudzinski's signs – are common in adults but not reliably present in children. Infants with meningitis and raised intracranial pressure (ICP) may have a bulging anterior fontanelle. In tuberculous meningitis, symptoms and signs may develop insidiously over several weeks. A characteristic petechial rash usually accompanies meningococcal meningitis if there is concomitant septicaemia.

Investigation

The diagnosis of meningitis is made by examination of CSF obtained by lumbar puncture. If ICP is raised, this procedure carries a risk (1–8%) of causing brain stem herniation, particularly in the presence of a focal space occupying lesion. If there are signs of raised ICP (e.g. reduced conscious level or papilloedema) or focal neurological signs, a CT scan may be useful to identify cerebral oedema, mass lesions or other differential diagnoses such as subarachnoid haemorrhage; however, a CT scan might appear normal in the presence of raised ICP. When there is clinical and/or CT scan evidence of raised ICP, the diagnostic benefits of lumbar puncture should be weighed against the risks. If the risk of brain stem herniation is high it may be safer to treat the patient empirically. In a few centres, rapid antigen testing and DNA PCR testing of blood may be available.

In bacterial meningitis, the CSF characteristically has a high neutrophil count, low glucose and high protein concentrations. A raised lymphocyte count is seen in early bacterial meningitis, *L. monocytogenes*, tuberculous and viral meningitis and, importantly, may be seen in partially treated bacterial meningitis.

If organisms are not seen on microscopy, culture may take days or even weeks in the case of tuberculosis.

Treatment

Antibiotic therapy is usually started empirically before the diagnosis and organism are confirmed. The choice of antibiotic is determined by the likely pathogen considering the patient's age. Microscopy, culture and sensitivity will later confirm the appropriateness of the antibiotic given. Expert microbiological advice should always be sought. In practice, a third-generation cephalosporin such as cefotaxime is appropriate for adults and children older than neonates.

Complications

1. Seizures. Treatment with benzodiazepines, phenytoin or phenobarbital alone or in combination is usually effective. Resistant seizures and status epilepticus may require thiopental or propofol, which necessitates intubation and ventilation.

2. Raised ICP. This may result from cerebral oedema and/or hydrocephalus, brain abscess, sterile subclinical effusion or empyema for which specific neurosurgical treatment may be indicated. Strategies for the management of raised ICP include intubation and control of ventilation to prevent hypercapnia and hypoxia, and resuscitation with fluids and vasoactive drugs to maintain blood pressure and cerebral perfusion pressure. Nursing the patient in a slightly head-up posture will reduce venous pressure and help enhance cerebral perfusion. Pyrexia should be controlled and active cooling may reduce the cerebral metabolic demand. Hyperglycaemia may worsen ischaemic brain damage and should be treated. Osmotic diuretics can reduce cerebral oedema but repeated administration in conditions such as meningitis where the blood–brain barrier is impaired may worsen cerebral oedema.

Various nerve palsies and learning difficulties may persist in patients recovering from meningitis. Nerve deafness is particularly common.

Since unfavourable outcomes are thought to be the result of inflammation in the subarachnoid space, several studies have been undertaken to assess the impact of steroids in the treatment of meningitis. A randomised, placebo-controlled trial of dexamethasone – 10 mg, 6-hourly for 4 days, started before or with the first dose of antibiotic, in adults with meningitis – demonstrated a significant reduction in mortality in the dexamethasone group. In this study, dexamethasone was particularly beneficial in patients with pneumococcal meningitis. The role of steroids in the treatment of children with meningitis is less clear. If started early, steroids may reduce the incidence of permanent hearing loss in children with *H. influenzae* or pneumococcal meningitis.

Prophylaxis

Prophylaxis is not usually considered necessary for contacts of patients with pneumococcal meningitis. For meningococcal meningitis, see p. 201.

Prognosis

With current antibiotic regimens and treatment strategies, the mortality of bacterial meningitis in the UK is 10% or less, with 10% of survivors suffering permanent neurological damage.

Further reading

De Gans J, Van de Beek D. Dexamethasone in adults with bacterial meningitis. *N Engl J Med* 2002; **347**: 1549–56.
Saez-Llorens X, McCracken GH. Bacterial meningitis in children. *Lancet* 2003; **361**: 2139–48.
Tauber MG. Management of bacterial meningitis in adults. *Curr Opin Crit Care* 1998; **4**: 276–81.

Related topics of interest

Infection control (p. 178)
Infection acquired in critical care (nonsocomial) (p. 182)
Meningococcal sepsis (p. 201)
SIRS, sepsis and multiple organ failure (p. 276)

Meningococcal sepsis

Jeff Handel

Meningococcal sepsis is caused by the Gram-negative coccus *Neisseria meningitidis*. The group B subtype causes two-thirds of cases and group C about one-third. Although 10% of the population have chronic asymptomatic nasopharyngeal carriage of pathogenic meningococci, invasive disease probably results from recent acquisition of the organism.

Meningococcal sepsis may occur at any age but it most commonly affects children and younger adults. It presents as a septicaemic illness that ranges in severity from a mild condition to fulminant septic shock with severe systemic inflammatory response and multiple organ failure (MOF). Death may occur in a matter of hours from intractable cardiovascular failure. Meningococcal meningitis and septicaemia can occur separately or as part of the same illness. The prognosis of meningococcal sepsis may be worse when meningitis is not present. Occasionally, meningococcal sepsis can present as a subacute condition with mild symptoms lasting several weeks. There may be a focus of infection, such as septic arthritis.

If meningitis is present, typical signs of meningism may occur.

Clinical features

Meningococcal sepsis usually begins as a non-specific illness with fever, influenza-like symptoms and sometimes diarrhoea. This may evolve rapidly into profound shock and (MOF).

The skin rash ('purpura fulminans') consists typically of spreading petechiae and ecchymoses. It is caused by capillary thrombosis and extravasation of red cells. It may cause large areas of skin infarction with loss of digits or limbs. Meningococci can often be detected in the skin lesions.

Management

Suspected meningococcal sepsis must be treated promptly and aggressively. Start antibiotic therapy immediately. The organism is almost always sensitive to penicillin G and cefotaxime. If there is a clear history of sensitivity to penicillin, chloramphenicol is an alternative. It has been suggested that antibiotics may increase endotoxin levels by lysing bacteria but treatment should not be delayed.

Aggressive cardiovascular resuscitation with fluids and inotropes is invariably necessary. Haemodynamic monitoring with a pulmonary artery flotation catheter may help to guide therapy. Alternatively, one of the non-invasive methods for measuring cardiac output can be used. Patients frequently require intubation and ventilation for cardiorespiratory and neurological failure.

Adrenocortical infarction (Waterhouse–Friderichsen syndrome, 'adrenal apoplexy') has been well described in meningococcal sepsis, and dysfunction with reduced glucocorticoid and mineralocorticoid production may occur as part of the systemic inflammatory response syndrome (SIRS). The role of steroid replacement therapy is controversial.

New therapies

Plasma exchange and haemofiltration to remove the mediators of septic shock and extracorporeal membrane oxygenation to treat intractable cardiovascular failure have both been recommended as adjunctive therapies. However, no benefit to outcome has been shown from either of these treatments.

A multicentre trial of recombinant bactericidal/permeability-increasing protein, an endotoxin-binding agent to block the inflammatory cascade, has not been shown to reduce mortality significantly. The effects of activated protein C, which may inhibit intravascular thrombosis and reduce organ damage, are currently being assessed.

Mortality

The mortality from meningococcal sepsis is approximately 19% overall and 40–50% in patients who are shocked. Scoring systems have been developed to predict mortality for groups of patients. The most common is the Glasgow meningococcal score, which uses seven weighted factors:

- Blood pressure.
- Skin/rectal temperature difference.
- Coma score.
- Absence of meningism.
- Rash.
- Base deficit.
- Deterioration in the last hour.

The maximum score is 15. A score of 8 predicts a 73% probability of death.

Vaccination

Effective vaccines have been developed against groups A and C meningococci. Unfortunately, group B meningococcus is not sufficiently immunogenic to produce an effective vaccine yet.

Meningococcal sepsis is a notifiable disease. Antibiotics (rifampicin or ciprofloxacin) to eradicate carriage are offered to household contacts of individual cases. In the case of a cluster (two cases in a community within a 4-week period) antibiotics are offered to all members of the community. Vaccine is offered to contacts of patients with disease due to group A or C meningococcus.

Further reading

Baines PB, Hart CA. Severe meningococcal disease in childhood. *Br J Anaesthesia* 2003; **90(1)**: 72–83.
Weir PM. Meningococcal septicaemia. *Curr Anaesthesia Crit Care* 1997; **8**: 2–7.

Related topics of interest

Myasthenia gravis

Myasthenia gravis (MG) is an autoimmune disease. The majority of patients (~90%) have antibodies to the nicotinic acetylcholine receptors in the postsynaptic membrane of the neuromuscular junction, although the correlation between absolute antibody levels and disease severity is weak. Muscarinic acetylcholine receptors, and thus the autonomic nervous system, are spared. Thymus disease is associated with MG; 75% of patients have histological evidence of an abnormality (e.g. germinal centre hyperplasia), whilst 10% have a benign thymoma. Other autoimmune disorders are associated with MG (e.g. thyroid disease, pernicious anaemia), as are certain HLA subgroups. The prevalence of MG is around five per 100000 population, with young women being affected most commonly (peak onset 20–30 years of age). Men over the age of 50 are the next most commonly affected, though most patients with a thymoma associated with MG fall in this group. Critical care may be required for patients with MG under the following circumstances:

- In crisis (myasthenic or cholinergic).
- With resultant respiratory failure.
- Following pulmonary aspiration.
- With a complication of immunosuppressive therapy.
- For postoperative care following a thymectomy.

Clinical features

The muscle weakness of MG is typically made worse by exertion and improved by rest. The characteristic distribution of affected muscles, in descending order, is extraocular, bulbar, cervical, proximal limb, distal limb and trunk. Thus, patients frequently complain of ptosis and diplopia, and dysphagia. Severe bulbar weakness leaves them at risk from frequent pulmonary aspiration.

The Eaton–Lambert syndrome, by contrast, is characterised by muscle weakness that improves on exertion and spares the ocular and bulbar muscles. It is a condition associated with small-cell carcinoma of the bronchus and sufferers, like myasthenics, are exquisitely sensitive to non-depolarising muscle relaxants.

Investigations

Edrophonium test

The diagnosis of MG is established by giving an intravenous dose of the short-acting anticholinesterase edrophonium. Anticholinesterases increase the amount of acetylcholine available at the neuromuscular junction. An improvement in muscle function following edrophonium thus supports the diagnosis. Before giving the drug, intravenous (i.v.) access, continuous ECG monitoring and full resuscitation facilities should be established, in particular, atropine for i.v. administration should be available in case of significant bradycardia following edrophonium. Patients who are weak due to cholinergic crisis may become apnoeic after edrophonium. Assess a muscle group appropriate for that specific patient (i.e. where they are weak). For those with respiratory weakness, forced vital capacity is measured. Give a test dose of 2 mg i.v. edrophonium, followed, in the absence of adverse effects, by 8 mg 1 min later. Assess muscle function before, and 1 and 10 min after giving edrophonium.

Electromyography
A decremental response in the size of the compound motor action potential after repeated electrical stimulation of a motor nerve can confirm the diagnosis. This is true even in the majority of those with only ocular symptoms.

Treatment

Anticholinesterases
Pyridostigmine bromide 60 mg is given four times a day and increased until an optimal response is achieved. It may not be possible to abolish all weakness and increasing the dose, even in small increments, in an attempt to do so may precipitate a cholinergic crisis.

Anticholinergics
Anticholinergics may be required to control side effects of anticholinesterase administration such as salivation, colic and diarrhoea. They are not used as a matter of routine in all patients.

Immunosuppression
Corticosteroids may benefit those patients with pure ocular symptoms and those whose response to anticholinesterases is suboptimal. Their administration may be associated with an initial deterioration, and improvement may take several weeks. Plasma potassium levels should be monitored to ensure that steroid-induced hypokalaemia (enhanced renal potassium loss) is not adding to muscle weakness. Azathioprine has been used in those with severe myasthenia unresponsive to other measures.

Plasma exchange
Some patients show a short-lived but dramatic improvement in weakness following plasma exchange. Maximum response is usually seen about a week after a series of about five daily exchanges. Improvement lasts for around a month. It may be a useful technique for those in severe myasthenic crisis or to enable weaning from ventilation.

Thymectomy
Thymectomy results in clinical improvement in around 80% of all myasthenics. It produces a more rapid onset of remission and is associated with a lower mortality than medical therapy alone. Patients due to undergo thymectomy should have their respiratory function optimised preoperatively. Plasma exchange and steroids may help with this. The dose of pyridostigmine should be reduced as much as possible without compromising respiratory function. This is because thymectomy often leaves patients more sensitive to the effects of anticholinesterases and cholinergic crisis may ensue after surgery. Also, the intraoperative management of neuromuscular blockade is easier in the presence of a mildly myasthenic patient. The response to thymectomy is

maximal by 3 years. The remission rate is ~35%, provided thymectomy is performed within the first 1–2 years after the onset of the disease.

Myasthenic crisis

This is a severe life-threatening worsening of MG. It can progress rapidly to respiratory failure, necessitating urgent tracheal intubation and respiratory support. Myasthenic crises can be precipitated by infection, pyrexia, surgical or emotional stress and certain drugs. These drugs include aminoglycosides (e.g. gentamicin) and polymyxin (e.g. neomycin) antibiotics, membrane stabilising antiarrhythmics (e.g. quinidine, procainamide lidocaine), anticonvulsants (e.g. phenytoin), and antidepressants (e.g. lithium). If the patient's forced vital capacity (FVC) falls below 10–15 ml kg^{-1} or they are unable to clear secretions, they require intubation and respiratory support. Many then withdraw all anticholinesterase therapy and rest the patient, believing that the sensitivity of the motor end plate to acetylcholine will increase under such circumstances.

Give subcutaneous heparin for prophylaxis against thromboembolism.

Plasma exchange or immunosuppressive therapy may be required to wean the patient from mechanical ventilation.

The differential diagnosis of an acutely weak patient with MG includes cholinergic crisis.

Cholinergic crisis

A cholinergic crisis is caused by an excess of acetylcholine available at the neuromuscular junction and usually follows excessive doses of anticholinergics. It, too, may present with respiratory failure, bulbar palsy and virtually complete paralysis. It may be difficult to distinguish from a myasthenic crisis but often includes an excess of secretions, which may worsen the respiratory failure. Other symptoms more likely during a cholinergic crisis include abdominal pain, diarrhoea and blurred vision. The differential may be made by giving a small dose of intravenous edrophonium. Patients in myasthenic crisis should improve whereas those with a cholinergic crisis will get worse.

Further reading

Drachman DB. Myasthenia gravis. *N Engl J Med* 1994; **330**: 1797–810.
Gajdos P, Chevret S, Toyka K. Plasma exchange for myasthenia gravis. *Cochrane Database Syst Rev* 2002; **4**: CD002275.
Vincent A, Palace J, Hilton-Jones D. Myasthenia gravis. *Lancet* 2001; **357**: 2122–8.

Related topics of interest

Weaning from ventilation (p. 331)

Nutrition

Martin Schuster-Bruce

Critically ill patients require nutritional support. Malnutrition is a common problem in critically ill patients and is associated with increased morbidity and mortality. It may be present on admission or can develop during the course of critical illness. In starvation, fat and protein are lost, but the protein loss is minimised and fat oxidation becomes the principal source of energy. However, in critical illness, with hypermetabolism, accelerated protein catabolism occurs. The rationale for providing nutritional support for critically ill patients is to prevent the breakdown of muscle and visceral protein.

Nutritional requirements

Energy
Existing body mass is the major determinant of total energy requirement. This can be measured directly using a metabolic cart or estimated using either a nutritional index (e.g. Harris–Benedict) or on a simple weight basis: $25–30\,kcal\,kg^{-1}$ body weight day^{-1} is adequate in most patients; 30–70% of the total energy can be given as carbohydrate, 15–30% as fat and 15–20% as protein sources.

Nitrogen
Nitrogen intake should be $0.1–0.3\,g\,kg^{-1}$ day^{-1} and can be given as protein $(1.2–1.5\,g\,kg^{-1})$ or amino acids.

Micronutrients
The precise requirements for vitamins, minerals and trace elements have yet to be determined. However, failing to include essential components of nutrition, whether administered enterally or parenterally, can result in severe complications, especially when recommencing nutritional support in the severely malnourished. This refeeding syndrome may manifest as severe electrolyte and fluid shifts associated with metabolic abnormalities. Clinical features are fluid-balance abnormalities, abnormal glucose metabolism, hypophosphataemia, hypomagnesaemia and hypokalaemia. In addition, thiamine deficiency can occur, producing Wernicke's syndrome.

Route of administration

Enteral
There is evidence that enteral nutrition (EN) has additional affects, beyond the supply of energy and protein. These include modulation of the host's immune response, improved splanchnic perfusion, maintenance of gut integrity and possibly

prevention of bacterial translocation and multiple organ dysfunction syndrome (MODS). Therefore, current data support the initiation of EN as soon as possible after resuscitation.

Standard 500ml proprietary feeds are iso-osmotic solutions containing 1–1.5 kcal ml^{-1} of energy, 45% of which is as carbohydrate, 20–35% as lipid and 15–20% as protein. Feeds are gluten- and lactose-free and contain substrates similar to those found in a normal diet (i.e. polymeric). They provide the normal requirements of electrolytes, vitamins and trace elements. Elemental feeds are available, but polymeric feeds are preferred since they are less likely to induce diarrhoea. Traditionally, feeds are given continuously with a daily 4h rest period to allow restoration of gastric pH and prevent bacterial overgrowth in the stomach. However, many critical care units are applying continuous insulin infusion protocols to enable very tight glycaemic control. These protocols require feed to be given without any rest period to avoid fluctuating calorie intact.

The nasogastric route is most commonly used, but impaired gastric emptying can limit infusion rates. Prokinetics may improve gastroparesis or alternatively, the small bowel can be fed directly via surgical jejunostomy or nasojejunal tubes. The latter may be placed at the bedside either endoscopically or blind with the assistance of prokinetic drugs that aid spontaneous passage of nasojejunal tubes through the pylorus. Some of the newer nasojejunal tubes can be placed blindly with remarkably high success rates.

Prokinetic agents

These are drugs that promote gastric emptying.

1. Erythromycin (200 mg i.v. tds) has a direct contractile effect via the motilin receptor. It has been shown to be an effective prokinetic in the critically ill and is the drug of choice.
2. Metoclopromide (10 mg i.v. tds) may promote gastric emptying by dopamine antagonism.
3. Neostigmine (2 mg i.v. given by infusion) is not a true prokinetic but can be an effective therapy for pseudo-obstruction, which can limit tolerance of EN due to bowel distension.

There are few absolute contraindications to EN (intestinal obstruction, anatomical disruption and severe intestinal ischaemia). Enteral nutrition can be successful in virtually all critically ill patients, even after major surgery and in acute pancreatitis. The main complications of EN are failure to achieve nutritional targets, abdominal pain, distension and diarrhoea. Nutritional targets are more likely to be met if EN is administered by strict protocol.

Enteral nutrition is no longer a therapy simply to prevent malnutrition.

Parenteral

Failure of EN alone is not an indication for parenteral nutrition. Parenteral nutrition does not share the additional benefits of EN and there is evidence that it may increase morbidity and mortality in critically ill patients. Parenteral nutrition is indicated only in the small group of patients who are unable to be fed enterally for up to 7 days. Patients who are malnourished before their critical illness and are unable to tolerate early EN may require parenteral nutrition immediately.

Intravenous fat emulsions have replaced glucose as the main energy source because they cause less metabolic derangement. Nitrogen is delivered as amino acids. Most hospitals use parenteral nutrition solutions which have been prepared aseptically in the hospital pharmacy and contain all the requirements for a 24 h period in a single bag. The feeds are non-physiological, hyperosmolar and irritant and are therefore infused into a central vein.

Complications include all those of central venous access. The risk of venous thrombosis and catheter-related sepsis is substantially increased. Catheter-related sepsis is reduced by the use of a dedicated lumen, minimising handling of the line and the use of antimicrobial coatings. Subcutaneous tunnelling does not seem to be of benefit. Other complications of parenteral nutrition include gut mucosal atrophy, hyperglycaemia requiring insulin therapy, and hepatobiliary problems, particularly fatty infiltration and intrahepatic cholestasis. Compared with EN, parenteral nutrition is nutritionally incomplete and dietary deficiencies can occur.

Immunonutrition

During severe illness, there is an alteration in the immune response, metabolic homeostasis and the inflammatory response. Specific dietary substrates have been evaluated for their individual effects on metabolic and immune functions.

Glutamine is an amino acid that facilitates nitrogen transport and reduces skeletal and intestinal protein catabolism. It is the major fuel for the enterocyte and preserves intestinal permeability and function. **Arginine** is an amino acid that improves macrophage and natural killer cell cytotoxicity, stimulates T-cell function and modulates nitrogen balance. **Omega-3-polyunsaturated fatty acids** are derived from fish oil and are potent anti-inflammatory agents and immune modulators. **Nucleotides** have immunostimulant properties on natural killer cells and T lymphocytes.

An enteral feed supplemented with arginine, nucleotides and omega-3-polyunsaturated fatty acids is commercially available. Randomised clinical trials of immune-enhanced feeds have failed to show a clear benefit in critically ill patients.

Further reading

Heyland DK, Dhaliwal R, Drover JW, *et al.* Canadian clinical practice guidelines for nutrition support in mechanically ventilated, critically ill adult patients. *J Parenter enteral nutr* 2003; **27**: 355–73.

Jolliet P, Pichard C, Biolo G, *et al.* Enteral nutrition in intensive care patients: a practical approach. *Intensive Care Med* 1998; **24**: 848–59.

Kennedy BC, Hall GM. Metabolic support of the critically ill patients: parenteral nutrition to immunonutrition. *Br J Anaesthesia* 2000; **85**: 185–7.

Pratt DS, Epstein SK. Recent advances in critical care gastroenterology. *Am J Respir Crit Care Med* 2000; **161**: 1417–20.

Related topics of interest

Obstetric emergencies – major haemorrhage

Jenny Tuckey

From the *Confidential Enquiries into Maternal Deaths in the United Kingdom 1997–1999*, seven deaths were directly due to obstetric haemorrhage (3.3 per million maternities): three cases of placental abruption, three cases of placenta praevia and one case of postpartum haemorrhage. Haemorrhage becomes life threatening when blood loss exceeds 40% of the blood volume.

Obstetric haemorrhage may occur antepartum (APH) or postpartum (PPH). Consideration of the fetus will be necessary in the case of APH. The principles of resuscitation are similar for APH or PPH. The obstetric intervention required will depend upon the cause of the blood loss.

Antepartum haemorrhage

APH is defined as bleeding from the birth canal after the 20th week of gestation and before the birth of the baby. The major causes may be diagnosed by ultrasound scan:

- Placental abruption.
- Placenta praevia.
- Uterine rupture.
- Placental conditions, e.g. vasa praevia.

Placental abruption

1. Definition. Separation of a normally implanted placenta (usually by haemorrhage into the decidua basalis) from the 20th week of pregnancy.

2. Incidence. Occurs in 1–1.5% of pregnancies and accounts for 20–25% APH. Major abruption occurs in about 0.2% of pregnancies, but may be associated with foetal mortality of 50%. Recurs in 10–15% of pregnancies.

3. Aetiology. The cause is identified in only the minority of cases. Causes include severe hypertensive disorders, trauma (e.g. road traffic accident (RTA), external cephalic version) and sudden reduction in the size of the uterus (e.g. after birth of first twin). Associations include smoking, cocaine abuse, low socioeconomic status, poor nutritional status, advancing age, advancing parity and thrombophilic conditions. These latter factors may be associated with degenerative changes in the basal arteries supplying the placenta or alternative mechanisms of placental ischaemia, which predispose to premature placental separation.

There appears to be an association between thrombophilic conditions and a number of adverse pregnancy outcomes, including placental abruption. There is presently insufficient evidence to determine whether screening for thrombophilias should be undertaken after a significant abruption, with a view to use of antithrombotic prophylaxis to improve the outcome in future pregnancies

4. Clinical features. Bleeding may be revealed, concealed or a mixture of the two. The fetus suffers as a direct reduction in the functioning intervillous space as well as indirect effects of maternal vasoconstriction and uterine spasm. If retroplacental haemorrhage > 500 ml occurs, foetal death is likely: if > 1000 ml, serious maternal sequelae are likely, including shock and disseminated intravascular coagulation (DIC).

With increasing placental separation and retroplacental haemorrhage, there is increasing abdominal tenderness, pain, rigidity and increased likelihood of foetal death. The uterine fundus may be higher than expected for gestational age.

Placenta praevia

1. Definition. The placenta is situated partly or wholly in the lower segment of the uterus.

2. Incidence. Placenta praevia accounts for 0.5–1.0% of pregnancies and is responsible for 15–20% APH.

3. Types of placenta praevia

- Major or complete praevia: if the placenta encroaches onto the cervical os, it is considered a major or complete praevia.
- Minor or partial praevia: if the lower segment placenta does not encroach on the cervical os, it is described as minor or partial praevia.

The significance of this grading is that the morbidity and mortality for mother and foetus increases the more the placenta encroaches upon the os. Because the endometrium is less well developed in the lower uterine segment, the placenta is more likely to become morbidly adherent (placenta praevia accreta). This may cause problems during the third stage when placental separation should occur. The risk of placenta accreta increases with the number of previous Caesarean deliveries: from 9% for placenta praevia with no previous lower segment Caesarean section (LSCS); 20–30% with one previous LSCS; to 40–50% with two–three previous LSCS. Placenta increta (where placenta invades myometrium) and percreta (where placental tissue fully penetrates the uterine wall) are rarer and more severe variants.

4. Aetiology. Implantation low in the uterine cavity increases with age, parity, multiple pregnancy, previous LSCS or termination and smoking.

5. Clinical Features. Painless vaginal bleeding occurs in the latter stages of pregnancy. The onset may be spontaneous or precipitated by coitus, coughing or straining. Any painless bleeding in the second half of pregnancy is placenta praevia until proved otherwise. Definitive diagnosis is by ultrasound scan. If there is a major degree of placenta praevia, Caesarean section will be required for safe delivery. There may be difficulty in delivering the placenta. This is because there is poorer contraction of the lower segment myometrium, and risk of placenta accreta. There is a higher than normal risk of PPH.

6. Management. After significant APH, hospitalise mothers with placenta praevia in the third trimester. Pursue conservative management until the foetus is mature. Deliver by LSCS by senior obstetric and anaesthetic personnel. An anterior placenta praevia may be directly under the uterine incision site. Cross-match 6 units of blood and insert two large-gauge intravenous cannulae. Use a fluid-warming device. If the placenta is anterior, and especially is there has been a previous LSCS and hence increased risk of placenta accreta, general anaesthesia is the technique of choice. Anticipate PPH.

Postpartum haemorrhage

PPH may be primary or secondary.

Primary PPH

1. Definition. Bleeding of 500 ml or more from the birth canal in the first 24 h after delivery. Major PPH is blood loss > 1000 ml in the 24 h after delivery.

2. Incidence. Occurs in approximately 2% of pregnancies.

3. Aetiology. Retained products of conception, uterine atony, trauma and bleeding diatheses. There is increased incidence if there is a precipitant or very prolonged labour, macrosomia, multiple gestation, operative delivery, LSCS, previous PPH, chorioamnionitis and obesity.

Retained products of conception

It is obvious if the entire placenta is retained. It is less obvious if the placenta is ragged and a small cotyledon retained. Treatment includes evacuation of the uterus under anaesthesia, regional or general. If there is placenta accreta, either wholly or in part, there will be no plane of cleavage. Haemorrhage may require embolisation or ligation of the uterine or iliac arteries. Hysterectomy may be necessary.

Uterine atony

Uterine atony is less common now with the routine use of oxytocic drugs at delivery. It is exacerbated by volatile anaesthetics, β-agonists used as tocolytics and magnesium sulphate. A full bladder, uterine sepsis, long labour and high parity inhibit normal uterine contraction.

Management
If obstetric manoeuvres such as uterine massage, bimanual compression, administration of oxytocin or ergometrinefail, intramuscular or intramyometrial injection of prostaglandin $F_{2\alpha}$ in 250 μg aliquots is appropriate. Compression of bleeding points is also possible by using uterine packing or extrinsic compression with a B-Lynch suture.

Trauma

1. Uterine rupture. Occurs in multiparous women with large foetus or malpresentation (e.g. brow), injudicious use of oxytocics, operative and other trauma (e.g. external version with uterine scar, mid forceps delivery). Symptoms include pain, tenderness on abdominal palpation and shock. Contractions decrease and there may be foetal distress. Symptoms are more extreme if the upper segment ruptures. Treatment includes uterine repair or, if necessary, hysterectomy.

2. Local trauma to the lower birth canal. Rarely causes life-threatening haemorrhage.

Coagulation defect

In obstetric practice, DIC is the commonest cause of failure of blood clotting. Predisposing factors include severe abruption, severe pre-eclampsia, amniotic fluid embolism, sepsis, shock and intrauterine death. Management should include early discussion with a senior haematologist.

Secondary PPH

Defined as excessive bleeding after the first 24 h postpartum until the end of the puerperium, secondary PPH is generally caused by retained products of conception which act as a nidus for infection.

Treatment

Antibiotics in the first instance. The uterus is friable at this time and great care must be taken not to perforate the uterus if surgical evacuation is required.

Unusual sequelae of obstetric haemorrhage

Sheehan (pathologist, England 1937) reported infarction of anterior and, occasionally, posterior lobe of pituitary gland. The first clinical manifestation is failure of lactation, then amenorrhoea. Later there will be failure of thyroid and adrenal axes.

Principles of management of obstetric haemorrhage

The principal goal is successful maternal resuscitation. All foetal issues are secondary to this. The aim is to maintain or restore adequate oxygen delivery to all organs, including the uteroplacental unit.

Further reading

Pargger H, Schneider MC. Major Haemorrhage. In: Russell IF, Lyons G (eds), *Clinical Problems in Obstetric Anaesthesia*. London: Chapman and Hall Medical, 1997, pp. 33–46.

The National Institute for Clinical Excellence, The Scottish Executive Health Department, The Department of Health, Social Services and Public Safety: Northern Ireland. Why Mothers Die 1997–1999. *The Confidential Enquiries into Maternal Deaths in the United Kingdom 1997–1999*. London: RCOG Press, 2001, pp. 94–103.

http://www.cemach.org.uk/publications/CEMDreports/cemdrpt.pdf

Obstetric emergencies – medical

Jenny Tuckey

Pulmonary thromboembolism

There were 35 deaths due to thromboembolism recorded in the *Confidential Enquiries into Maternal Deaths (CEMD) in the United Kingdom 1997–1999* (rate 16.5 per million pregnancies). Of the 35 deaths, 31 were from pulmonary embolism (PE) and four from cerebral thrombosis.

The 31 deaths from pulmonary embolism is a substantial reduction from the 46 cases reported in 1994–1996. This was due mainly to the dramatic fall in deaths after lower segment Caesarean section (LSCS), following the publication, in 1995, of the Royal College of Obstetricians and Gynaecologists guidelines on prophylaxis at Caesarean section. Thromboembolism is the commonest cause of direct maternal death in the UK. Further reduction in death from this cause will only be possible by examining risk factors for all mothers (i.e. including vaginal deliveries) and giving prophylaxis appropriately.

Pregnancy-induced hypertension

There were 15 direct deaths due to pregnancy-induced hypertension reported to the CEMD during 1997–1999 (rate 7.1 per million pregnancies). It is the second major cause of maternal death in the UK. Pre-eclampsia is defined as 'gestational proteinuric hypertension developing during pregnancy or for the first time in labour'. It occurs in approximately 10% of pregnancies, most commonly between 33 and 37 weeks of gestation. The only cure is delivery of the placenta. Pre-eclampsia generally resolves within 48–72h of delivery. The commonest causes of death due to hypertensive diseases of pregnancy (CEMD 1997–99) were intracranial haemorrhage, HELLP (*h*aemolysis, *e*levated *l*iver enzymes, *l*ow *p*latelet count) syndrome and hepatic rupture.

The American College of Obstetricians and Gynecologists use any one of the following to define severe pre-eclampsia: systolic blood pressure (BP) >160mmHg, diastolic BP >110mmHg, mean arterial pressure >120mmHg, proteinuria (5g in 24h or 3+/4+ on semi-quantitative 'dipstick' testing), oliguria (<500ml in 24h), headache or cerebral disturbance, visual disturbance, epigastric pain or raised liver enzymes (transaminases), pulmonary oedema, cyanosis or HELLP syndrome.

Pre-eclampsia is a multisystem disease with a variable clinical presentation. Placental ischaemia is associated with widespread endothelial damage, which may involve all maternal organ systems. Mild pre-eclampsia has a good prognosis, but severe pre-eclampsia is associated with morbidity and mortality.

Eclampsia

Eclampsia is diagnosed if one or more grand mal convulsions (not related to other conditions) occur in pre-eclampsia. Eclampsia is more common in teenagers and in cases of multiple pregnancy. In the UK, 40% of eclamptic fits occur after delivery, most commonly within the first 3 days.

HELLP

The HELLP syndrome is one form of severe pre-eclampsia and is associated with a maternal mortality of up to 24%. HELLP syndrome presents with malaise in 90%, epigastric pain (90%) and nausea and vomiting (50%). Physical signs include right upper quadrant tenderness (80%), weight gain and oedema. Blood pressure may be normal and proteinuria may be absent. Resolution of symptoms following delivery may be slow. Corticosteroids may hasten the normalisation of platelets and liver enzymes and hence recovery.

Management of pre-eclampsia

The general aims are to minimise vasospasm, improve perfusion of the uterus, placenta and maternal vital organs and assess fetal maturity. The ultimate cure is delivery of the baby and placenta.

1. Antihypertensive agents. These drugs (e.g. labetalol, nifedipine or hydralazine) are given if the diastolic blood pressure persistently exceeds 100 mmHg.

2. Clinical assessment. Foetal growth, proteinuria, urate and platelet count are measured.

3. Steroids. For example, two doses of betamethasone 12 mg at 24 h interval, are given to aid maturation of the foetal lungs if the pregnancy is < 34 weeks. Delivery is ideally delayed for 48 h for maximal benefit.

4. Magnesium sulphate. This may be given as prophylaxis against convulsions. The results of the Collaborative Eclampsia Study and the Magpie Trial support its use as prophylaxis and treatment of convulsions. It is a central nervous system depressant, cerebral vasodilator and mild antihypertensive. It increases prostacyclin release by endothelial cells, increases uterine and renal perfusion and decreases platelet aggregation. Conversely, its tocolytic effect may prolong labour and increase blood loss.

5. Fluid management. In severe pre-eclampsia, careful fluid management is crucial. Mothers are susceptible to pulmonary oedema due to leaky pulmonary capillaries and low colloid osmotic pressure because of renal protein loss. In severe cases, central venous pressure (CVP) correlates poorly with left ventricular end-diastolic pressure.

Amniotic fluid embolism (AFE)

Between 1997 and 1999 there were eight maternal deaths due to AFE (3.8 per million maternities). It occurs in 1 in 8000 to 1 in 80 000 live births. Mortality is as high as 86%, with 50% dying within the first hour. AFE can occur in early pregnancy, at the time of termination of pregnancy or amniocentesis or following closed abdominal trauma. It can also occur during Caesarean section or artificial rupture of the membranes, and in the elderly, multiparous parturient undergoing a vigorous labour driven by oxytocin.

Pathophysiology

Amniotic fluid or foetal matter enters the maternal circulation. This can occur asymptomatically. The presence of meconium worsens the prognosis. If there is 'collapse', the haemodynamic changes are biphasic. Initially, amniotic fluid causes pulmonary vasoconstriction, which results in transient pulmonary hypertension and profound hypoxia due to mechanical obstruction to the pulmonary arteries. A degree of pulmonary vasospasm may be due to production of vasoactive substances such as leukotrienes. Later, left ventricular (LV) dysfunction causes secondary pulmonary hypertension. This LV dysfunction may be secondary to an initial period of hypoxia, or depression of the myocardium by components of amniotic fluid.

Clinical features

Typically, there is a sudden onset of dyspnoea, cyanosis and hypotension out of proportion to blood loss, followed quickly by cardiorespiratory arrest. Up to 20% have seizures and up to 40% develop disseminated intravascular coagulation (DIC) with bleeding from the vagina, surgical incisions and intravenous cannula sites. Non-cardiogenic pulmonary oedema will follow in up to 70% of initial survivors.

Management is supportive.

Intracranial bleed

Between 1997 and 1999 there were 16 maternal deaths due to intracranial haemorrhage (11 subarachnoid and five intracerebral bleed).

Cardiac arrest in pregnancy

This is almost always an unexpected event and attendant personnel usually have little experience of resuscitation or cardiac arrest. Hypoxia develops rapidly due to the reduced functional residual capacity (FRC) and increased oxygen consumption of pregnancy. Caval compression must be avoided and chest compressions performed with a wedge beneath the mother's right hip, or else the gravid uterus displaced manually. Early intubation is essential to prevent aspiration. If spontaneous circulation is not restored rapidly, the foetus should be delivered by immediate LSCS to minimise aortocaval compression and optimise the chance of maternal survival.

Local anaesthetic toxicity

Typical complaints are circumoral numbness, tinnitus, light-headedness, confusion and a sense of impending doom. Muscle twitching and grand mal convulsion may occur. All these symptoms and signs are exacerbated by acidosis and hypoxia. Central nervous system symptoms usually occur before cardiovascular collapse.

Further reading

Duley L, Altman D, Carroli G, *et al*. Do women with pre-eclampsia, and their babies, benefit from magnesium sulphate? The Magpie trial: a randomised placebo-controlled trial. *Lancet* 2002; **359**: 1877–90.

The National Institute for Clinical Excellence, The Scottish Executive Health Department, The Department of Health, Social Services and Public Safety, Northern Ireland. Why Mothers Die 1997–1999. *The Confidential Enquiries into Maternal Deaths in the United Kingdom 1997–1999*. London: RCOG Press, 2001, pp. 49–93, 104–110.

http://www.cemach.org.uk/publications/CEMDreports/cemdrpt.pdf

Pancreatitis

Inflammation associated with acute pancreatitis may also involve tissues around the pancreas and/or remote organs. Approximately 80% of cases of acute pancreatitis are mild and resolve with simple fluid and electrolyte replacement and analgesia. However, the remaining 20%, representing those with severe acute pancreatitis, are subject to organ failure and/or local complications (e.g. necrosis, pseudocysts, fistulae). Severe disease carries a mortality of 10–20%.

Causes

Alcohol abuse and gallstones cause 80% of cases of acute pancreatitis, with the latter accounting for the majority of these. Acute idiopathic pancreatitis occurs in about 10% of cases. However, biliary sludge can be found in two-thirds of these and they often respond to endoscopic sphincterotomy. Many other conditions make up the remaining 10% of causes (e.g. drugs, trauma, infections and tumours).

Pathogenesis

For reasons that remain incompletely understood (possibly related to duodenopancreatic reflux), pancreatic trypsin is activated inappropriately. This results in auto-digestion of pancreatic tissue. In severe cases, circulating enzymes cause a systemic inflammatory response syndrome (SIRS).

Clinical features

Continuous, epigastric pain that radiates through to the back is a typical presentation of acute pancreatitis. It is often accompanied by nausea and vomiting and a low-grade fever. Abdominal distension, due to an associated ileus, is common. Evidence of retroperitoneal bleeding in the form of periumbilical (Cullen's sign) or flank (Grey Turner's sign) bruising is rare and indicates severe disease. There may be evidence of basal pleural effusions and atelectasis.

There are two phases in the clinical course of severe acute pancreatitis. The early toxaemic phase (0–15 days) is characterised by SIRS associated with marked fluid shifts. In the later, necrotic phase, intra-abdominal necrosis with or without subsequent infection causes local and systemic complications.

Investigations

Amylase
The appropriate clinical features in combination with a serum amylase of >1000 U will confirm the diagnosis of acute pancreatitis. If the upper limit of the normal range for serum amylase is used as the cut-off value, the specificity is reduced to 70%. Amylase is a small molecule and is cleared rapidly by the kidneys; renal impairment will exacerbate the increase in serum amylase. Serum amylase is not always raised in acute pancreatitis; normoamylasaemic pancreatitis occurs in up to 10% of cases,

probably because of unusually rapid urinary clearance of amylase. Serum lipase takes longer to clear and may be a better historical indicator of pancreatitis; it rises within 4–8h of an episode of acute pancreatitis, peaks at 24h, and returns to normal after 8–14 days. The combination of both serum amylase and lipase will provide sensitivity and specificity of 90–95% for detecting acute pancreatitis.

Ultrasound

Abdominal ultrasound will identify gallstones although bowel gas associated with an accompanying ileus may make the examination technically difficult.

Computed tomography

Contrast-enhanced computed tomography (CT) of the abdomen is the best method of imaging the pancreas. It may show pancreatic necrosis, and/or pseudocysts. CT is indicated:

- Where the initial diagnosis is in doubt.
- In the presence of severe pancreatitis, fever and leucocytosis, CT-guided fine-needle aspiration will help with the diagnosis of infected pancreatic necrosis.

Prognostic indicators

A number of scoring systems have been used to help to assess the severity of pancreatitis. The APACHE II system (p. 266) enables rapid determination of prognosis but is relatively complex. Ranson's criteria form the most popular system. They are divided into five criteria that are assessed on admission and a further six that are evaluated at 48 hours:

On admission

- Age > 55 years.
- White blood count $> 16\,000\,\text{mm}^{-3}$.
- Glucose $> 11\,\text{mmol}\,\text{l}^{-1}$.
- Lactate dehydrogenase $> 350\,\text{IU}\,\text{l}^{-1}$.
- Aspartate aminotransferase $> 250\,\text{U}\,\text{l}^{-1}$.

During initial 48 hours

- Haematocrit decrease $> 10\%$.
- Blood urea increase $> 1.8\,\text{mmol}\,\text{l}^{-1}$.
- Serum calcium $< 2\,\text{mmol}\,\text{l}^{-1}$.
- $PaO_2 < 8\,\text{kPa}$.
- Base deficit $> 4\,\text{mmol}\,\text{l}^{-1}$.
- Fluid sequestration $> 6\,\text{l}$.

The presence of fewer than three Ranson's criteria indicates a mild pancreatitis and a mortality of $< 1\%$. The mortality increases to 16% in the presence of three or four criteria and $> 40\%$ with five or more criteria. The presence of three or more of Ranson's criteria indicates a likely need for admission to a critical care unit. The

Imrie score reduces the number of Ranson's criteria by three (LDH, base deficit and fluid deficit) without losing predictive power.

Management

The general principles of management are metabolic and nutritional support, control of symptoms and prevention and treatment of organ dysfunction.

Resuscitation

Patients with acute pancreatitis will require aggressive fluid resuscitation with guidance from invasive monitoring, and correction of hyperglycaemia and electrolyte disorders. Patients with SIRS associated with severe pancreatitis will often require inotropic support. Abdominal distension, basal pleural effusions and atelectasis all contribute to significant respiratory embarrassment even in the absence of ARDS. The level of respiratory support required will range from simple oxygen therapy to intubation and mechanical ventilation.

Calcium

The rationale for correcting hypocalcaemia associated with pancreatitis is not entirely clear. Total serum calcium does not correlate well with ionised calcium and any replacement should be titrated against the latter. Correction of hypocalcaemia will improve arterial pressure but may not enhance cardiac index and oxygen delivery.

Nutrition

Oral feeding is withheld and nasogastric drainage is usually instituted, although there is little hard data to support either of these therapies. Most patients with mild uncomplicated pancreatitis do not benefit from nutritional support; they can usually begin oral refeeding within a few days of the onset of their pain. However, patients who have moderate to severe pancreatitis should receive early nutritional support. Enteral feeding has been shown to be safe, as effective as parenteral nutrition, and well tolerated in severe acute pancreatitis. It is less expensive than parenteral feeding and preserves mucosal function. Nasojejunal placement of the feeding tube will avoid pancreatic stimulation and will enable successful feeding even in the presence of gastric stasis. In the absence of a nasojejunal tube, nasogastric feeding is worth attempting; it is thought to be safe and may be successful. Parenteral nutrition should be started only if enteral feed is not tolerated.

Analgesia

The severe pain associated with acute pancreatitis will require systemic opioids or thoracic epidural analgesia. The latter is more effective and in the absence of contraindications is the method of choice. Theoretical concern that morphine causes spasm of the sphincter of Oddi has led to the recommendation of pethidine for systemic analgesia. In reality, morphine is probably a better choice.

Antibiotics

Prophylactic antibiotics are indicated for those patients who are predicted to develop severe pancreatitis. Bacterial infection of necrotic pancreatic tissue occurs in 40–70%

of patients with acute necrotising pancreatitis. Prophylactic high-dose cefuroxime, a quinolone or a carbapenem have been shown to reduce morbidity, though not mortality.

Gallstone extraction
Endoscopic retrograde cholangiopancreatography (ERCP) and extraction of gallstones is indicated in the acute setting only when increasing jaundice or cholangitis complicates severe pancreatitis.

Surgery
The precise role of surgery in acute pancreatitis remains controversial. It is usually reserved for one or more of the complications discussed below.

Complications

The systemic complications of multiple organ dysfunction or failure are well-recognised sequelae of SIRS. Local complications include pancreatic necrosis, pseudocysts and fistulas.

Pancreatic necrosis
Pancreatic necrosis is detected by lack of enhancement of the pancreatic tissue on contrast-enhanced CT scan. Once necrosis develops, the presence of bacterial contamination and the general condition of the patient will determine the outcome. Necrosectomy is usually reserved for persistently febrile patients who fail to respond to broad-spectrum antibiotics with or without percutaneous drainage of fluid collections over 3 days or more.

Pseudocyst
A pseudocyst is a collection of pancreatic secretions that lacks an epithelial lining. Pseudocysts complicate acute pancreatitis in fewer than 5% of cases. Drainage should be considered in the following circumstances:

- Larger than 5–6 cm in diameter and increasing in size.
- Pain.
- Gastric outlet obstruction.
- Infection or haemorrhage into the cyst.

Drainage may be undertaken percutaneously or at laparotomy. Ultrasound- or CT-guided percutaneous drainage is an effective method for decompression although there is a significant risk of recurrence.

Fistulae
Disruption of the pancreatic duct may cause pancreatic fistulae. A pancreaticopleural fistula will result in an extensive pleural effusion. A pancreaticoperitoneal fistula should be suspected in patients with massive ascites. Persistent pancreatic fistulae will require surgery.

Further reading

Baron TH, Morgan DE. Acute necrotizing pancreatitis. *N Engl J Med* 1999; **340**: 1412–17.

Mergener K, Baillie J. Acute pancreatitis. *BMJ* 1998; **316**: 44–8.

Mitchell RMS, Byrne MF, Baillie J. Pancreatitis. *Lancet* 2003; **361**: 1447–55.

Wyncoll DL. The management of severe acute necrotizing pancreatitis: an evidence based review of the literature. *Intensive Care Med* 1999; **25**: 146–56.

Pneumonia – community acquired

Pneumonia is an acute septic episode with respiratory symptoms and radiological shadowing that was neither pre-existing nor of other known cause. Community-acquired infection is defined as an infection that occurs in a patient who has not been hospitalised in the preceding 2 weeks or an infection that occurred within 48h of admission to hospital.

Approximately 60–80% of adults with pneumonia are treated at home by general practitioners, whereas 1–4 per 1000 of the population are admitted to hospital with pneumonia annually. The mortality is 5–15% among those requiring hospital admission and 35–50% for those admitted to a critical care unit. Community-acquired pneumonia (CAP) occurs more commonly in those over 65, in smokers and in those with other non-respiratory illnesses. The pathogenesis of CAP differs from pneumonia acquired while the patient is in hospital (nosocomial pneumonia, see p. 227). Although antibiotic strategies differ, the general approach to critical care management of pneumonia is the same regardless of the aetiology.

Epidemiology

Streptococcus pneumoniae is the commonest cause of CAP. It is isolated in about 30% of cases and probably accounts also for the third of cases in which no causative organism is found. Other organisms commonly found are listed in Table 13. Among patients admitted to a critical care unit, *Legionella* is the second commonest cause of CAP.

Table 13 Pathogens causing adult community-acquired pneumonia in the UK by site of care (%)

	Community	Hospital	Critical care unit
Streptococcus pneumoniae	36	36.1	21.6
Haemophilus influenzae	10.2	4.5	3.8
Legionella spp	0.4	3.7	17.8
Staphylococcus aureus	0.8	2.1	8.7
Mycoplasma pneumoniae	1.3	13.1	2.7
Viral (mainly influenza)	13.1	9.1	5.4

Haemophilus influenzae is the commonest cause of bacterial exacerbation of chronic obstructive pulmonary disease (COPD). The possibility of *Staphylococcus aureus* should be considered during an influenza epidemic, particularly if there is radiological evidence of cavitation. *Mycoplasma* is commonly associated with cough, sore throat, nausea, diarrhoea, headache and myalgia. Generally, clinical features are not sensitive or specific enough to predict the microbial aetiology. As legionellosis has become increasingly recognised, and less severely ill patients are seen earlier in the course of the disease, clinical features of unusual severity once considered distinctive of *Legionella* infection are now known to be non-specific. However, hyponatraemia does occur more frequently with infections with *Legionella* spp. than in other types of pneumonia.

Assessment of severity

The British Thoracic Society (BTS) recommends an assessment of severity based on adverse prognostic features.

Pre-existing adverse prognostic features
- Age ≥ 50 years.
- Presence of coexisting disease.

Core clinical adverse prognostic features (CURB)
- **C**onfusion: new mental confusion.
- **U**rea: raised $>7\,\text{mmol}\,l^{-1}$.
- **R**espiratory rate: raised $\geq 30\,\text{min}^{-1}$.
- **B**lood pressure: low blood pressure (systolic blood pressure $<90\,\text{mmHg}$ and/or diastolic blood pressure $\leq 60\,\text{mmHg}$).

Additional clinical adverse prognostic features
- Hypoxaemia ($SaO_2 < 92\%$ or $PaO_2 < 8\,\text{kPa}$, regardless of FiO_2).
- Bilateral or multilobe involvement on the chest radiograph.

Patients with two or more core adverse prognostic features are defined as having severe pneumonia and are at high risk of death. These patients may need treatment in a critical care unit.

Investigations

Investigations should be undertaken to assess severity and identify aetiology:

- Chest X-ray.
- Arterial blood gas analysis.
- Full blood count: a white cell count $>15\,000 \times 10^9\,l^{-1}$ makes a bacterial pathogen likely. A normal count is often seen in atypical or viral infection, but this is not specific enough to be of diagnostic value.
- Urea, electrolytes and liver function tests.
- Sputum Gram stain, culture and sensitivity. The presence of Gram-positive diplococci implies pneumococcal infection. Results of sputum culture must be interpreted cautiously; many of the organisms responsible for pneumonia are normal upper respiratory tract commensals.
  Pneumococcal antigen may be identified in the sputum, blood or urine, even in patients who have already received antibiotics.
- Urine antigen test. Antigens of *Streptococcus pneumoniae* and *Legionella* spp. can be detected in urine. The test for *Legionella* has a sensitivity of 70% and a specificity of almost 100%. The sensitivity for pneumococcal urinary antigen in defining invasive pneumococcal disease is 60–90%, with a specificity close to 100%.
- Blood culture.

- Serology is available for influenza A and B viruses, respiratory syncytial virus, adenovirus, *Coxiella burnetti*, *Chlamydia psittaci*, *Mycoplasma pneumoniae* and *Legionella pneumophila*, but does not often provide diagnostic changes early enough to be clinically useful. However, the majority of patients with *Mycoplasma* pneumonia will have a positive *Mycoplasma*-specific immunoglobulin M titre on admission to hospital.
- Influenza can be confirmed by culture or immunofluorescence of nasopharyngeal aspirates.
- Bronchoscopy is normally reserved for those with very severe pneumonia. This will enable sampling by protected specimen brush (PSB) or by bronchoalveolar lavage (see Pneumonia – hospital acquired, p. 227). Legionella culture should be undertaken on these samples. Bronchoscopy will also enable the diagnosis of any underlying lung disease such as a bronchial tumour.

Management

All patients with severe CAP should be given oxygen to maintain $PaO_2 > 8\,kPa$, and antibiotics as indicated below. On the ward, the minimum monitoring should include regular pulse, blood pressure and respiratory rate, pulse oximetry and repeat blood gas sampling. Physiotherapy is helpful for those patients with copious secretions. These patients will often be dehydrated and may require intravenous fluid replacement. Patients with persisting indicators of severe CAP should be admitted to a critical care unit. Mask CPAP and/or non-invasive positive pressure ventilation (NIPPV) will improve oxygenation and may prevent the need for tracheal intubation. If the patient's admission to the critical care unit has been delayed until they are exhausted, non-invasive techniques are unlikely to be successful.

Antibiotic therapy

The infecting organism is usually unknown when treatment is initiated. Empirical therapy should always cover *Streptococcus pneumoniae*. Penicillin-resistant pneumococci are increasing worldwide, although less so in the UK. In two recent multinational studies, the worldwide prevalence of penicillin-resistant and macrolide-resistant *S. pneumoniae* was 18–22 and 25–32%, respectively. In the UK, a second- or third-generation cephalosporin (e.g., cefuroxime or cefotaxime) combined with clarithromycin remains appropriate empirical therapy. Antibiotic treatment should be continued for 7 days and then reviewed. If *Legionella* is suspected, clarithromycin should be combined with rifampicin or ciprofloxacin and given for 14–21 days. Staphylococcal pneumonia is treated with flucloxacillin for 14–21 days. Patients with severe, microbiologically undefined, pneumonia require 10 days of antibiotic therapy. Patients admitted to a critical care unit with severe CAP and who have influenza identified in nasopharyngeal aspirate are often given oseltamivir 75 mg twice daily for 5 days, although there is little evidence for its efficacy in critically ill patients.

Severe acute respiratory syndrome (SARS)

Severe acute respiratory syndrome (SARS) emerged from Guangdong Province, China, in November 2002. It was responsible for the first pandemic of the 21st

Century, affecting 8000 patients in 26 countries and causing 774 deaths. It is caused by a novel coronavirus (SARS-CoV), which probably originated in animals. It has an incubation period of 2–10 days and is transmitted primarily in health care settings. The primary mode of transmission is through direct or indirect contact of mucous membrane with infectious respiratory droplets or via contaminated objects or surfaces (fomites).

The initial manifestations of SARS are not specific, and it cannot be clinically differentiated from other causes of CAP. Infected persons present initially with myalgia, malaise, rigors and cough. Shortness of breath and tachypnoea occurs only later in the course of the illness. Lymphocytopenia is common. The initial chest radiograph is abnormal in 60–100% of cases and shows ground-glass opacifications. Diagnosis can be made using reverse transcriptase polymerase chain reaction (RT-PCR) testing, but the sensitivity and specificity of this test has yet to be defined.

In patients older than 65 years, the mortality rate exceeds 50%. About 20–30% of patients need admission to a critical care unit and most require intubation and mechanical ventilation. Non-invasive ventilation and mask CPAP should not be used because they increase the risk of spreading the virus. Staff undertaking invasive airway procedures, such as intubation and bronchoscopy, should wear personal protective equipment, as indicated by local policy. Some health care organisations specify the use of full protective suits, including positive pressure hoods, by staff undertaking these high-risk procedures. Treatment of SARS is supportive. As yet, there is no proven specific treatment.

Further reading

File TM. Community-acquired pneumonia. *Lancet* 2003; **362**: 1991–2001.

Halm EA, Tierstein AS. Management of community-acquired pneumonia. *N Engl J Med* 2002; **347**: 2039–45.

Peiris JSM, Yuen KY, Osterhaus ADME, Stohr K. The severe acute respiratory syndrome. *N Engl J Med* 2003; **349**: 2431–41.

The British Thoracic Society. Guidelines for the management of community-acquired pneumonia in adults. *Thorax* 2001; **56(Suppl 4)**: iv, 1–65:
www.brit-thoracic.org.uk/

Related topics of interest

Arterial blood gases – analysis (p. 31)
Chronic obstructive pulmonary disease (p. 114)
Infection control (p. 178)
Infection acquired in critical care (nosocomial) (p. 182)
Pneumonia – hospital acquired (p. 227)
Respiratory support – non-invasive techniques (p. 254)
Respiratory support – invasive (p. 260)

Pneumonia – hospital acquired

Nosocomial infection is defined as an infection occurring more than 48 h after hospital admission, or within 48 h of discharge. Nosocomial pneumonia accounts for 15% of all hospital-acquired infections and 31% of infections acquired in the intensive therapy unit (ITU). It is a cause of considerable morbidity and mortality.

Pathogenesis

The aetiology of nosocomial pneumonia is influenced significantly by the patient's length of stay in hospital. The early-onset (<5 days) hospital-acquired pneumonias are likely to be caused by potentially pathogenic microorganisms (PPM) that were carried by the patient at the time of hospital admission. Patients admitted to hospital with a reduced conscious level and impaired airway reflexes (e.g. trauma) are most likely to succumb to this 'primary endogenous infection'. The organisms concerned are likely to be upper respiratory tract commensals such as *Streptococcus pneumoniae*, *Haemophilus influenzae* and *Staphylococcus aureus*.

In health, an intact mucosal lining, mucus, normal gastrointestinal motility, secretory IgA and resident anaerobes inhibit colonisation of the gastrointestinal tract by aerobic bacteria. In the critically ill, impairment of these protective mechanisms leads to colonisation of the gastrointestinal tract by aerobic Gram-negative bacteria (e.g. *Escherichia coli*, *Pseudomonas aeruginosa*, *Klebsiella* spp., *Proteus* spp.), *Staphylococcus aureus* and yeasts (e.g. *Candida* spp.). Secondary endogenous infection is caused by PPMs acquired in the critical care unit. These have variable patterns of resistance and are a significant cause of pneumonia developing after 5 days in hospital (late onset). There are several risk factors for colonisation and infection by abnormal flora:

- Prolonged intubation bypasses the natural mechanical host defences, causes mucosal damage and facilitates entry of bacteria into the lung. Nasotracheal intubation increases the risk of sinusitis. Approximately two-thirds of ITU patients with sinusitis will develop pneumonia.
- Mechanical ventilation for more than 24 h is a significant risk factor for nosocomial pneumonia (ventilator-associated pneumonia or VAP). There is a cumulative risk of VAP with duration of mechanical ventilation: 3% per day in the first week, 2% per day in the second week and 1% per day in the week.
- Nasogastric tubes encourage gastro-oesophageal reflux, bacterial migration and sinusitis.
- Opiates, high FiO_2, inadequate humidification and tracheal suctioning impair mucociliary transport.
- A gastric pH > 4.0 encourages colonisation by Gram-negative organisms. Thus, H_2-blockers are more likely than sucralfate to contribute to nosocomial pneumonia; however, the difference between these drugs is small. In a multicentre Canadian study, ranitidine was more effective than sucralfate in reducing gastrointestinal bleeding, with no differences in the rates of respiratory tract infection.
- The supine position encourages microaspiration.
- Patients over the age of 60 years and those with chronic lung disease are more likely to develop nosocomial pneumonia.

Diagnosis

Several clinical criteria have been used for diagnosis of nosocomial pneumonia but the most popular are:

1. New or progressive consolidation on the chest radiograph.
2. Fever.
3. Leucocytosis.
4. Purulent tracheobronchial secretions.

There are significant limitations in using these criteria alone to diagnose nosocomial pneumonia:

- Purulent tracheal aspirates are commonly produced by colonisation of the upper airway alone.
- The radiological appearances of pneumonia are non-specific.
- There are many causes of fever in the critically ill.

The use of clinical signs alone will lead to overdiagnosis of nosocomial pneumonia. Excessive use of antibiotics will encourage the selection of multi-resistant organisms.

Diagnostic techniques

Simple aspiration of the tracheal tube or tracheostomy has good sensitivity but poor specificity for diagnosing pneumonia. Although these specimens are less likely to be contaminated than expectorated sputum, there will still be frequent false-positive cultures from organisms colonising the upper airway and tracheal tube. Quantitative cultures of tracheal aspirates using 10^5–10^6 colony-forming units per ml ($cfu\,ml^{-1}$) as the cut off may have an acceptable diagnostic accuracy.

There are several techniques that bypass the upper respiratory tract and enable a relatively uncontaminated sampling of the lower airways. This may improve diagnostic accuracy. The protected specimen brush (PSB) is passed through a fibreoptic bronchoscope, enabling collection of uncontaminated specimens from suspected areas of infection. Bacteria cultured in concentrations higher than $10^3\,cfu\,ml^{-1}$ are considered pathogenic. Alternatively, with the bronchoscope wedged in a distal airway, bronchoalveolar lavage (BAL) with 20 ml aliquots of saline will sample a larger area of lung. This method is more sensitive than the PSB, but contamination of the bronchoscope with organisms from the upper airway reduces its specificity. Thus, following BAL, only cultures of $>10^4\,cfu\,ml^{-1}$ are considered significant. The protected mini-BAL technique combines attributes from the PSB and BAL techniques and has excellent sensitivity (97%) and specificity (92%) in diagnosing pneumonia. The ultimate invasive diagnostic technique, open lung biopsy, is rarely indicated in the diagnosis of nosocomial pneumonia, except for immunosuppressed patients.

Prevention

Every effort must be made to minimise colonisation by PPM and reduce spread of infection. Enteral nutrition started early will reduce colonisation of the gastrointestinal tract. Maintain mechanically ventilated patients in a 30–45° head-up position; this reduces the rate of nosocomial pneumonia by 75%. Closed suction systems may reduce contamination of the patient's airway. Avoid long-term nasotracheal intubation. Selective decontamination of the digestive tract (SDD) was developed to reduce the incidence of Gram-negative pneumonia in the critically ill (see Infection Control, p. 178). The frequency of nosocomial pneumonia is reduced with SDD and one study has shown reduced mortality with this therapy. However, few critical care units use SDD because it is relatively expensive and there is a theoretical risk of selecting resistant organisms.

Treatment

Seriously ill patients with nosocomial pneumonia are treated with empirical therapy after samples have been taken. An immediate Gram-stain of the sample may be helpful. Some critical care units run a programme of microbiological surveillance. Regular samples are taken from all patients in the unit and sent for culture. This helps to define the local flora and will direct empirical therapy for severe nosocomial pneumonia. Early onset pneumonia can be treated with a second- or third-generation cephalosporin (e.g. cefuroxime or cefotaxime). Metronidazole is added if aspiration is a possibility. If the patient has previously received a cephalosporin, or the nosocomial pneumonia is late in onset (>5 days), therapy may be changed to ciprofloxacin and amoxicillin. This will cover Gram-negatives and *S. aureus* as well as many community-acquired organisms. Other possibilities are a carbapenem (imipenem or meropenem) or piperacillin/tazobactam combined with an aminoglycoside.

Prognosis

The European Prevalence of Infection in Intensive Care (EPIC) study showed that pneumonia acquired in the critical care unit almost doubled the risk of death. Most of this contribution to increased mortality comes from late-onset nosocomial pneumonia.

Further reading

Johanson WG, Dever LL. Nosocomial pneumonia. *Intensive Care Med* 2003; **29**: 23–9.
Vincent J-L. Nosocomial infections in adult intensive care units. *Lancet* 2003; **362**: 2068–77.

Related topics of interest

Post-resuscitation care

The objective of cardiopulmonary resuscitation (CPR) is to produce a patient with normal cerebral function, no neurological deficit, a stable cardiac rhythm and normal haemodynamic function resulting in adequate organ perfusion. The return of a spontaneous circulation (ROSC) is just the first step in what may be a long process in some patients.

Aims of post-resuscitation care

- Prevent a further cardiac arrest (secondary prevention).
- Define the underlying pathology.
- Limit organ damage.
- Predict non-survivors.

Secondary prevention

To stabilise a patient who has survived initial resuscitation as many variables as possible should be corrected. Oxygenation should be optimised. Following all but the briefest cardiac arrest (e.g. ventricular fibrillation responding to immediate precordial thump or early defibrillation), this will require assisted ventilation via a tracheal tube. Even after an immediate return to full consciousness following a short cardiac arrest, patients should be given additional oxygen via a facemask.

Electrolyte disturbances, in particular of the cations K^+, Mg^{2+} and Ca^{2+}, should be corrected. Acidaemia (high blood H^+ ion concentrations) should be corrected by addressing the underlying cause (e.g. poor peripheral perfusion) rather than by the administration of alkali such as bicarbonate. Bicarbonate is converted to carbon dioxide, which will enter cells and may cause intracellular acidosis. Exceptions, when small amounts of bicarbonate may be given following cardiac arrest, are profound acidaemia (pH < 7.1, base excess > −10) when the excess H^+ ions may depress myocardial function, cardiac arrest associated with hyperkalaemia or following tricyclic antidepressant overdose. Bicarbonate (or other alkalis) should be administered against known blood acid–base status and its effect monitored by frequent arterial blood gas analysis.

Blood glucose must be controlled tightly, even in the non-diabetic. Blood glucose of greater than $7\,\text{mmol}\,l^{-1}$ should be treated with insulin and maintained in the range $4–7\,\text{mmol}\,l^{-1}$.

Define the underlying pathology

The patient's pre-arrest medical condition should be established.

Assessment of the current status requires a thorough physical examination, seeking, in particular, evidence of correct placement of tracheal tube (bilateral, equal signs of air entry), broken ribs and pneumothorax. Listen to the heart for evidence of murmurs (valvular damage, septal rupture) and seek evidence of ventricular failure. A brief neurological assessment should be made and the Glasgow Coma Scale (GCS) score recorded. Investigations to support the physical findings include a CXR, 12-lead ECG, arterial blood gas analysis and baseline creatinine and electrolytes.

Limit organ damage

In those patients whose cardiac arrest is associated with myocardial ischaemia, a supply of oxygenated blood needs to be restored to all parts of the myocardium as soon as possible. This will help prevent myocardial necrosis and limit the size of any associated acute infarct. Coronary artery reperfusion using thrombolytic agents carries its own risk of the development of arrhythmias.

At least a third of patients who achieve ROSC following cardiac arrest eventually die a neurological death, whereas one-third of long-term survivors have motor or cognitive deficit.

The extent of damage to other organs, especially the brain, after ROSC depends greatly on the ability of the heart to deliver adequate amounts of oxygenated blood to them. This, in turn, may influence the occurrence of a secondary hypoxic insult consequent upon microcirculatory changes. A variety of inflammatory mediators (TNF, IL-1, IL-6) may contribute to this 'post-resuscitation syndrome'.

Therapeutic hypothermia after cardiac arrest

Two prospective, randomised trials have compared treatment with mild hypothermia versus normothermia after cardiac arrest. The entry criteria for these trials were similar: ROSC with persistent coma after out-of-hospital ventricular fibrillation (VF) arrest. Both studies excluded patients whose arrests were probably of non-cardiac aetiology or those with severe cardiogenic shock. Patients randomised to the hypothermia group were cooled to a target temperature of 32–34°C for up to 24h, followed by passive rewarming. Patients allocated to the control group were maintained at 'normothermia'.

The primary outcome measure defined prospectively in both studies was a favourable neurological outcome. The results of these two studies and of previous animal studies suggest that mild therapeutic hypothermia after cardiac arrest results in a statistically significant improvement in neurological outcome.

Predict non-survivors

Staff working in critical care have a moral, ethical and fiscal responsibility to treat only those patients who will benefit from it. Despite years of research, survival from cardiac arrest remains disappointing. Short duration of cardiac arrest and CPR correlates with more rapid ROSC and better neurological outcomes. Prognostication in unconscious patients after more protracted CPR remains unreliable in the first 24h and possibly for as long as 72h after ROSC. Myocardial, neurological and other organ function may all improve slowly given appropriate support over a period of time. Intensive care is indicated while evidence of improvement is sought. Failure to show signs of neurological improvement and myoclonus are associated with a poor long term prognosis.

Long-term management

All patients who have survived an acute myocardial infarction require rehabilitation and lifestyle counselling.

Automatic implantable cardioverter defibrillators (AICDs) reduce mortality in those patients at risk of recurrent cardiac arrest due to ventricular tachycardia or fibrillation. Such patients should be identified using electrophysiological testing and considered for implantation of an AICD.

Care of the resuscitation team

All attempts at resuscitation should be audited formally and the team debriefed at the earliest opportunity after cessation of the acute resuscitation, regardless of the outcome. Audit data should be recorded on a standard Utstein template so that comparable multicentre information can be gathered. Examination of the performance of the team should take the form of a positive critique and not develop into a fault/blame culture. Whether the attempts at resuscitation were successful or not, the relatives of the patient will require considerable support. Equally, the pastoral needs of all those associated with the arrest, no matter how hardy they may seem, should not be forgotten.

Further reading

Craft TM. Post resuscitation care. In: Bossaert L (ed.), *European Resuscitation Council Guidelines for Resuscitation*. Amsterdam: Elsevier, 2000.

The Hypothermia after Cardiac Arrest Study Group. Mild therapeutic hypothermia to improve neurologic outcome after cardiac arrest. *N Engl J Med* 2002; **346**: 549–56.

Related topics of interest

Cardiac chest pain (acute coronary syndrome) (p. 81)
Cardiac pacing (p. 96)
Cardiopulmonary resuscitation (p. 104)

Potassium

Potassium is the major intracellular cation. A 70 kg adult has 3500 mmol potassium, of which about 60 mmol (2%) is extracellular. The normal extracellular concentration ranges from 3.5 to 5.1 mmol l^{-1}. The intracellular concentration is 150 mmol l^{-1}. Large changes in total body potassium can occur without significant effect on plasma potassium concentration.

Potassium therapy should take account of both maintenance and replacement requirements. The daily requirement for potassium is approximately 1 mmol kg^{-1}.

Hypokalaemia: < 3.5 mmol

Hypokalaemia occurs in more than 20% of in-hospital patients and is severe (<3.0 mmol l^{-1}) in a quarter of these cases. Mild hypokalaemia is usually well tolerated in healthy patients but may be associated with increased morbidity and mortality in those with severe cardiovascular disease.

Causes

1. Gastrointestinal. Prolonged severe diarrhoea, prolonged vomiting/nasogastric suction, laxative abuse, malabsorption/malnutrition, ureterosigmoidostomy, fistulae, colonic mucus-secreting neoplasms.

2. Renal. Drugs (thiazide and loop diuretics, steroids, carbenoloxone), hyperaldosteronism, Cushing's syndrome, renal tubular acidosis type 1, diuretic phase of acute renal failure (ARF), nephrotic syndrome, metabolic alkalosis, hypomagnesaemia.

3. Other. Intravenous fluids with inadequate supplements. β_2 agonists (e.g. salbutamol), xanthines (e.g. aminophylline, caffeine), glucose/insulin infusions, metabolic alkalosis, congestive cardiac failure, cirrhosis, liver failure, hyperthyroidism.

Clinical features

Mild hypokalaemia is usually asymptomatic; the diagnosis is made on blood analysis. Tachycardia, e.g. SVT (especially with digoxin therapy), ventricular arrhythmias and cardiac arrest may occur. There may be increased blood pressure secondary to sodium retention. Muscle weakness may cause cramps, an ileus and constipation. There may be loss of tendon reflexes and the patient may be easily fatigued, complaining of apathy and sleepiness. There may be polyuria.

Early ECG changes include large U waves and later there may be flattened or inverted T waves. The ST segments may be depressed. Loss of hydrogen ions in exchange for potassium may cause a metabolic alkalosis.

Management

Eliminate artefactual causes, for example contamination by intravenous infusion fluid. Minimise unnecessary potassium-wasting drugs and consider the use of potassium sparing diuretics (amiloride, spironolactone).

Potassium chloride may be given by intravenous infusion at a rate of

20–$30 \, \text{mmol} \, \text{h}^{-1}$, repeated according to measured concentrations. In profound hypokalaemia ($< 2 \, \text{mmol} \, \text{l}^{-1}$), more rapid rates under continuous EGG monitoring will be required. Potassium phosphate is used to provide both potassium and phosphate replacement.

If the patient is asymptomatic and the potassium is low–normal (3.6–$4.0 \, \text{mmol} \, \text{l}^{-1}$), it may be sufficient to provide oral supplements or to add potassium to maintenance fluids or parenteral nutrition. Oral potassium is safer, as it is slower to enter the circulation.

On average, a reduction in serum potassium of $0.3 \, \text{mmol} \, \text{l}^{-1}$ requires a reduction in total body potassium of $100 \, \text{mmol}$. Magnesium will need to be supplemented at the same time.

Hyperkalaemia: $> 5.5 \, \text{mmol} \, \text{l}^{-1}$

Causes

1. Impaired renal excretion. For example, in ARF, advanced chronic renal failure, due to potassium-sparing diuretics or in steroid deficiency (Addison's disease or hypoaldosteronism).

2. Potassium shift from cells. This occurs in acidosis, haemolysis, massive blood transfusion, tumour lysis following chemotherapy, rhabdomyolysis, suxamethonium (especially in patients with neurological disease or denervation), malignant hyperthermia and following cardiac arrest.

3. Other causes. These include giving too much potassium and familial hyperkalaemic periodic paralysis.

Clinical features

Most patients will be asymptomatic until the potassium is $> 6.0 \, \text{mmol} \, \text{l}^{-1}$.

Arrhythmias are related more closely to the rate of rise than the absolute values but may progress to cardiac arrest. There may be muscle weakness and loss of tendon reflexes. The patient may be confused. ECG changes include peaked T waves, flattened P waves, and wide QRS complexes.

Management

Ensure that the finding of hyperkalaemia is not an error. Stop giving all potassium-containing fluids. Depending on the level of potassium and urgency, the treatment options are:

- Intravenous calcium to antagonise the cardiotoxic effects of hyperkalaemia. Calcium chloride 10% contains $0.68 \, \text{mmol} \, \text{ml}^{-1}$ and an initial dose of $10 \, \text{ml}$ can be repeated if the effect is inadequate. It has an immediate onset and lasts up to $60 \, \text{min}$ Calcium gluconate 10% contains $0.225 \, \text{mmol} \, \text{ml}^{-1}$.
- Bicarbonate 50–$100 \, \text{mmol}$ given over 10–$20 \, \text{min}$. Onset of action is around $5 \, \text{min}$ and lasts up to $2 \, \text{h}$.
- 50% glucose $50 \, \text{ml}$ with 20 units soluble insulin, which will increase cellular uptake of potassium.

- Infusion of a β_2 agonist may also be used to drive potassium into the cells but there is a risk of arrhythmias.
- Ion exchange resins, e.g. calcium resonium can be used orally (15 g, 6-hourly) or rectally (30 g, 12-hourly).

Renal losses of potassium may be increased with the use of a loop diuretic and dialysis can be used to both decrease plasma potassium and correct acidosis.

Further reading

Gennari F. Hypokalemia. *N Engl J Med* 1998; **339**: 451–8.
Halperin M, Kamel K. Potassium. *Lancet* 1998; **352**: 135–40.

Related topics of interest

Adrenal disease (p. 9)
Calcium, magnesium and phosphate (p. 65)
Fluid repacement therapy (p. 156)
Sodium (p. 281)

Psychological aspects of critical care

Jas Soar

The critical care environment can be psychologically stressful for patients, relatives and staff. Inevitably, care focuses on the physical needs of the patient. The psychological, social and spiritual aspects of care are often overlooked. The needs of the family and staff must also be acknowledged and addressed.

Patient problems

Patient problems can be considered as problems associated with the disease resulting in admission, specific aspects unique to the critical care environment and, long-term effects manifesting after discharge.

Problems associated with the disease resulting in admission

Patients may present to the critical care unit with the whole range of organic and functional psychiatric disorders. Distress, anxiety and depression are associated with physical disease. Pathological anxiety and depression are common in those with life-threatening illness or chronic disease. Unpleasant and demanding medical treatments exacerbate depression. Syndromes associated with delirium ('ICU psychosis') have been described in patients after cardiopulmonary bypass and major surgery. Symptoms include disorientation, hallucinations, paranoia, restlessness and combativeness. Drugs, hypoxia and metabolic abnormalities contribute. Psychological impairment usually resolves but can contribute to increased morbidity and mortality, especially in elderly patients.

Careful use of sedation and analgesia is needed to minimise distress. Patients may benefit from treatment with antidepressants. Selective serotonin reuptake inhibitors (SSIRs) are well tolerated in the critically ill. The use of small increments of intravenous haloperidol (0.5–2 mg) is helpful for agitation and delirium. Haloperidol can cause QT interval prolongation with risk of arrhythmia and extra-pyramidal side effects with excessive dosage.

Specific aspects unique to the critical care environment

The high-technology environment of the critical care unit can cause patient fear, anxiety, vulnerability and dependency. Psychological stressors include the following factors:

Physical factors

Exposure to multiple uncomfortable/painful procedures. Preparing and warning the patient (e.g. before suctioning) and appropriate analgesia and sedation for procedures may be beneficial. Noise levels of less than 35 decibels (dB) are required to facilitate restful sleep. This rarely occurs in the critical care environment, where noise levels range from 55–65 dB, with peaks reaching 90 dB. Sudden noises above 80 dB cause arousal from sleep. Alarms, pagers and staff conversation have been rated as highly annoying. Lighting around the clock disrupts normal circadian rhythms. Odours are also troublesome.

Psychological factors

These include loss of privacy and invasion of personal space. Sensory disturbance occurs due to lack of familiar sights and sounds together with an increase in abnormal stimuli. Isolation from friends and family, if visiting is limited, can cause worry.

Sleep disturbance

Sleep disturbance and sleep fragmentation results in disorientation and fatigue. Alterations in the amount of REM and non-REM sleep are detrimental to the patient's medical condition. Non-pharmacological measures should be tried first to promote sleep, including privacy, noise control (ear plugs) and disturbance-free rest periods. Lighting that gives a day–night orientation also helps. Keeping the patient orientated in time and space as well as adequately informed of what is happening is beneficial. Benzodiazepines improve sleep latency and sleep time but may have little effect on sleep architecture.

Long-term effects manifesting after discharge

A large number of patients have little recall of events while on the critical care unit. Lack of sleep, pain, anxiety and noise are common complaints. Physical disability will have an ongoing psychological impact. Many hospitals now have an intensive care follow-up clinic. These clinics have highlighted the post-discharge burden on patient and family. Problems include fatigue, weakness, anxiety, sleep disturbance, sexual problems (reduced libido and impotence), mood swings, memory and concentration difficulties.

A small but significant proportion of patients have recurrent and frightening memories of the critical care unit. For example, up to one third of patients who survive ARDS may develop post-traumatic stress disorder (PTSD). Traumatic events are persistently re-experienced. This may result in terror, guilt, hostility, anxiety and depression. Symptoms may result in significant impairment of daily function. In motor vehicle accident victims, chronic PTSD was related to the severity of trauma, ongoing medical problems, perceived threat, dissociation during the accident, female gender, previous emotional problems and litigation. Education, social support, cognitive therapy and antidepressant drugs may benefit these patients.

Family-related issues

These include anxiety and depression and presence of relatives during resuscitation and invasive procedures.

Anxiety and depression

Relatives visiting patients in the intensive care unit often suffer from symptoms of anxiety or depression. This is associated with patient factors (acute illness, young age), family-related factors (spouse, female, pre-existing psychological problems, overseas descent) and care issues (no regular meetings with staff, absence of dedicated meeting room, contradictions in information provided). This can often be helped by good communication, and counselling from social workers and support staff. Some relatives may need to contact their own doctor if problems persist.

The presence of relatives during resuscitation and invasive procedures

This is controversial, although becoming more widespread. Relatives may wish to be present and there is some benefit from their presence. Relatives can see that everything is being done for their loved one. If the patient dies, it may help their grieving process. To achieve this and to overcome the worries of staff, protocols are needed to ensure that relatives are briefed about what they will see, hear and, possibly, smell. Otherwise, they may find events disturbing and bewildering. A competent member of staff needs to advise the relative and offer support and reassurance. Ideally, the same member of staff should spend some time with them after the proceedings to discuss their reactions and to answer any questions.

Staff issues

The critical care environment can place a physical and emotional burden on staff. Staff 'burnout' and 'compassion fatigue' are recognised risks. Units must ensure welfare, physical and emotional support for their staff. Individuals may benefit from different kinds of support. Many staff prefer and benefit from informal peer support, whereas others may require organised activities such as debriefing or counselling after traumatic events. Trained persons must carry out debriefing and counselling.

References

American website with background information and links on post-traumatic stress disorder: http://www.ncptsd.org/index.html

Brown TM, Boyle MF. ABC of psychological medicine: delirium. *BMJ* 2002; **325**: 644–7.

Cochrane review on the value of debriefing after traumatic events: http://www.update-software.com/abstracts/ab000560.htm

Gill D, Hatcher S. Antidepressants for depression in medical illness (Cochrane Review). In: *The Cochrane Library,* Issue 2. Oxford: Update Software, 2002.

Jones C, Griffiths RD, Humphries GM, Skirrow PM. Memory, delusions and the development of acute PTSD related symptoms after intensive care. *Crit Care Med* 2001; **29**: 573–80.

Lange PM. Family stress in the intensive care unit. *Crit Care Med* 2001; **29(10)**: 2025–6.

Peveler P, Carson A, Rodin G. ABC of psychological medicine: depression in medical patients. *BMJ* 2002; **325**: 149–52.

Related topics of interest

Analgesia in critical care – basic (p. 17)
Analgesia in critical care – advanced (p. 22)
Sedation (p. 270)

Pulmonary aspiration

Andrew Padkin

Pulmonary aspiration is the passage of foreign liquids or solids into the lower respiratory tract. The incidence of aspiration of gastric contents associated with anaesthesia is approximately 3 per 10 000 anaesthetics; however, this complication is responsible for up to 20% of all anaesthetic-related deaths. Mortality associated with aspiration varies widely between 3.8 and 85%, depending on the aspirate (type and volume), the number of pulmonary lobes involved and the patient's underlying clinical condition and treatment.

Predisposing factors

Impaired cough and gag reflexes
1. Decreased conscious level, e.g. overdose, anaesthesia, head injury, meningitis, seizures, metabolic coma, cerebrovascular accident, severe illness.
2. IX and X cranial nerve disease:
   - Brain stem, e.g. motor neurone disease, syringobulbia, polio.
   - Pressure effects/invasion near the jugular foramen, e.g. glomus tumour, nasopharyngeal carcinoma.
   - Demyelination, e.g. Guillain–Barré syndrome, diphtheria.
   - Neuromuscular junction disease, e.g. myasthenia gravis.

Increased risk of vomiting/regurgitation
1. Increased intra-abdominal pressure (pregnancy, bowel obstruction, obesity).
2. Slow gastric emptying (labour, trauma, opiates, alcohol, intra-abdominal sepsis, pyloric stenosis).
3. Abnormal lower oesophageal sphincter (reflux disease, pregnancy, hiatus hernia, presence of nasogastric tube).
4. Abnormal oesophageal anatomy (oesophagectomy, oesophageal stricture, tracheo-oesophageal fistula).
5. Abnormal oesophageal motility (achalasia, scleroderma).

Substances aspirated

Solids
1. Large solids (e.g. meat in adults, peanuts in children) may cause large airway obstruction that is immediately life threatening. These must be removed immediately (e.g. by back blows).
2. Smaller solids (e.g. teeth, peanuts in adults) can cause lower airway obstruction. If partial obstruction occurs, a monophonic wheeze may be heard. Atelectasis

distal to the obstruction may be followed by persistent infection, abscess formation and bronchiectasis. Vegetable matter causes particular problems by producing a localised inflammatory reaction.

Liquids

Non-infected fluids
Sterile acid   Gastric acid causes lung damage within minutes. Injury severity increases with increasing acidity and volume, although critical values for these are difficult to determine. Many authors suggest that a pH <2.5 and volume greater than 25 ml (or $0.4\,ml\,kg^{-1}$) are associated with severe injury, though the evidence for these values is weak.

Four effects may occur early:

1. Laryngospasm.
2. Vagally-mediated bronchospasm.
3. Surfactant dysfunction, leading to patchy atelectasis.
4. Alveolar-capillary breakdown, leading to interstitial oedema and haemorrhagic pulmonary oedema. Following aspiration, lung volume is decreased, pulmonary compliance is decreased, there is an increase in pulmonary vascular resistance and a large intrapulmonary shunt develops. The initial acute inflammatory process usually starts to resolve by 72 h, but may be followed by a fibroproliferative phase.

A prolonged clinical course with the development of ARDS occurs in 15%. Aspiration of acid particulate matter causes the most severe damage.

Non-acidic fluids (e.g. blood, saliva)   Although alveolar damage and acute inflammatory changes are usually less severe, severe hypoxia due to laryngospasm, bronchospasm and surfactant dysfunction may be life threatening.

Infected fluids
Immediate effects are similar to those caused by non-infected fluids. In previously healthy patients, gastric contents are sterile and infection is unusual in the early stages following aspiration. In contrast, the upper gastrointestinal (GI) tract often becomes colonised by Gram-negative aerobes and anaerobes in those who are hospitalised, use antacids or use H_2 antagonists. This is thought to be due to a lack of the normal protective acidic gastric environment. If pulmonary infection develops in these patients following aspiration, it is likely to be due to the above organisms.

Clinical presentation

In acute aspiration there may be soiling of the pharynx or trachea. Dyspnoea, coughing, wheeze and severe hypoxaemia all occur. If large volumes of acid have been aspirated, signs of hypovolaemia may be present. Fever and leucocytosis may occur in the absence of infection.

Diagnosis

Usually clinical, though tracheal suction can be used to detect acid pH. Testing tracheal samples for glucose is unreliable.

CXR may reveal a small solid if it is radiopaque, or simply show distal collapse or consolidation.

Acid aspiration usually leads to diffuse bilateral pulmonary infiltrates. Isolated right upper lobe changes may be seen after supine aspiration, and right middle/lower lobe changes after semi-recumbent aspiration.

Management

Prevention of aspiration of gastric contents is achieved in four ways.

1. Posture. All spontanously breathing unconscious patients should be placed in the recovery position unless contraindicated until airway protection is achieved.

2. Airway protection. Tracheal intubation or tracheostomy provides the best airway protection for patients at risk of aspiration.

3. Reduction of volume of gastric contents. Nasogastric tubes are used for aspiration of gastric contents in those patients with gastric stasis though they impair oesophageal sphincter function.

4. Anaesthesia. Anaesthesia should be planned carefully in those at risk of aspiration. Preoperatively, gastric contents are minimised and neutralised by nasogastric suction or by using a prokinetic drug, an H_2 antagonist or proton pump inhibitor and sodium citrate. Regional anaesthesia may be possible, enabling surgery without compromising the airway. If general anaesthesia is necessary, tracheal intubation should be performed after a rapid sequence induction with cricoid pressure.

Treatment

1. Position. If the airway is not protected and there are no contraindications, position the patient laterally and head down.

2. Airway clearance. Suck out any material from the pharynx. If the patient is intubated, the trachea can be suctioned to clear semi-solid material (liquid disperses quickly). Physiotherapy will aid clearance of the lower airways.

3. Oxygen. Give high-concentration oxygen to maintain oxygen saturation.

4. Tracheal intubation. If the patient is at risk of further aspiration, intubate the trachea.

5. Mechanical ventilation. If mechanical ventilation is required, the use of positive end-expiratory pressure (PEEP) will maintain alveolar recruitment and diminish shunt. It also decreases pulmonary vascular resistance (unless excessive PEEP is used, which causes overdistension).

6. Cardiovascular support. Monitor fluid balance carefully because hypovolaemia is common. Inotropes are often necessary.

7. Bronchodilators. Bronchospasm may be severe; bronchodilators are given although they may not be very effective.

8. Bronchoscopy. Small particles may be removed by flexible fibreoptic bronchoscopy. Lavage is not useful unless the aspirated matter is particulate. Even then only small amounts of saline should be used. Rigid bronchoscopy enables wide-bore suctioning and the passage of large grasping forceps, and is the procedure of choice for the removal of most inhaled objects.

9. Antibiotics. Early treatment with antibiotics should be considered only when infected fluid has been aspirated (e.g. faecal aspiration in bowel obstruction). Secondary bacterial infection occurs in 20–30% and antibiotics should be directed at the responsible organism. Antibiotics with specific anaerobic activity are not routinely necessary; however, they are required in patients with severe periodontal disease, putrid sputum or evidence of lung abscess on CXR.

10. Steroids. Steroids have no proven benefit after aspiration, and may slow pulmonary healing.

Microaspiration

Microaspiration is thought to be a major cause of ventilator-associated pneumonia (VAP). It occurs in intensive care patients when colonised secretions pool in the subglottic area above the tracheal cuff space then leak around the cuff along longitudinal folds in the wall.

Prevention

1. Decreasing the bacterial colonisation of upper GI secretions. H_2-blockers or sucralfate (which appears to be less popular) are used as prophylaxis against upper GI bleeding in critically ill patients. Sucralfate is protective to gastric cells without altering gastric pH, so would be expected to be associated with less upper GI and tracheobronchial colonisation with pathogenic bacteria, and hence fewer episodes of VAP. This has been confirmed in some observational studies. However, a recent large multicentre randomised controlled trial has shown no significant difference in the incidence of VAP in patients treated with ranitidine compared with those treated with sucralfate, with ranitidine providing greater protection against GI bleeding.

2. Decreasing reflux of gastric contents. Providing enteral nutrition by gastrostomy or jejunostomy rather than via a nasogastric tube may decrease the incidence of VAP, although it doesn't completely prevent it.

3. Decreasing the amount of fluid that leaks past the cuff. Nursing intensive care patients semi-recumbent rather than supine decreases microaspiration.

Further reading

Leroy O, Vandenbussche C, Collinier C, *et al.* Community-acquired aspiration pneumonia in intensive care units. Epidemiological and prognosis data. *Am J Respirat Crit Care Med* 1997; **156**: 1922–9.

Lomotan JR, George SS, Brandselter RD. Aspiration pneumonia. Strategies for early recognition and prevention. *Postgrad Med* 1997; **102**: 225–31.

Marik PE. Aspiration pneumonitis and aspiration pneumonia. *N Engl J Med* 2001; **344**: 665–71.

Ng A, Smith G. Gastroesophageal reflux and aspiration of gastric contents in anesthetic practice. *Anesth Analg* 2001; **93**: 494–513.

Related topics of interest

Renal failure – rescue therapy

Aggressive treatment of prerenal failure may avoid the onset of established renal failure and the requirement for renal replacement therapy (RRT). Every factor contributing to prerenal failure must be addressed.

Nephrotoxic drugs

Non-steroidal anti-inflammatory drugs (NSAIDs) inhibit the synthesis of renal prostaglandins that would normally dilate the afferent arterioles. In the presence of low renal blood flow, NSAIDs may cause acute renal failure (ARF). These drugs are contraindicated in patients with impending renal failure. Angiotensin-converting enzyme (ACE) inhibitors are also contraindicated in these patients; they reduce the production of angiotensin-2 that normally constricts the efferent arterioles, thus maintaining glomerular perfusion pressure.

Circulating volume

Fluid loading will tend to reverse many of the physiological mechanisms that maximise fluid retention (e.g. release of aldosterone and antidiuretic hormone). Single, independent central venous pressure (CVP) measurements are poor indicators of intravascular volume; differences in myocardial compliance and venous tone make interpretation very difficult. The dynamic process of assessing the response of the CVP to a fluid challenge (e.g. 200 ml of colloid) is more useful, but high venous tone will still tend to mask hypovolaemia. A low dose nitrate infusion (e.g. glyceryl trinitrate (GTN) $2 \, mg \, h^{-1}$) will reduce venous tone and may reveal hypovolaemia. Simple clinical signs, such as rewarming of the peripheries, will also help to indicate restoration of adequate circulating volume.

Cardiac output and oxygen delivery

If oliguria persists despite adequate circulating volume, an inotrope such as dobutamine can be added to increase cardiac output. A haemoglobin concentration of $>8 \, g \, dl^{-1}$ and appropriate oxygen saturation will help to ensure adequate renal oxygen delivery.

Renal perfusion pressure

Renal blood flow and glomerular filtration rate (GFR) are normally autoregulated over a wide range of mean arterial pressure. However, in the presence of ischaemic acute tubular necrosis (ATN) and/or sepsis, autoregulation may be impaired significantly. Thus, in the critically ill, adequate renal blood flow may depend on achieving the patient's normal premorbid systolic blood pressure. In the presence of an adequate circulating volume and cardiac output, a noradrenaline (norepinephrine) infusion can be titrated to achieve this 'normal' blood pressure. The increase in urine output often seen with this approach may be accounted for by (a) the increase in renal perfusion pressure and (b) the relatively greater increase in arteriolar resistance on the efferent side of the glomerulus in comparison with the afferent side (increasing filtration fraction).

Furosemide

Oxygen tension is particularly low in the outer medulla. At this point, blood flow is slow to maintain the medullary osmotic gradient. The ion pumps in the medullary thick ascending limb of the loop of Henle (mTAL) are high oxygen consumers. Furosemide reduces the activity of the sodium–potassium–chloride co-transporter in the tubular cell, thus reducing oxygen consumption. Animal studies have shown that furosemide increases renal medullary oxygen tension.

Furosemide also stimulates production of vasodilator prostaglandins, thereby increasing afferent arteriolar flow. A bolus of 10 mg of furosemide, followed by an infusion of 1–10 mg h^{-1}, may produce an adequate urine output. Continuous infusion of furosemide may be more effective than bolus injections. Although the use of furosemide in this way undoubtedly enhances urine output and is theoretically sound, there is little evidence that it prevents renal failure. However, the conversion of oliguric renal failure to polyuric renal failure may make the management of fluid balance easier, which might postpone or prevent the need for RRT in some critically ill patients.

Dopamine

A low-dose dopamine infusion (0.5–2 µg kg^{-1} min^{-1}) used to be the most popular treatment for oliguria in the presence of an adequate circulating volume. The increase in renal blood flow was thought to be a specific effect mediated through dopamine receptors. In reality, this dose of dopamine has significant inotropic and chronotropic effects and the increase in renal blood flow is probably secondary to a general increase in cardiac output. There are several risks associated with low-dose dopamine infusions. These include the induction of gut mucosal ischaemia, cardiac arrhythmia, myocardial ischaemia, a decrease in T-cell function and inhibition of virtually all anterior pituitary-dependent hormones in critically ill patients. Like furosemide, dopamine will often induce a diuresis but is not 'protective' against the onset of acute renal failure. As dopamine has potentially harmful effects, in the presence of an adequate circulating volume and appropriate blood pressure, a low-dose furosemide infusion is a more logical choice for the treatment of oliguria.

Fenoldopam

Fenoldopam is a highly selective dopamine type-1 agonist that preferentially dilates the renal and splanchnic vasculature. Some studies have shown that it prevents radio-contrast-induced nephropathy and further research is being undertaken to quantify its potential role in the prevention of acute renal failure in the critically ill.

Acetylcysteine

N-acetylcysteine scavenges reactive oxygen metabolites and there is limited evidence that it reduces the incidence of radiocontrast-induced nephropathy. Its role in the critical care unit has to be determined.

Abdominal compartment syndrome

Intra-abdominal hypertension (>20–25 mmHg) has several causes, including:

- Severe acute pancreatitis.
- Faecal peritonitis.
- Retroperitoneal haematoma (aortic aneurysm, pelvic fracture).
- Intestinal obstruction.
- Postoperative intra-abdominal surgery.
- Patients with multiple injuries and massive fluid resuscitation.

High intra-abdominal pressure (IAP) may cause oliguria by reducing total renal blood flow (increased venous resistance) or by direct compression of renal parenchyma. If other causes of oliguria have been eliminated and the IAP (measured from the bladder) exceeds 20 mmHg, surgical decompression of the abdomen should be considered.

Further reading

Lameire NH, De Vriese AS, Vanholder R. Prevention and nondialytic treatment of acute renal failure. *Curr Opin Crit Care* 2003; **9**: 481–90.

Related topics of interest

Fluid replacement therapy (p. 156)
Renal failure – acute (p. 247)
Renal replacement therapy (p. 251)

Renal failure – acute

There are several definitions for acute renal failure (ARF): 'a recent, reversible or potentially reversible deterioration in renal function' is one of the most practical.

Incidence

Approximately 1% of patients have ARF at the time of admission to hospital. The incidence increases to 5–7% during hospitalisation.

Causes

In most cases ARF is multifactorial but the classification of potential causes encourages a systematic approach to investigation and treatment.

Prerenal

Inadequate perfusion of otherwise normal kidneys:

- Hypovolaemia (haemorrhage, sepsis, gastrointestinal losses, burns, inadequate intake).
- Hypotension (hypovolaemia, cardiac failure, vasodilatation).
- Functional acute renal failure (non-steroidal anti-inflammatory drugs (NSAIDs), hepatorenal syndrome).
- Abdominal compartment syndrome.

Renal

Intrinsic parenchymal renal disease can be classified according to the primary site of injury:

- Acute tubular necrosis (ATN) accounts for 85% of the intrinsic causes of renal failure. The pathophysiology of ATN is complex. The term ATN is a misnomer because microscopic examination of renal biopsy specimens from patients with ARF usually reveals little histological damage. The damage is focal and localised only to certain areas of the nephron. The worst affected area is the straight (S3) segment of the proximal tubule and not the thick ascending limb of Henle's loop as was thought previously. The S3 segment is particularly vulnerable because the inner cortical/outer medullary region in which it lies is relatively hypoxic. S3 cells exposed to either an ischaemic or toxic injury will develop a sublethal injury or will die. Under these circumstances, it was thought that cell death was due to necrosis – a chaotic, unregulated process. However, it is now recognised that these cells may undergo programmed cell death, or apoptosis. Apoptotic cells are removed cleanly by phagocytes and this accounts for the relative lack of histological damage in the presence of ARF. Renal ischaemia can occur despite normal or raised global renal blood flow (e.g. sepsis); this reflects intrarenal redistribution of blood flow away from the outer medulla. Toxins causing ATN include inflammatory mediators, aminoglycosides, paracetamol, heavy metals and myoglobin. Renal ischaemia, caused by a global reduction in blood flow or intrarenal redistribution of blood, and toxic insults act synergistically to invoke ATN. NSAIDs compound the problem by blocking the production of prostaglandin, a substance that offers renal protection during low-flow states.

- Interstitial nephritis accounts for fewer than 10% of the causes of intrinsic ARF. It may be caused by an allergic reaction to a drug or by autoimmune disease, infiltrative diseases (e.g. sarcoidosis) or infection.
- Glomerulonephritis is an infrequent cause of ARF (5%) and may be related to systemic illness such as systemic lupus erythematosus (SLE) or Goodpasture's syndrome.
- Small- or large-vessel renal vascular disease is another cause of ARF. The vascular disorder may be embolic or thrombotic.

Postrenal

Obstruction to both urinary outflow tracts will cause ARF. The obstruction, which can be at any level within the urinary tract, must be detected and resolved quickly. This optimises the likelihood of complete recovery.

- Intrarenal obstruction may be caused by proteins (e.g. haemoglobin, myoglobin) or drugs (e.g. methotrexate).
- Renal pelvis – calculi, tumours or blood clot.
- Ureter – stones, accidental ligation.
- Bladder – prostatic enlargement, bladder tumour.
- Urethra – stricture.

Diagnosis and investigations

History

The patient's history and examination will indicate the likely cause of ARF. The patient's recorded observations may reveal a period of hypovolaemia and/or hypotension. In critical care patients, oliguria ($<0.5\,ml\,kg^{-1}\,min^{-1}$) is usually the first indication of acutely impaired renal function.

Plasma biochemistry

Rising blood urea and creatinine levels, and a metabolic acidosis, with or without hyperkalaemia, confirm the diagnosis. Prerenal factors are excluded by ensuring normovolaemia and a mean arterial pressure within the patient's normal range (see Renal failure – rescue therapy, p. 244).

Exclude urinary outflow obstruction

Urinary outflow obstruction must also be excluded, particularly if the patient is anuric. Check that the urinary catheter is positioned correctly. Ultrasound may reveal a dilated urinary system. Small kidneys indicate a degree of chronic renal disease. If the patient is anuric following any recent surgery that could conceivably involve the renal arteries, renography is indicated.

Urinalysis

Plasma and urine osmolality, urine sodium and protein content and urine microscopy are valuable investigations for ARF. Typical urine findings in prerenal ARF and ATN

Table 14 Typical urine findings in prerenal acute renal failure (ARF) and acute tubular necrosis (ATN)

Parameter	Prerenal ARF	ATN
Urine osmolarity (mosm l^{-1})	>500	<350
Urine sodium (mmol l^{-1})	10–20	>20
Urine urea (mmol l^{-1})	>250	<150
Urine: plasma ratio osmolarity	>1.5	<1.1
Urine: plasma ratio urea	>20	<10
Fractional excretion of sodium	<1%	>1%

are listed in Table 14. In prerenal ARF the tubules attempt to 'restore intravascular volume' by reabsorption of salt and water. Loss of tubular-concentrating ability in intrinsic ARF results in urine and plasma that are iso-osmolar. Urinary sodium concentration is high. Pigmented granular casts are associated with ATN, and red cell casts with glomerulonephritis.

Renal biopsy

Renal biopsy is rarely necessary in the evaluation of ARF. It may be indicated if the history, clinical features and laboratory and radiological investigations have excluded pre- and postrenal causes and an intrinsic cause, other than ATN, is likely.

Rhabdomyolysis

Crush injury, compartment syndrome and burns cause myocyte necrosis, which releases myoglobin, creatine kinase (CK) and other cellular contents. The diagnosis of rhabdomyolysis is made when serum CK exceeds 600 IU l^{-1} or six times the upper limit of normal. Severe rhabdomyolysis is accompanied by a CK level of many thousands. The CK begins to rise 2–12 h after injury and reaches its peak value at 1–3 days.

Rhabdomyolysis causes ARF by three mechanisms:

- Tubular obstruction: myoglobin precipitates in the renal tubules; cast formation is enhanced by acidic conditions and poor washout.
- Tubular damage by oxidant injury: the haem group of myoglobin causes lipid peroxidation, particularly in the proximal tubule.
- Vasoconstriction: movement of fluid into damaged muscle causes hypovolaemia and reduced renal blood flow.

Fluid and, if necessary, inotropes are given to restore cardiac output and renal perfusion. Give intravenous bicarbonate to maintain the urine pH >7.0; alkalinisation will improve tubular washout of myoglobin and prevent lipid peroxidation and renal vasoconstriction. Mannitol has no advantage over volume expansion alone. If these measures fail to prevent ARF, start renal replacement therapy early. Twenty per cent of patients who develop ARF from rhabdomyolysis will die. Survivors will nearly always recover their renal function within 3 months.

Further reading

Singri N, Ahya SN, Levin ML. Acute renal failure. *JAMA* 2003; **289**: 747–51.
Wan L, Bellomo R, Di Giantomasso D, Ronco C. The pathogenesis of septic acute renal failure. *Curr Opin Crit Care* 2003; **9**: 496–502.

Related topics of interest

Renal failure – rescue therapy (p. 244)
Renal replacement therapy (p. 251)

Renal replacement therapy

Indications

In critically ill patients, renal replacement therapy (RRT) is generally started early after the onset of acute renal failure. It simplifies fluid and nutritional management and early use of RRT may improve outcome. Indications for RRT include:

- Fluid overload.
- Hyperkalaemia ($>6.0\,\mathrm{mmol\,l^{-1}}$).
- To create space for drugs and nutrition.
- Creatinine rising $>100\,\mu\mathrm{mol\,l^{-1}day^{-1}}$.
- Creatinine $>300\text{–}600\,\mu\mathrm{mol\,l^{-1}}$.
- Urea rising $>16\text{–}20\,\mathrm{mmol\,l^{-1}\,day^{-1}}$.
- Metabolic acidosis (pH <7.2) caused by renal failure.
- Clearance of dialysable nephrotoxins and other drugs.
- Encephalopathy.

Principles of dialysis and filtration

Dialysis describes the *diffusion* of solute across a semi-permeable membrane and down a concentration gradient. Filtration is the movement of solute by *convection* across a semi-permeable membrane. Dialysis is particularly efficient for small molecules such as K^+, Na^+ and urea. Dialysis can be undertaken by using an artificial membrane or the peritoneum. It can be performed continuously or intermittently. The size of the molecules removed by filtration will depend on the cut-off point (size of the holes) of the artificial membrane. Membranes designed for dialysis or filtration are most commonly made of polyacrylynitrile. This is a biocompatible material and is unlikely to cause significant complement activation.

Renal replacement therapy techniques

Methods of renal replacement include:

- Peritoneal dialysis.
- Intermittent haemodialysis.
- Continuous haemodialysis and/or haemofiltration.

Peritoneal dialysis
In critical care units peritoneal dialysis (PD) has been largely replaced by more advanced techniques of RRT. It may be used where haemodialysis is contraindicated or where the appropriate equipment is unavailable.

Intermittent haemodialysis
Intermittent haemodialysis (IHD) is undertaken rarely in critical care units within the United Kingdom. Continuous techniques (described below) are more widely available and, in the critically ill patient with multiple organ failure, cause less haemodynamic

instablity. Critically ill patients do not tolerate the rapid changes in plasma osmolality and intravascular volume that can occur with IHD. Renal units treating patients with 'single-organ' acute renal failure or chronic renal failure typically use IHD. Many American critical care physicians also prefer to use IHD for managing renal failure in the critical care unit.

Continuous renal replacement therapies
The following techniques are used for continuous RRT in the critical care unit:

- Continuous venovenous haemofiltration (CVVH).
- Continuous venovenous haemodialysis (CVVHD) or haemodiafiltration (CVVDF).

Venous access is obtained with a single, wide-bore, double-lumen cannula placed in the subclavian, internal jugular or femoral vein. A pump delivers blood to the filter. The excellent urea clearance achieved with CVVHDF is sufficient for even the most catabolic patients. Modern machines enable control of blood, dialysate, filtrate and replacement fluid flows, thus providing good control of the patient's fluid balance. The rate of fluid replacement is determined by the desired fluid balance. Many critical care physicians use the CVVH mode alone. This produces adequate urea and creatinine clearance in most patients and omission of the dialysis mode reduces the risk of significant intravascular fluid shifts.

In a recent study, critically ill patients with acute renal failure were randomly assigned to CVVH at $20 \, \mathrm{ml \, kg^{-1} h^{-1}}$, $35 \, \mathrm{ml \, kg^{-1} h^{-1}}$ or $45 \, \mathrm{ml \, kg^{-1} h^{-1}}$. Survival in the group assigned to $20 \, \mathrm{ml \, kg^{-1} h^{-1}}$ was significantly lower than the other two groups and there was no difference in survival between the $35 \, \mathrm{ml \, kg^{-1} h^{-1}}$ and the $45 \, \mathrm{ml \, kg^{-1} h^{-1}}$ groups. Based on this study, it has become common practice to undertake CVVH using $35 \, \mathrm{ml \, kg^{-1} h^{-1}}$. Recent evidence suggests that CVVH does not remove inflammatory mediators in clinically significant quantities.

Replacement fluid

Bicarbonate is unstable in solution and many replacement fluids contain either lactate or acetate instead of bicarbonate. In the presence of significant liver dysfunction, lactate or acetate may not be metabolised adequately and the use of standard replacement fluids may cause an increasing metabolic acidosis. Bicarbonate replacement solutions are now available and are used when there is any doubt about the patient's capacity to metabolise lactate. If prepared immediately before use, the bicarbonate will remain in solution for about $12 \, \mathrm{h}$.

Anticoagulation

Unless the patient has a significant coagulopathy, anticoagulant therapy is necessary to prevent clotting of the filter and extracorporeal circuit. Following a bolus of 3000 units, a heparin infusion is started at $10 \, \mathrm{U \, kg^{-1} h^{-1}}$ and adjusted to maintain an APTT at 1.5–2 times the control value. In those few patients who develop heparin-induced thrombocytopenia and in other high-risk cases, epoprostenol ($2.5–5 \, \mathrm{ng \, kg^{-1} min^{-1}}$), danaparoid or citrate infusions are alternatives.

Nutrition

Renal replacement therapy enables critically ill patients to receive protein and calories in quantities required by their catabolic state. Wherever possible, this is given by the enteral route. A significant quantity of non-urea nitrogen is lost across the filter; thus it may be appropriate to increase the nitrogen content of feeds given to patients receiving RRT.

Diuretic phase

The oliguric or anuric phase of ATN lasts typically for 2–4 weeks, although there is considerable variation in this period. The return of renal function presents with a diuresis. At this stage urine output is high, but renal function may still be poor. A rising urea and creatinine may indicate the need for a few more days of RRT.

Further reading

Ronco C, Bellomo R, Homel P, *et al*. Effects of different doses in continuous veno-venous haemofiltration on outcomes of acute renal failure: a prospective randomised controlled trial. *Lancet* 2000; **355**: 26–30.

Van Biesen W, Vanholder R, Lameire N. Dialysis strategies in critically ill acute renal failure patients. *Curr Opin Crit Care* 2003; **9**: 491–5.

Related topics of interest

Renal failure – rescue therapy (p. 244)
Renal failure – acute (p. 247)

Respiratory support – non-invasive techniques

Jas Soar

Impairment of pulmonary gas exchange causes hypoxaemia with or without hypercarbia. Non-invasive respiratory support techniques aim to produce adequate oxygenation and acceptable carbon dioxide excretion. Invasive methods of respiratory support, which require tracheal intubation, are covered elsewhere. Respiratory failure can be defined as type I or type II.

Acute hypoxaemic (type I) respiratory failure

This is the commonest form of respiratory failure and is associated with virtually all acute diseases of the lung, which generally involve fluid filling or collapse of alveoli.

Hypoxaemia is due ventilation/perfusion (V/Q) mismatch, true shunt (areas of zero V/Q) or, most often, a combination of the two. True shunt occurs when alveoli are completely collapsed, totally consolidated or filled with oedema fluid. V/Q mismatch is caused by regional variations in compliance and perfusion abnormalities.

Ventilatory (type II) respiratory failure

Inadequate alveolar ventilation (ventilatory failure) with resultant hypercarbia may be due to:

- Central nervous system depression: drugs, head injury, stroke, infection.
- Neuromuscular disease: Guillain–Barré syndrome, myasthenia gravis, spinal trauma.
- Chest wall/pleural disease: pneumothorax, flail chest, pleural effusion.
- Upper airway obstruction: laryngeal oedema, infection, foreign body.
- Small airway disorders: asthma, chronic obstructive pulmonary disease (COPD).
- Failure to compensate for increased carbon dioxide production.
- Failure to compensate for an increase in dead space and rebreathing.
- A combination of these factors.

In the patient breathing room air, hypoventilation will cause hypoxaemia (alveolar gas equation). This is easily corrected by increasing fractional inspired oxygen concentration (FiO_2). In the patient breathing air, pulse oximetry is a fair monitor of alveolar ventilation; when oxygen is being given, pulse oximetry will not reflect hypoventilation and arterial blood gas analysis is required to assess carbon dioxide tension ($PaCO_2$) and pH. An increase in dead space, either physiological dead space or dead space due to inappropriate breathing system design, will result in hypercarbia if the patient is unable to increase minute ventilation to compensate. It is important to consider excessive equipment dead space when hypercarbia occurs in a patient receiving any form of respiratory support.

Assessment

Acute respiratory failure causes life-threatening derangements in arterial blood gases and acid–base status, whereas the effects of chronic respiratory failure are often less dramatic and not as readily apparent. Shortness of breath (dyspnoea) often accompanies respiratory failure. An increase in respiratory rate (tachypnoea) is a good indicator of critical illness. Once respiratory failure is suspected on clinical grounds, an arterial blood gas analysis will confirm the diagnosis and assist in the distinction between acute and chronic forms. This helps to assess the severity of respiratory failure and guide management. Visible cyanosis is present when the concentration of deoxygenated haemoglobin in the capillaries or tissues is at least $5\,g\,dl^{-1}$. Confusion and somnolence may occur in respiratory failure. Myoclonus and seizures may occur with severe hypoxaemia. Polycythaemia is a complication of long-standing hypoxaemia.

Simple measures to improve respiratory function

Prevention of respiratory complications is important. Particular groups of patients at high risk include those with known respiratory disease, depressed level of consciousness, impaired cough, chest trauma and postoperative upper abdominal and thoracic surgery. Attention should be directed to:

1. **Treating the underlying condition.** In practice, there may be difficulties in identifying underlying pathology. For example, in theory, differentiating infection from heart failure should be easy but in practice it can be very difficult. Empirical treatment in these situations may be justifiable.

2. **Airway opening manoeuvres.** Airway obstruction may be subtle and must always be corrected.

3. **Posture.** Sitting the patient up reduces the weight of the abdominal contents on the diaphragm, increases functional residual capacity (FRC), reduces the central blood volume, improves ventilation and reduces left ventricular diastolic pressure. Early mobilisation and sitting out in a chair will help prevent atelectasis. One exception to this is the quadriplegic patient, in whom ventilation is improved by a supine or slightly head-down position.

4. **Analgesia.** Pain after thoracic or abdominal surgery or trauma inhibits diaphragmatic movement, deep breathing and sighing resulting in a reduced FRC and lung collapse. Inhibition of coughing leads to sputum retention. Treat pain aggressively with a multiple modality approach using paracetamol, opioids, non-steroidal anti-inflammatory drugs (NSAIDs) and neural blockade as appropriate.

5. **Physiotherapy.** Physiotherapy is an important part of respiratory support. Deep

breathing exercises, particularly in conjunction with incentive spirometry, improve lung expansion and FRC. Coughing improves sputum clearance.

6. Humidification. Humidification with oxygen therapy will preserve mucociliary clearance, reduce viscosity of secretions and reduce collapse and infection.

7. Infection control. This should be scrupulous to reduce the chances of cross-infection and nosocomial pneumonia.

Oxygen therapy

Hypoxic patients should be given supplementary oxygen. Titrate the inspired concentration (FiO_2) to normalise the patient's oxygen saturation. In some patients with severe COPD, giving oxygen may reverse hypoxic pulmonary vasoconstriction and increases V/Q mismatch. The subsequent increase in dead space may then cause hypercarbia. This mechanism, and not the removal of 'hypoxic drive', explains why some COPD patients become progressively hypercarbic with high-concentration oxygen.

Variable performance devices

These devices comprise the facemask (e.g. 'MC' mask, 'Hudson' mask) and nasal prongs. They do not deliver a constant FiO_2. Most oxygen delivery systems enable a maximum flow of $15\,l\,min^{-1}$. The patient's peak inspiratory flow may reach more than $30\,l\,min^{-1}$, even during quiet breathing. Thus, a variable amount of room air is inspired along with the delivered oxygen.

In the acutely dyspnoeic patient, peak inspiratory flow may be many times that of the normal subject and the actual FiO_2 will be lower and even less predictable. Despite this, these devices are safe as long as oxygenation is being monitored. They have the advantage of being simple and inexpensive.

Nasal prongs are well tolerated and do not interfere with eating and drinking. They are not as effective in mouth-breathing patients. A flow of more than $4\,l\,min^{-1}$ is uncomfortable.

Fixed performance devices

A constant FiO_2 can be achieved by delivering the air/oxygen mixture at flows that exceed the patient's peak inspiratory flow, or by providing a reservoir bag of gas mixture from which the patient breathes. These devices may not perform as expected in the presence of high peak inspiratory flows or abnormal breathing patterns.

The Venturi mask uses the Bernoulli principle: a moving gas has a lower pressure than stationary gas. Oxygen is forced through a small orifice, producing a high-velocity jet which 'sucks' ambient air into the entrainment chamber. The volume of air entrained, and thus the FiO_2, is a fixed function of the oxygen flow and the characteristics of the Venturi.

The Ventimask has separate Venturis for each FiO_2 and the correct oxygen flow must be given. Other systems employ a fixed Venturi but with a variable aperture to regulate air intake. Typically, to achieve an FIO_2 of 0.6, the oxygen flow is set at $15 \, l \, min^{-1}$ and the total gas mixture flow is $30 \, l \, min^{-1}$, which exceeds peak inspiratory flow for the normal patient.

The 'reservoir' mask uses a collapsible bag into which high-flow fresh oxygen is delivered and from which the patient inspires. Valves prevent inspiration from ambient air and prevent expiration into the reservoir bag. The system is designed to provide as high a FIO_2 as possible. In practice, there is inspiratory leakage of ambient air and thus a FIO_2 of 1.0 cannot be achieved.

Continuous positive airway pressure

Continuous positive airway pressure (CPAP) is indicated in any patient with hypoxia unresponsive to simple methods of oxygen delivery. Failure of alveolar ventilation may also be an indication for CPAP if improvement in compliance and reduction in the work of breathing improve alveolar ventilation significantly. Patients with profound hypoventilation require mechanical ventilation. CPAP does not benefit the apnoeic patient and is often inappropriate in patients with reduced consciousness.

Advantages of CPAP

1. Increase in FRC. A low FRC causes atelectasis and lung collapse, leading to V/Q mismatch and reduced pulmonary compliance with increased airway resistance, which increases the work of breathing. Restoration of a normal FRC will improve oxygenation and reduce the work of breathing.

2. Reopening closed alveoli (recruitment). This occurs as part of the general improvement in FRC.

3. Reduction in left ventricular transmural pressure. This is of value in left ventricular failure and may be the main way in which CPAP improves oxygenation in acute cardiogenic oedema. CPAP does not necessarily drive pulmonary oedema fluid back into the circulation and total lung water may not change despite clinical improvement.

4. Reducing threshold work. In patients experiencing auto-PEEP or dynamic hyperinflation, the inspiratory muscles have to work to drop the alveolar pressure from its positive, end-expiratory value to less than the upper airway pressure (normally zero) before inspiratory gas flow occurs. This is termed threshold work and may be significant. By increasing the airway pressure, CPAP reduces the work required to initiate inspiratory flow.

5. Airway splinting. CPAP is a specific treatment for obstructive sleep apnoea and is often of value in patients with temporary airway problems.

6. Delivery of high FIO_2. Because CPAP systems are closed, with no rebreathing, the chosen inspired oxygen concentration can be delivered reliably, up to and including 100% oxygen.

Adverse effects of CPAP

1. Hypotension. An increase in intrathoracic pressure reduces right ventricular end-diastolic volume and can precipitate hypotension in the presence of hypovolaemia.

2. Barotrauma. As with any form of pressure therapy, overinflation and gas trapping are possible, although frank barotrauma is rare.

3. Discomfort. Patients frequently find the CPAP mask uncomfortable and claustrophobic; patient refusal of mask CPAP is common.

4. Gastric distension. When CPAP is delivered by facemask, gastric inflation can occur. Although this is an indication for gastric decompression, prophylactic placement of a nasogastric tube is not required in every patient.

5. Pulmonary aspiration. Vomiting or regurgitation into a tight-fitting CPAP mask may result in massive aspiration.

6. Pressure necrosis. This may be helped by the use of a hydrocolloid or similar dressing placed over vulnerable areas such as the bridge of the nose.

When used in the treatment of obstructive sleep apnoea, a nasal mask is often effective and is better tolerated by the patient. In patients with manifest respiratory failure, a full facemask is usually necessary.

Airway pressure is kept at a specified level (typically 5–15 cmH$_2$O) throughout the respiratory cycle of spontaneously breathing patients. This requires inspiratory gas at flows in excess of the patient's maximal inspiratory flow capacity and a threshold resistor in the expiratory limb of the breathing system. Check the continuity of the positive pressure by examining the expiratory valve; it should stay open throughout the respiratory cycle. An alternative, but less efficient, method for providing CPAP utilises a pressurised reservoir of fresh gas such as a spring-loaded concertina-style reservoir bag.

Non-invasive ventilation

Non-invasive ventilation (NIV) via a facemask, nasal mask or helmet mask can be used instead of conventional ventilation via a tracheal tube. The technique and problems are similar to those described for CPAP. The indications and timing for NIV include:

- Prevent the need for tracheal intubation and invasive ventilation in acute respiratory failure.
- Alternative to tracheal intubation and conventional ventilation in established respiratory failure.
- Weaning tool in resolving respiratory failure.
- Prevention of re-intubation of trachea after weaning from conventional ventilation.

Several studies have shown a benefit of NIV in acute exacerbations of COPD.

There is also increasing evidence that NIV may be useful in patients with other causes of acute respiratory failure.

Non-invasive ventilation augments tidal volume by sensing inspiratory effort and providing pressure support to the patient. When flow stops, the pressure returns to the preset CPAP level. This results in a decrease in respiratory rate, decreased work of breathing improved alveolar ventilation and possible avoidance of tracheal intubation. However, NIV has limitations and is not successful in every patient. Patient comfort and compliance are critical for success.

Non-invasive ventilation can be provided by conventional ventilators and by simpler, specifically designed, ventilators. The preferred mode is CPAP with pressure support. Pressure support ventilation minimises peak inspiratory mask pressure and air leakage, and is better tolerated. It may be necessary to try several masks to provide effective ventilation that is comfortable for the patient. The level of medical and nursing care required initially to establish and maintain NIV is often much higher than required for conventional ventilation.

The benefits of avoiding the need for tracheal intubation include:

- Lower incidence of ventilator-associated pneumonia.
- Avoidance of sedative drugs.
- Allows patient to talk.

Further reading

Guidelines on non-invasive ventilation in acute respiratory failure. British Thoracic Society Standards of Care Committee. *Thorax* 2002; **57**: 192–211. Available on-line at:
http://www.brit-thoracic.org.uk/pdf/NIV.pdf

Lightowler JV, Wedzicha JA, Elliott MW. Non-invasive positive pressure ventilation to treat respiratory failure resulting from exacerbations of chronic obstructive pulmonary disease: Cochrane systematic review and meta-analysis. *BMJ* 2003; **326**: 185.

Mehta S, Hill NS. Noninvasive ventilation. *Am J Respir Crit Care Med* 2001; **163(2)**: 540–77. Available on-line at:
http://ajrccm.atsjournals.org/cgi/content/full/163/2/540

Thomson AJ, Webb DJ, Maxwell SR, Grant IS. Oxygen therapy in acute medical care. *BMJ* 2002; **324**: 1406–7.

Related topics of interest

Arterial blood gases – analysis (p. 31)
Chronic obstructive pulmonary disease (p. 114)
Respiratory support – invasive (p. 260)
Tracheal intubation (p. xx)
Tracheostomy (p. 307)
Weaning from ventilation (p. 331)

Respiratory support – invasive

Stephen Fletcher

The provision of respiratory support by positive pressure ventilation is a core function of the critical care unit. As ventilator technology has progressed, new, and often more complex, modes of ventilation have been developed. Using the equipment available, and in the light of current knowledge, the clinician must attempt to select the safest and most appropriate mode of ventilation for each patient.

Indications for mechanical ventilation

Despite didactic lists of indications for ventilation and trigger values of PaO_2 and $PaCO_2$, in practice, the combination of respiratory failure, patient fatigue and conscious level dictate the need for mechanical ventilation.

Complications of mechanical ventilation

Although mechanical ventilation often improves oxygenation and carbon dioxide removal, it has several adverse effects:

- The increase in pleural pressure reduces right ventricular diastolic volume and cardiac output, and therefore causes hypotension. Thus, tissue oxygen delivery may fall despite an increase in red blood cell oxygen content. Transmission of airway pressure to the pleural space depends on lung and chest wall compliance. In the presence of low lung compliance (e.g. ARDS) there is little transmission. There is increased pressure transmission in patients with low chest wall compliance (e.g. COPD, abdominal distension); thus, these patients sustain significant cardiovascular impairment from positive pressure ventilation.
- High airway pressures, particularly when transmitted to the distal airways can cause barotrauma. Peak pressure may be a poor indicator of risk of barotrauma. End-inspiratory plateau pressure reflects alveolar pressure and may be a better indicator of risk of barotrauma. Changes in alveolar volume are dependent on the transpulmonary pressure; in the presence of low chest wall compliance, a high inspiratory plateau pressure may be necessary to produce an adequate tidal volume. Pulmonary damage is related more closely to changes in alveolar volume, which cause high shear forces between open and closed lung units and loss of surfactant ('volutrauma'). Alveolar overdistension and subsequent disruption will result in pneumomediastinum and pneumothorax. Volutrauma will also cause pulmonary interstitial oedema.

Recent trends in ventilatory techniques have emphasised the importance of reducing distal airway pressure by encouraging the patient to maintain some spontaneous respiratory effort while gaining a degree of assistance from the ventilator. Keeping the alveoli open and eliminating large swings in alveolar pressure reduces shear forces and limits parenchymal damage.

Modes of ventilation

Mechanical ventilation can be pressure-targeted ('pressure control') or flow-controlled volume-cycled ('volume control'). The addition of positive end-expiratory pressure (PEEP) can improve oxygenation by preventing alveolar collapse. Excessive PEEP will compromise venous return and may cause hypotension.

Volume-controlled ventilation

Standard volume-controlled mechanical ventilation is the most unsophisticated mode. Breaths are delivered at a preselected rate and volume. Lung compliance determines the airway pressures generated. The main limitation of this mode is that it does not enable any contribution from the patient. Volume-targeted modes provide a preset volume unless a specified pressure limit is exceeded. Depending on the precise ventilator, the clinician may select either tidal volume and flow delivery pattern or flow delivery pattern and minimum minute ventilation. Older ventilators provided only a constant flow. A decelerating flow will improve distribution of ventilation to the lungs.

Pressure-controlled ventilation

Inspiratory pressure is limited to a level selected by the clinician, while inspiratory flow will vary with the resistance and compliance of the patient's respiratory system. Tidal volume depends on the inspiratory flow rate and inspiratory time. The decelerating flow pattern reduces peak airway pressure but mean airway pressure is increased. Oxygenation can be enhanced dramatically by prolonging inspiratory time. Inverse ratio ventilation is defined by an I:E ratio greater than 1:1 and can be used in conjunction with volume controlled or pressure controlled modes. The longer inspiratory time reduces peak airway pressures. The short expiratory time will not enable complete lung deflation, and there may be a significant increase in end-expiratory alveolar pressure (auto-PEEP or intrinsic-PEEP ($PEEP_i$)) even when external PEEP is zero. Mean airway pressure is increased. High $PEEP_i$ may cause overdistension of the lung, and will impair venous return and reduce cardiac output.

Assisted mechanical ventilation

During mechanically assisted ventilation, inspiration is initiated by the patient and then supplemented by the ventilator. Assisted modes enable much better ventilator–patient synchrony and reduce respiratory muscle atrophy. This enhances patient cooperation and should eliminate the need for heavy sedation. Older ventilators have pressure triggers, which require the patient to generate negative pressure below the set level of end-expiratory pressure to initiate the machine's inspiratory phase. Modern ventilators have much improved, sensitive, flow triggers, which will enable initiation of the inspiratory phase without a negative-pressure deflection.

The patient-initiated breaths can be pressure supported (to a predetermined peak inspiratory pressure) or volume supported (to a predetermined tidal volume). During pressure support ventilation (PSV), inspiration ends when the inspiratory flow reaches a threshold value (e.g. 25% of peak flow), which theoretically coincides with the end of the inspiratory muscle effort. This method of cycling is one of the most comfortable for the patient. The level of pressure support is adjusted to enable the patient's respiratory rate to be between 25 and 30 breaths min^{-1}.

Synchronised intermittent mandatory ventilation (SIMV) forces a number of mandatory breaths (to a preset tidal volume or pressure) in addition to the patient's own efforts. The mandatory breaths are synchronised to the patient's own inspiratory effort. SIMV ensures a minimum minute volume but there may be substantial variation in tidal volume between the mandatory breaths and the patient's unassisted breaths.

Strategies for mechanical ventilation

When initiating mechanical ventilation, typical settings might be:

PEEP	5 cmH$_2$O
Tidal volume (VC mode)	6–8 ml kg^{-1} predicted body weight
Inspiratory pressure (PC mode)	20 cmH$_2$O (15 above PEEP)
Frequency	10–15 min^{-1}
I:E ratio	1:2
Pressure trigger	−1 to −3 cmH$_2$O
Flow trigger	1–2 l min^{-1}
Pressure support	20 cmH$_2$O (15 above PEEP)

These settings are titrated against the patient's PaO_2 and $PaCO_2$ and comfort. Carbon dioxide elimination can be improved by increasing the tidal volume (or peak pressure) or by increasing the respiratory rate. Oxygenation of arterial blood can be improved by increasing fractional inspired oxygen concentration (FIO_2), increasing external PEEP, by prolonging the inspiratory time or by recruiting collapsed lung units (e.g. prone ventilation). Prolonging the inspiratory time will raise mean airway pressure and create PEEP$_i$. Prolonged exposure to an $FIO_2 > 0.5$–0.6 may cause pulmonary oxygen toxicity and it may be better to increase PEEP and/or prolong the inspiratory time once this concentration is required. The optimum level of PEEP in relation to the FIO_2 has yet to be determined. It is not necessary to achieve 'normal' arterial blood gases; in the absence of lactic acidosis or a marked base deficit, a PaO_2 of 8 kPa or an SaO_2 of 88% may be adequate. Use a tidal volume of 6–8 ml kg^{-1} predicted body weight. Where possible, inspiratory plateau pressure should be limited to < 35 cmH$_2$O (higher pressures are acceptable if the chest wall compliance is low). This should reduce overdistension of relatively compliant areas of lung. This protective ventilation strategy may cause hypercarbia. If renal function is adequate, the rising $PaCO_2$ will be compensated adequately and the pH will remain near normal. In patients with ARDS, ventilation with low tidal volumes (6–8 ml kg^{-1} predicted body weight) improves survival compared with ventilation using tidal volumes of 12 ml kg^{-1}.

Adjuncts to mechanical ventilation

Prone ventilation

In ARDS, the lung comprises discrete healthy and diseased portions. Dependent areas become consolidated, causing a large V/Q mismatch. Placing the ventilated patient prone improves the distribution of ventilation and improves V/Q matching. In practice, around 60% of patients will show improvement in oxygenation. This improvement may be sustained by changing periodically from front to back. It is common practice to leave the patient prone for periods of up to 20 h. The main disadvantage of prone positioning is the likelihood of tube and catheter displacement, difficulty nursing and pressure effects on the face. A prospective randomised controlled trial in patients with acute respiratory failure demonstrated that prone ventilation improved oxygenation compared with conventional ventilation but did not improve survival.

Nitric oxide (NO)

In ARDS, NO causes vasodilatation in ventilated lung areas, secondarily reducing perfusion to poorly ventilated regions. V/Q matching improves and oxygenation increases in 60–70% of patients. Use of NO does not improve outcome from ARDS and its use in the treatment of adults is now uncommon.

Epoprostenol (PGI$_2$)

Nebulised epoprostenol 2–10 ng kg^{-1} min^{-1} will improve oxygenation as effectively as NO and is easier to monitor and deliver. It may be useful as a means of improving oxygenation in patients unresponsive to prone ventilation.

Specialist modes of ventilation

High-frequency ventilation

There are three modes of high-frequency ventilation:

- High-frequency ventilation (HFV). Although some conventional ventilators can achieve the frequency that defines HFV (60–120 breaths min^{-1}), this mode is rarely used.
- High-frequency oscillation ventilation (HFOV). Until recently, most of the clinical experience with this mode had been obtained in small children. A diaphragm oscillating at 3–20 Hz (3–9 Hz in adults) induces CO$_2$ elimination and a system of CPAP provides the oxygenation. In theory, HFOV is ideal for lung-protective ventilation; peak airway pressures are reduced, mean airway pressure is increased and lung volume is maintained throughout the respiratory cycle. A recent prospective randomised clinical trial in adults with ARDS demonstrated improved oxygenation using HFOV compared with conventional ventilation but no difference in mortality.
- High-frequency jet ventilation (HFJV). Jet ventilation requires both a special ventilator and a specific design of tracheal tube. High-pressure gas (1–2 bar) is directed into the distal trachea at frequencies of 1–5 Hz. A T-piece system attached to the tracheal tube provides the desired inspiratory gas mixture (termed the bias flow). Altering the bias flow controls CO$_2$ elimination. Tidal volumes are usually

unmeasurable; gas exchange occurs via poorly defined mechanisms thought to include facilitated diffusion.

In comparison with conventional ventilation, none of these modes has increased survival in adults. Difficulty in humidifying inspired gases, barotrauma and other technical problems limit the usefulness of HFV.

Independent lung ventilation

The lungs of patients with severe asymmetric lung disease have marked differences in compliance, causing unevenly distributed ventilation. By placing a double-lumen endobronchial tube and attaching two ventilators, one to each lumen, it is possible to optimise the ventilation settings for each lung individually. The endobronchial tube can be difficult to position initially, and later can migrate out of position. The relatively narrow lumina of the double-lumen tube can make aspiration or suction difficult.

Tracheal gas insufflation (TGI)

The simple act of infusing oxygen by catheter into the airway at the level of the carina improves oxygenation (partly by simply increasing the mean FIO_2) and CO_2 elimination. The main benefit comes from an effective reduction in dead space.

Cuirass ventilation

The airtight placement of a rigid shell on the anterior thorax enables ventilation by negative pressure. The Hayek oscillator enables very high-frequency cuirass ventilation. Although there are theoretical advantages, including haemodynamic stability and improved sputum clearance, in practice, the cuirass systems are rarely used.

Partial liquid ventilation (PLV)

Perfluorocarbon solutions, such as Perflubron, have a high solubility for oxygen. In PLV these solutions are instilled into the lungs until a meniscus is seen in the tracheal tube. Oxygenation improves by a combination of improved distribution of perfusion (a function of the solution's weight) and improved alveolar stability. The technique remains experimental.

Extracorporeal CO_2 removal (ECCO$_2$R)

ECCO$_2$R is a modification of full extracorporeal membrane oxygenation (ECMO). The lower extracorporeal blood flow enables smaller vascular catheters to be used while still maintaining high gas flows across the membrane. This optimises CO_2 removal but oxygenation is still partly dependent on the lungs. Low-frequency ventilation enables the lungs to 'rest'. Although these extracorporeal techniques are undoubtedly beneficial in neonates, their contribution to the management of adult ARDS is controversial. The only prospective randomised trial completed to date shows no improvement in outcome in comparison with conventional respiratory support. Another trial is ongoing.

Further reading

Malarkkan N, Snook NJ, Lumb AB. New aspects of ventilation in acute lung injury. *Anaesthesia* 2003; **58**: 647–67.

The Acute Respiratory Distress Syndrome Network. Ventilation with lower tidal volumes as compared with traditional tidal volumes for acute lung injury and the acute respiratory distress syndrome. *N Engl J Med* 2000; **342**: 1301–8.

Tobin MJ. Advances in mechanical ventilation. *N Engl J Med* 2001; **344**: 1986–96.

Related topics of interest

Scoring systems

Data collected in the critical care unit can facilitate research and quality assurance. Severity of illness scoring systems enable these data to be adjusted for case mix. Scoring systems can provide:

- Case-mix adjustment for evaluative research.
- A tool for comparative audit.
- A mechanism to decide resource allocation.
- An aid for the clinical management of patients.

Scoring systems used in the critical care unit are either specific or generic and they may be either anatomical or physiological. Anatomical scoring systems assess the extent of injury (e.g. abbreviated injury score, injury severity score), whereas physiological systems assess the impact of injury on function (e.g. Glasgow Coma Scale (GCS)).

Scoring system development

Patient variables that influence survival are collected either by consensus or by statistical analysis. A scoring model is developed from a large cohort of patients and then validated on another cohort. The discrimination of the model describes how well it distinguishes between survivors and non-survivors. Calibration describes how closely predictions correlate with actual outcome across the spectrum of risk.

Glasgow Coma Scale

The GCS was introduced in 1974 as a means of quantifying the neurological status of head-injured patients. Conscious level is assessed by eye opening and verbal and motor responses. The assessment is easily repeatable and can be used for continuous monitoring of the patient's neurological status. The GCS is also an indicator of outcome.

The maximum score is 15 and is calculated in adult patients according to the responses in Table 15. In the unconscious patient, motor response is elicited by applying pressure to the superior orbital rim; localisation is then defined as raising of the patient's hand above shoulder level. In young children and babies the responses are defined differently. The minimum score is 3 and coma is defined as GCS of 8 or less.

Table 15 Glasgow Coma Scale

Score	Eye opening	Verbal response	Motor response
6	–	–	Obeys commands
5	–	Orientated	Localises to pain
4	Spontaneous	Confused	Normal flexion to pain
3	To speech	Inappropriate	Abnormal flexion to pain
2	To pain	Incomprehensible	Extends to pain
1	None	None	None

Injury Severity Score – ISS

The Injury Severity Score (ISS) is derived from the Abbreviated Injury Scale (AIS), which assigns a score from 0 (no injury) to 6 (fatal injury) for over 1200 injuries. The body is divided into six regions:

- Head and neck.
- Abdomen and pelvic contents.
- Bony pelvis and limbs.
- Face.
- Chest.
- Body surface area.

The ISS is calculated by individually squaring and then summing the AIS values for the three most severely injured body regions. The maximum value possible is $3 \times 5^2 = 75$. An AIS of 6 is automatically assigned an ISS of 75. The ISS can be used to predict prognosis in individual patients, and mortality in cohorts of trauma patients. The new ISS (NISS) has been developed from the ISS. It enables more than one injury to be included from a single body region and may predict outcome more accurately.

Therapeutic Intervention Scoring System – TISS

TISS is a method of measuring sickness severity of critically ill patients based on the type and amount of treatment received. It has both clinical and administrative applications:

- Assessing severity of illness.
- Determining resource requirements (nursing ratios, number of critical care beds).
- Assessing use of critical care facilities and function.

Unfortunately, TISS is not standardised and score allocations vary in different hospitals. Daily data are collected from every patient on 76 possible clinical interventions. Ideally, data are collected at the same time(s) each day and by the same observer. Each intervention is rated from 1 to 4 points and points are awarded only for the highest-scoring intervention where several related interventions have been undertaken in the assessment period.

Based on the TISS score, four classes of patients are recognised:

Class I	< 10 points	does not require critical care
Class II	10–19 points	1:2 nurse:patient ratio
Class III	20–39 points	1 critical care nurse
Class IV	> 40 points	1:1 nurse:patient ratio (+ more nursing assistance)

TISS can provide an estimate of the cost of an episode of care. The total cost of running the unit is divided by the total number of TISS points allocated. A typical figure is around £25 per TISS point. A simplified version based on 28 therapeutic activities (TISS 28) has been published.

Measuring severity by patient characteristics and physiological measurements

Examples of these systems include Acute Physiology and Chronic Health Evaluation (APACHE II and APACHE III), the Simplified Acute Physiology Score (SAPS I and SAPS II) and Mortality Probability Models (MPM II).

APACHE II is the system in most common use in the UK. It was developed in 1985 from a database of 5815 admissions to 13 critical care units in the United States. The worst values of 12 physiological variables in the first 24 h after admission to the critical care unit are used to derive an Acute Physiology Score (APS):

- Temperature.
- Mean arterial pressure.
- Heart rate.
- Respiratory rate.
- Oxygenation.
- Arterial pH.
- Serum sodium.
- Serum potassium.
- Serum creatinine.
- Haematocrit.
- White cell count.
- GCS.

Points are added for age and for chronic health or immunosupression in the 6 months before admission. Age points are assigned as follows:

< 44 years	0
45–54 years	2
55–64 years	3
65–74 years	5
> 75 years	6

Non-operative or emergency postoperative care scores an additional 5 points; elective postoperative scores 2 points. Possible APACHE II scores range from 0 to 71 and the risk of hospital death increases with increasing score. The probability of death is calculated by entering the APACHE II score into an equation that includes a weighting factor for the diagnostic category. APACHE III uses 17 physiological variables, co-morbidity and age to produce an APS. However, its predictive equation is not in the public domain.

The standardised mortality ratio (SMR) is the ratio of observed deaths in the cohort to the number of deaths predicted by a scoring system. An SMR greater than 1 implies excess mortality. The SMR should reflect the performance of a critical care unit.

Other methods to measure severity and response to treatment have focused on sequential assessments of organ dysfunction and organ failure. These include the Multiple Organ Dysfunction Score (MODS), the Logistic Organ Dysfunction Score (LODS), the Sequential Organ Failure Assessment (SOFA) and the Brussels Score.

Further reading

Gunning K, Rowan K. Outcome data and scoring systems. *BMJ* 1999; **319**: 241–4.

Knaus WA, Draper EA, Wagner DP, *et al.* APACHE II: a severity of disease classification system. *Crit Care Med* 1985; **13**: 818–29.

Pappachan J. Severity of illness scoring systems. *Anaesthesia and Intensive Care Med* 2004; **5**: 29–31.

Related topics of interest

Sedation

Sedatives help to relieve anxiety, encourage sleep, help the patient to synchronise with the ventilator and permit therapeutic procedures. The requirements for sedation vary greatly depending on the patient's pathology, psychological state and intensity of the medical and nursing procedures being undertaken. Improving the patient's environment may help to reduce the need for drugs. Effective communication and appropriate reassurance will help to relieve the patient's anxiety. Many patients receiving mechanical ventilation will require sufficient sedation to keep them comfortable yet rousable to voice. Patients with a tracheostomy who are receiving assisted modes of ventilation may not require any sedation. Where indicated, epidural analgesia will prevent the need for large doses of systemic analgesia. Those requiring unphysiological modes of ventilation (e.g. inverse ratio), prone ventilation or control of intracranial hypertension or seizures, for example, will need heavy sedation.

The ideal sedative

The ideal sedative would possess the following properties:

- Anxiolysis.
- Analgesia.
- Hypnosis.
- Amnesia.
- Titratability.
- Predictable effect.
- Rapid elimination.
- Lack of cardiovascular and gastrointestinal side effects.
- No development of tolerance.
- Low cost.

No single drug meets all of these ideals and for this reason it is common practice to use a combination of drugs. However, even this approach rarely achieves all of the objectives.

Drug administration

Sedatives are given usually by bolus or by continuous intravenous infusion (Table 16). Inhalational sedation with isoflurane has been described but is rarely used. Continuous infusion is a convenient method of drug administration but may produce oversedation if the patient's conscious level is not assessed frequently. Bolus dosing will reduce the incidence of oversedation but is less convenient for nursing staff. In patients who are receiving mechanical ventilation, daily interruption of sedative drug infusions decreases the duration of mechanical ventilation and the length of stay on the critical care unit. Unless there are specific contraindications, stopping sedative drug infusions each morning should be routine practice.

Table 16 Drugs used for sedation, analgesia and paralysis

Drug	Bolus	Infusion	Comments
Midazolam	$25–50\,\mu g\,kg^{-1}$	$50–100\,\mu g\,kg^{-1}\,h^{-1}$	Prolonged effects in the critically ill
Propofol	$0.5–2\,mg\,kg^{-1}$	$1–3\,mg\,kg^{-1}\,h^{-1}$	Causes hypotension
Clonidine		$0.05–0.4\,\mu g\,kg^{-1}\,h^{-1}$	Can cause hypotension
Morphine	$0.1–0.2\,mg\,kg^{-1}$	$40–80\,\mu g\,kg^{-1}\,h^{-1}$	Active metabolites accumulate in renal failure
Fentanyl	$1–5\,\mu g\,kg^{-1}$	$2–7\,\mu g\,kg^{-1}\,h^{-1}$	Cumulative with prolonged infusion
Alfentanil	$15–30\,\mu g\,kg^{-1}$	$20–120\,\mu g\,kg^{-1}\,h^{-1}$	Relatively expensive
Remifentanil	$0.5–1\,\mu g\,kg^{-1}$	$6–12\,\mu g\,kg^{-1}\,h^{-1}$	Ultra short acting, but expensive
Atracurium	$0.5\,mg\,kg^{-1}$	$0.1–0.5\,mg\,kg^{-1}\,h^{-1}$	Metabolised independently of renal/hepatic function

Drugs

Sedative drugs

Propofol and benzodiazepines are the commonest sedatives used in critical care. Benzodiazepines produce excellent sedation, anxiolysis and amnesia. Midazolam is the most commonly used benzodiazepine in critical care. All benzodiazepines are extensively metabolised in the liver. Sepsis will reduce blood flow to the liver and will impair the metabolism of benzodiazepines. The active metabolite of midazolam is α-hydroxy-midazolam. This is shorter acting than the metabolites of diazepam but nevertheless will accumulate with prolonged infusion and will add to the sedative effects of midazolam.

Propofol is an intravenous anaesthetic. It is eliminated rapidly from the central compartment and full recovery of consciousness is achieved very quickly (minutes) even after infusions for many days. Hepatic and renal dysfunction have no clinically significant effect on the metabolism of propofol. Propofol reduces systemic vascular resistance and will tend to cause hypotension. Anecdotal reports of severe cardiovascular depression after prolonged propofol infusions in critically ill children have prevented its widespread use in patients under 16 years. When propofol is used in combination with an opioid, typical infusion rates to achieve adequate sedation are $1.5–3\,mg\,kg^{-1}\,h^{-1}$. The lipid carrier can cause lipaemia after prolonged infusions of higher doses.

Clonidine is an α_2-adrenoceptor agonist. It has analgesia, sedative and anxiolytic properties and can be given by continuous infusion (up to $4\,\mu g\,kg^{-1}\,h^{-1}$). It is particularly suitable for sedating patients withdrawing from chronic alcohol abuse, during weaning from long-term ventilation or in patients with tetanus. Dexmedetomidine, a highly selective α_2-agonist, has recently been approved for use as a sedative in the United States.

Analgesic drugs

Opioids produce effective analgesia and anxiolysis, and reduce respiratory drive. The respiratory depression produced by opioids may help the patient to synchronise with the ventilator. Excessive doses will cause apnoea and prevent the use of patient-triggered modes of ventilation. They also cause gastrointestinal stasis, which impairs absorption of enteral feed. Morphine is cheap and remains a popular choice for analgesia and sedation in critical care. It is metabolised mainly in the liver to morphine-3-glucuronide and morphine-6-glucuronide. The latter is a potent analgesic and is excreted in the urine. Considerable accumulation of this metabolite occurs in patients with renal impairment and for this reason morphine is normally avoided in patients with renal failure.

Fentanyl is a synthetic opioid that is commonly used in anaesthetic practice. In single doses, fentanyl has a short duration of action. However, redistribution rather than the clearance determines duration of action. Thus, after a prolonged infusion, recovery from fentanyl can take a considerable time, i.e. the context-sensitive half-life is prolonged. Alfentanil is shorter acting than fentanyl. The action of alfentanil is terminated by clearance rather than distribution; thus following a prolonged infusion, accumulation is less likely (short context-sensitive half-life). However, in critically ill patients even the clearance of alfentanil can be variable. Remifentanil is an ultra-short acting opioid and is now licensed for use as a sedative in the critical care unit. It has a very short context-sensitive half-life. No residual opioid activity is present within about 10 min of stopping its infusion. The high cost of remifentanil is deterring more widespread use.

Assessment of sedation

It may be possible to simply ask the patient whether or not their sedation is adequate. In most cases, however, the patient's illness, the presence of a tracheal tube and the effects of sedation itself may make this impossible. There are a variety of sedation scoring systems but the most widely used is that described by Ramsay:

Awake levels:

1. Patient anxious and agitated or restless, or both.
2. Patient cooperative, orientated and tranquil.
3. Patient responds to commands only.

Asleep levels dependent on response to glabellar tap or loud auditory stimulus:

4. Brisk response.
5. Sluggish response.
6. No response.

Levels 2–4 are appropriate for most patients. The level of sedation must be assessed regularly, particularly when the sedatives are given by infusion. Physical methods of measuring sedation have been described. Most are used primarily for assessing depth of anaesthesia and many are based on electroencephalography. None of these systems are in routine clinical use.

Neuromuscular blocking drugs

In most critical care units neuromuscular blocking drugs are used only occasionally, typically for those patients who are otherwise difficult to ventilate or to prevent rise of intracranial pressure with coughing in head-injured patients. Atracurium and cisatracurium are non-cumulative and are the neuromuscular blockers of choice in the critically ill. Serious myopathies and neuropathies have been described with prolonged infusions of aminosteroid drugs (e.g. vecuronium).

Further reading

Hogarth DK, Hall J. Management of sedation in mechanically ventilated patients. *Curr Opin Crit Care* 2004; **10**: 40–6.

Kress JP, Pohlman AS, O'Connor MF, Hall JB. Daily interruption of sedative infusions in critically ill patients undergoing mechanical ventilation. *N Engl J Med* 2000; **342**: 1471–7.

Related topics of interest

Analgesia in critical care – basic (p. 17)
Analgesia in critical care – advanced (p. 22)
Psychological aspects of critical care (p. 236).

Sickle cell disease

Sickle cell disease is an autosomal dominant haemoglobinopathy found in Negroes, in non-Negroes from around the Mediterranean, and in parts of India. The β chain of haemoglobin A (HbA) has valine substituted for glutamine in position 6 to produce HbS. In the heterozygous form (sickle cell trait) this provides some protection against falciparum malaria. Ten per cent of Negroes in the UK have sickle cell trait. This is associated with a normal life expectancy, an Hb greater than $11\,g\,dl^{-1}$, no clinical signs or symptoms and sickling only if the SaO_2 is less than 40%. There is, however, an increased risk of pulmonary infarcts. Co-dominant expression of the haemoglobin gene allows normal and abnormal haemoglobin to coexist. Haemoglobin S may be produced with mutant haemoglobins such as haemoglobin C (giving SC disease), and with β thalassaemia. In the homozygote, deoxygenated HbS becomes insoluble and causes red blood cells to become rigid and sickle shaped. This is more likely if hypoxia, acidosis, low temperature or cellular dehydration occurs. Sickling is initially reversible, but when potassium and water are lost from the cell it becomes irreversible. Sickled cells result in decreased microvascular blood flow, causing further local hypoxia, acidosis and thus more sickling. Local infarction causes the symptoms and signs of a sickle cell crisis. Chest symptoms (pleuritic pain, cough and fever), musculoskeletal complaints (bone pain, muscle tenderness, erythema), abdominal pain, splenic sequestration (acute anaemia and aplastic crisis), haematuria, priapism and cerebrovascular events (transient ischaemic attacks (TIAs) and strokes) may occur during a crisis. Chronic haemolytic anaemia, increased infection risk and specific organ damage such as 'autosplenectomy', gallstones, renal and pulmonary damage occur as the result of long-term sickling. Osteomyelitis and meningitis are more common and prophylactic antibiotics are often given. Homozygotes usually present in early childhood when HbF levels fall and HbS predominates. Survival beyond the fourth or fifth decade is rare.

Problems

1. Anaemia. Anaemia may present as an acute illness in the very young. Children as young as 10 weeks may suffer acute splenic sequestration. The spleen enlarges rapidly and traps large numbers of red blood cells. This may result in a sudden and progressive anaemia and circulatory failure. Death may ensue in as little as 5 h. Episodes are frequently recurrent with the third or fourth ending in death. The child must be resuscitated with blood and fluid to maintain tissue oxygenation. This may then be followed by release of the sequested red cells from the spleen and subsequent polycythaemia as the spleen returns to its normal size. Acute sequestration is increasingly uncommon after 5 years of age by which age children who survive have usually undergone autosplenectomy and rendered the spleen functionally useless.

2. Infection risk. Below the age of 2 years there is an increased risk of pneumococcal septicaemia and meningitis. The increased risk of pneumococcal meningitis may be between 20 and 600 times normal. Splenomegaly suggests an at-risk child. Prophylactic penicillin and pneumococcal vaccine should be given.

Prevention of sickle crisis

Normothermia, good hydration and oxygenation prevent the development of a sickle crisis. A high FiO_2 is used. Hyperventilation (respiratory alkalosis) shifts the oxygen dissociation curve to the left and oxygen is more readily bound to haemoglobin, thus preventing sickling. Cardiac output is maintained to prevent microvascular sludging and vasoconstrictors are avoided. Monitoring includes pulse oximetry, temperature, urine output and the state of hydration. Regional anaesthesia may be used for patients in pain after surgery or those in an acute crisis. Tourniquets are avoided and patients nursed carefully to prevent venous stasis. Excessive sedation may cause hypoventilation, and hypoxia and should be avoided.

At-risk patients should have a Sickledex test, which detects HbS by causing sickling when the cells are exposed to sodium metabisulphite. It does not differentiate between the homozygote and the heterozygote and, if positive, formal electrophoresis must be performed. This will quantify the types and amounts of each haemoglobin. In the homozygote HbA concentrations $>40\%$ with a total $Hb > 10\,g\,dl^{-1}$ but $< 12\,g\,dl^{-1}$ should be achieved by exchange transfusion. This optimises oxygen delivery and blood viscosity. Patients are assessed for pre-existing organ damage and other pathologies consequent upon tissue infarction.

Further reading

Harrison JF, Davies SC. Acute problems in sickle cell disease. *Hospital Update*, 1992; **18**: 709–16, 751.

Vijay V, Cavenagh JD, Yate P. The anaesthetist's role in acute sickle cell crisis. *Br J Anaesthesia* 1998; **80**: 820–8.

Related topics of interest

Anaemia (p. xx)
Blood transfusion and complications (p. 50)
Hypothermia (p. 174)

SIRS, sepsis and multiple organ failure

Matt Oram

Most critically ill patients will exhibit the systemic inflammatory response syndrome (SIRS). There are many causes of SIRS, including infection (sepsis), trauma, burns, pancreatitis and cardiopulmonary bypass. The most severely affected patients may develop shock and the multiple organ dysfunction syndrome (MODS). Definitions of these terms have been agreed by expert consensus and are detailed below.

Definitions

1. Infection. The inflammatory response to the presence of microorganisms or the invasion of normally sterile host tissue by those organisms.

2. Bacteraemia. The presence of viable bacteria in the blood.

3. The systemic inflammatory response syndrome. Diagnosed when the patient exhibits two of the following four abnormalities:

- Temperature $>38°C$ or $<36°C$.
- Heart rate >90 beats min^{-1}.
- Respiratory rate >20 breaths min^{-1} or $PaCO_2 < 4.3$ kPa.
- White blood cell count >12000 cells mm^{-3} or <4000 cells mm^{-3} or $>10\%$ immature cells (band forms).

4. Sepsis. SIRS resulting from infection.

5. Severe sepsis. Sepsis associated with organ dysfunction, hypoperfusion or hypotension. Hypoperfusion and perfusion abnormalities may include, but are not limited to, lactic acidosis, oliguria or an acute alteration in mental status.

6. Septic shock. Sepsis with hypotension (systolic blood pressure <90 mmHg or a reduction of >40 mmHg from baseline) and perfusion abnormalities (see severe sepsis above) or the requirement for vasoactive drugs despite adequate fluid resuscitation in the absence of other causes of hypotension.

7. The multiple organ dysfunction syndrome. Altered organ function in an acutely ill patient such that homeostasis cannot be maintained without intervention. Although there are no universally agreed definitions of organ dysfunction, there are several organ failure assessment scores (e.g. the Sequential Organ Failure Assessment (SOFA) score (see Scoring systems p.266) or the MODS score), which define the severity of organ dysfunction in cardiovascular, respiratory, renal, hepatic, neurological and coagulation systems.

Classifying sepsis

PIRO (Predisposing factors, Infection, Response to the infection and Organ dysfunction) is a new system for classifying septic patients, which is similar to the TNM (Tumour, Node, Metastasis) system for describing malignancies. In comparison with the previous definitions it gives a more precise description of the patient and how they are affected by their illness.

Pathophysiology of the inflammatory cascade

The trigger

Inflammation requires a trigger, which may be infective or non-infective. Infective triggers include endotoxin from Gram-negative cell membranes, components of Gram-positive cell walls (e.g. peptidoglycans and lipoteichoic acid), viral DNA or fungal antigens.

Recognition

Recognition of the trigger by the body involves several cell surface receptors, part of the innate immune system, such as the family of Toll-like receptors or the CD14 receptor on macrophages.

Mediator release

- Having recognised the trigger, various inflammatory mediators are released from leucocytes, including cytokines (small polypeptides, e.g. tumour necrosis factor (TNF) and interleukins (IL) such as IL-1 and IL-8), platelet activating factor, leukotrienes, thromboxane and prostaglandins. The complement system is activated.
- These inflammatory mediators cause leucocyte proliferation (with further mediator release) as well as systemic effects such as increased capillary permeability (causing oedema), fever, raised metabolic rate and catabolism.
- Inducible nitric oxide synthase (iNOS) causes increased nitric oxide production from the endothelium, resulting in vasodilatation.
- Neutrophils adhere to the endothelium and migrate into the tissues releasing various toxic substances, including reactive oxygen species (e.g. superoxide).
- Coagulation is activated, causing microvascular thrombosis, clotting factor consumption and sometimes bleeding.

Compensatory anti-inflammatory response syndrome (CARS)

Various anti-inflammatory substances are released, which counteract the excess pro-inflammatory mediators. These include anti-inflammatory cytokines (e.g. IL-4 and IL-10), soluble TNF receptors, IL-1 receptor antagonist and naturally occurring anticoagulants (e.g. protein C). An excessive CARS may cause sepsis-induced immunosuppression.

Tissue hypoxia

Tissues may become hypoxic for several reasons, including hypotension (vasodilatation, hypovolaemia and, in some patients, myocardial depression), microvascular thrombosis (due to activation of coagulation), tissue oedema acting as a barrier to oxygen diffusion, and shunting past some capillary beds. This results in anaerobic metabolism and lactic acidosis. In sepsis, despite adequate oxygen delivery, lactic acidosis may also be caused by mitochondrial dysfunction. Reperfusion of previously hypoxic tissues can cause further release of damaging reactive oxygen species.

Organ dysfunction

The combination of tissue hypoxia and cellular damage by reactive oxygen species may precipitate organ dysfunction. The clinical presentation will depend on the organ system involved and the severity of the dysfunction. All organ systems can be affected by the inflammatory response, including:

- Cardiovascular system – hypotension with either a high or sometimes a low cardiac output.
- Respiratory system – acute lung injury and the acute respiratory distress syndrome (ARDS).
- Renal function – acute, usually oliguric, renal failure.
- Hepatic function – intrahepatic cholestasis and jaundice.
- Gastrointestinal system – stress ulceration, failure of enteral nutrition and possibly translocation of intestinal bacteria into the systemic circulation.
- Nervous system – critical illness polyneuropathy and 'septic encephalopathy'.
- Coagulation – disseminated intravascular coagulation (DIC) and thrombocytopenia.

Genetic susceptibility to sepsis

Genetic polymorphisms cause variability in the production of cytokines between individuals. For example, individuals who are homozygous for high production of TNF have a higher mortality from sepsis than heterozygotes who produce less TNF.

Treatment of SIRS and sepsis

The principles of treatment are organ support and correction of the underlying disorder: for example, in gallstone pancreatitis, endoscopic retrograde cholangiopancreatography (ERCP) may be necessary. The management of sepsis will include identification of the source of infection, antibiotic therapy and surgical drainage or debridement if indicated.

Monitoring of organ function involves careful clinical assessment, invasive arterial and central venous pressure monitoring, and occasionally cardiac output measurement. Hourly urine output is measured. Blood is taken for regular assessment of arterial gases, acid–base status, lactate, electrolytes, blood glucose, renal and liver function as well as haematological and coagulation profiles.

Organ support may involve giving intravenous fluid and vasoactive drugs, mechanical ventilation, haemofiltration, enteral nutrition and correction of coagulation factor deficiencies.

Goal-directed therapy (GDT)

In high-risk surgery, mortality can be reduced by optimising cardiac output, oxygen delivery and oxygen consumption before, during and after surgery. When these principles of management were applied to critically ill patients there was either no benefit or an increase in mortality. This may be because the inflammatory cascade has been activated hours or days earlier and tissue hypoxia/organ dysfunction is already established. Recently, a randomised trial of GDT (using central venous oxygen saturation as a marker of adequacy of oxygen delivery) showed a mortality benefit when applied to a group of patients with early severe sepsis or septic shock. One of the key differences between the control and GDT groups was the early use of additional intravenous (i.v.) fluid in the latter. The difference between this trial and the previous trials of GDT in critically ill patients was that the optimisation took place soon after admission to the emergency department before the patient was transferred to the intensive care unit.

Specific therapies for sepsis

Numerous trials of specific therapies for sepsis have been undertaken. Despite promising animal studies, until recently, none has shown a mortality benefit in randomised trials in humans. These therapies have included antibodies to endotoxin, antibodies to various inflammatory cytokines, antithrombin, heparin, high-dose corticosteroids, antioxidants, nitric oxide synthase inhibitors, granulocyte colony-stimulating factor, growth hormone and attempts to remove mediators by haemofiltration. The reasons why these therapies have resulted in either no improvement in outcome or even increased mortality may be explained by the complexity of the inflammatory cascade, the heterogeneity of critically ill patients and the timing of the insult relative to the timing of the therapy. Recently, however, two therapies have improved outcome: low-dose corticosteroids and activated protein C.

Low-dose corticosteroids

High-dose steroids (e.g. methylprednisolone $30\,mg\,kg^{-1}$), given early in sepsis, increase mortality. Recently, several trials of low-dose corticosteroids (e.g. hydrocortisone 50 mg i.v., 6-hourly) have shown improved shock reversal and decreased vasopressor dose and mortality. This benefit may be due to reversal of a relative adrenal insufficiency caused by sepsis, decreased production of inflammatory mediators or an improvement in adrenoceptor response to catecholamines. In one study, giving low-dose steroids to patients who were later found not to have adrenal insufficiency tended to increase mortality, although this was not statistically significant. It is probably best to do a tetracosactrin test (see Adrenal disease p.9), start steroids and then stop them if the result is normal.

Activated protein C (APC)

The inflammatory and coagulation cascades are linked closely in sepsis. Inflammatory mediators such as the cytokines TNF and IL-1 can trigger coagulation by release of tissue factor from monocytes and the endothelium. They may also inhibit fibrinolysis. The procoagulant thrombin can stimulate various inflammatory pathways. Protein C is a naturally occurring anticoagulant which also promotes fibrinolysis and may reduce the production of inflammatory cytokines. Reduced concentrations of protein

C occur in many patients with sepsis and are associated with increased mortality. In a recent randomised trial, recombinant human APC reduced mortality significantly when given to patients with severe sepsis and septic shock. Most benefit was seen in the sickest patients. The main disadvantages of recombinant human APC are increased bleeding and high cost.

Further reading

2001 SCCM/ESICM/ACCP/ATS/SIS. International sepsis definitions conference. *Crit Care Med* 2003; **31**: 1250–6.

Annane D, Sebille V, Charpentier C, *et al.* Effect of treatment with low doses of hydrocortisone and fludrocortisone on mortality in patients with septic shock. *JAMA* 2002; **288**: 862–71.

Bernard GR, Vincent J-L, Laterre P-F, *et al.* Efficacy and safety of recombinant human activated protein C for severe sepsis. *N Engl J Med* 2003; **344**: 699–709.

Bochud P-Y, Calandra T. Pathogenesis of sepsis: new concepts and implications for future treatment. *BMJ* 2003; **326**: 262–6.

Dellinger RP, Carlet JM, Masur H, *et al.* Surviving sepis campaign guidelines for management of severe sepsis and septic shock. *Crit Care Med* 2004; **32**: 858–73.

Hotchkiss RS, Karl IE. The pathophysiology and treatment of sepsis. *N Engl J Med* 2003; **348**: 138–50.

Rivers E, Nguyen B, Havstad S, *et al.* Early goal-directed therapy in the treatment of severe sepsis and septic shock. *N Engl J Med* 2001; **345**: 1368–77.

Related topics of interest

Adrenal disease (p. 9)
Fluid replacement therapy (p. 156)
Inotropes and vasopressors (p. 186)
Scoring systems (p. 266)

Sodium

Sodium is the principal extracellular cation. Normal plasma values are in the range $133–145\,mmol\,l^{-1}$ with a requirement of $1–2\,mmol\,kg^{-1}\,day^{-1}$.

Hyponatraemia

Hyponatraemia is the most common electrolyte abnormality seen in hospitalised patients. It is associated most commonly with increased total body water and sodium, and is compounded by giving hypotonic intravenous (i.v.) fluids.

Pathophysiology

Hyponatraemia may occur in the presence of low, normal or high total body sodium and may be associated with a low, normal or high serum osmolality. Basic mechanisms involve:

- Shift of water out of cells secondary to osmotic shifts (hyperglycaemia, mannitol, alcohol).
- Shift of sodium into cells to maintain electrical neutrality (hypokalaemia).
- Excessive water retention (renal failure, oedematous states (congestive heart failure, nephrotic syndrome, cirrhosis, hypoalbuminaemia), syndrome of inappropriate antidiuretic hormone (SIADH)).
- Excessive water administration (glucose infusions, absorption of irrigation solutions).
- Excessive sodium loss (renal, bowel loss).
- Translocational hyponatraemia.
- Hyperglycaemia accounts for up to 15% of cases of hyponatraemia; every $5.6\,mmol\,l^{-1}$ increase in serum glucose causes the serum Na^+ to fall by $1.6\,mmol\,l^{-1}$.

Causes of hyponatraemia associated with volume depletion are:

- Renal loss: diuretics, osmotic diuresis (glucose, mannitol), renal tubular acidosis, salt-losing nephropathy, mineralocorticoid deficiency/antagonist.
- Non-renal loss: vomiting, diarrhoea, pancreatitis, peritonitis, burns.

Causes of hyponatraemia associated with normal or increased circulating volume include:

- Water intoxication: postoperative 5% glucose administration, TURP (transurethral resection of the prostate) syndrome, SIADH, renal failure.
- Oedematous states (congestive heart failure, cirrhosis, nephrotic syndrome).
- Glucocorticoid deficiency, hypothyroidism.

Clinical features of hyponatraemia

The rate of change of serum sodium is more important than the absolute concentration. Symptoms are rare with serum sodium $> 125\,mmol\,l^{-1}$.

- Mild: confusion, nausea, cramps, weakness.
- Severe (Na^+ usually $< 120\,mmol\,l^{-1}$): headache, ataxia, muscle twitching, convulsions, cerebral oedema, coma, respiratory depression.

Diagnosis

Assess the patient's urine volume and level of hydration (circulating volume), the nature of any i.v. fluid replacement and recent administration of diuretics. Exclude hyperglycaemia and measure simultaneous urine and plasma osmolalities. The urine osmolality is inappropriately high with SIADH and advanced renal failure. In SIADH, the serum osmolality is $<270\,mosmol\,kg^{-1}$ and the urine osmolality is inappropriately high $(>100\,mosmol\,kg^{-1})$. There should also be an absence of renal disease and no recent diuretic administration. The urine sodium will be increased despite a normal salt and water intake. The signs of SIADH improve with fluid restriction.

Management

Follow the ABC priorities and treat the underlying disorder. The rate of correction of the hyponatraemia depends on the underlying condition and the clinical features. In chronic causes with mild or no symptoms, hyponatraemia should be corrected slowly over a period of days; rapid correction may precipitate osmotic demyelination. There is increased risk of demyelination in the presence of malnutrition, alcoholism, hypokalaemia and severe burns and in elderly females taking thiazides.

Rapid partial correction of hyponatraemia may be accomplished by:

- Stopping all hypotonic fluids.
- Fluid restriction.
- Giving demeclocycline or lithium (ADH antagonists).
- Giving furosemide.

The rate of correction of acute and symptomatic hyponatraemia is more difficult to dictate. The morbidity from acute cerebral oedema is worse in children, females (particularly during menstruation and elderly females on thiazides) and psychiatric patients. Acute hyponatraemia developing over less than 48h carries a high risk of permanent neurological damage and rapid partial correction of the hyponatraemia is indicated. Depending on the underlying cause, rapid partial correction of hyponatraemia may be accomplished by:

- Stopping all hypotonic fluids.
- Hypertonic saline (e.g. 3% sodium chloride solution at $1\,ml\,kg^{-1}\,h^{-1}$).
- Use of diuretics (furosemide is best given by low-dose infusion).
- Frequent measurement of electrolytes with adjustment of therapy.

For acute symptomatic hyponatraemia, the aim is to increase the serum sodium by $2\,mmol\,l^{-1}\,h^{-1}$ until symptoms resolve (correction may need to be more rapid if severe neurological signs are present). In the acute setting an increase of serum sodium of up to $20\,mmol\,l^{-1}\,day^{-1}$ is probably safe. For chronic symptomatic hyponatraemia, aim for a correction rate of $<0.5\,mmol\,l^{-1}\,h^{-1}$ for the first 24h and $<0.3\,mmol\,l^{-1}\,h^{-1}$ thereafter.

The main causes of morbidity associated with hyponatraemia are cerebral oedema, respiratory failure and hypoxia. The relation and risk of central pontine myelinolysis associated with rapid correction is unclear. The risks of rapid correction must be weighed against the risk of continued symptomatic hyponatraemia.

Hypernatraemia

Hypernatraemia results from inadequate urine concentration, losses of hypotonic fluids by various routes or from excessive administration of sodium. Patients who are unable to drink have lost their major defence against hypernatraemia. High-risk groups include infants and the elderly and patients on hypertonic infusions and osmotic diuretics.

Pathophysiology

Hypernatraemia may be seen in the context of low, normal or high total body sodium.

Low total body sodium and hypernatraemia results from loss of both sodium and water, but the water loss is proportionately greater. It is caused by hypotonic fluid loss from the kidney or gut and is accompanied by signs of hypovolaemia.

Increased total body sodium and hypernatraemia usually follows administration of hypertonic sodium-containing solutions.

Normal total body sodium and hypernatraemia is caused by loss of water in greater proportion than sodium. This usually results from renal losses due to central or nephrogenic diabetes insipidus (DI). Initially, euvolaemia is maintained, but uncorrected water loss will lead eventually to severe dehydration and hypovolaemia.

Diabetes insipidus

Diabetes insipidus (DI) is caused by impaired reabsorption of water by the kidney. Water reabsorbtion is regulated by ADH, which is secreted by the posterior pituitary. Cranial DI is caused by lack of ADH production or release, while nephrogenic DI results from renal insensitivity to the effects of circulating ADH.

Causes of cranial DI
- Head injury.
- Neurosurgery.
- Pituitary tumour (primary: pituitary, craniopharyngioma, pinealoma; secondary: breast).
- Pituitary infiltration (sarcoid, histiocytosis, tuberculosis).
- Meningitis/encephalitis.
- Guillain–Barré syndrome.
- Raised intracranial pressure.
- Drugs (ethanol, phenytoin).
- Idiopathic.

Causes of nephrogenic DI
- Drugs (lithium, demeclocycline).
- Congenital nephrogenic DI.
- Chronic renal failure.
- Sickle cell disease.
- Hypokalaemia.
- Hypercalcaemia.

Diagnosis

Polyuria (may be $>400\,\text{ml}\,\text{h}^{-1}$) in the presence of a raised serum osmolality (>300 $\text{mosmol}\,\text{kg}^{-1}$) is suggestive of DI. The diagnosis is confirmed by measuring urine and plasma osmolalities simultaneously. In DI the urine osmolality is inappropriately low (often $<150\,\text{mosmol}\,\text{kg}^{-1}$) in the presence of an abnormally high serum osmolality. The effects of osmotic and loop diuretics must be excluded.

Psychogenic polydipsia (compulsive water drinking) is differentiated by the presence of a low serum osmolality ($<280\,\text{mosmol}\,\text{kg}^{-1}$).

Clinical features

Signs and symptoms of hypernatraemia are often non-specific and include lethargy, irritability, confusion, nausea and vomiting, muscle twitching, hyper-reflexia and spasticity, seizures and coma.

Management

Treatment of DI follows the ABC priorities. Treat the underlying pathology and replace water (usually as 5% i.v. glucose). Vasopressin may be given (caution in coronary artery disease and peripheral vascular disease). Desmopressin (DDAVP) has a longer half-life and less vasoconstrictor effect.

In nephrogenic DI, administration of the causative drug should be stopped. Thiazides (e.g. chlortalidone) have a paradoxical antidiuretic effect. Chlorpropamide and carbamazepine may be beneficial.

Morbidity and mortality tend to be higher in acute severe hypernatraemia than in chronic hypernatraemia. Mortality associated with chronic severe hypernatraemia (serum sodium $>160\,\text{mmol}\,\text{l}^{-1}$) can be as high as 60%, while acute severe hypernatraemia is associated with mortality rates of up to 75%. Neurological damage is common in those surviving severe hypernatraemia. Correction should be slow ($<2\,\text{mmol}\,\text{l}^{-1}\,\text{h}^{-1}$) to avoid the risk of cerebral oedema.

Further reading

Arieff AI, Ayus JC. Pathogenesis and management of hypernatraemia. *Current Opinion in Critical Care* 1996; **2**: 418–23.

Kumar S, Berl T. Sodium. *Lancet* 1998; **325**: 220–8.

Related topics of interest

Calcium, magnesium and phosphate (p. 65)
Fluid replacement therapy (p. 156)
Potassium (p. 233)
Status epilepticus (p. 291)

Spinal injuries

Claire Fouque

Management of patients who have sustained multiple trauma or localised spinal trauma requires careful assessment for spinal injury. Failure to immobilise, investigate and manage these patients may result in the worsening of existing spinal cord injury or the production of a new cord injury. The incidence of spinal cord injuries is around 15–20 per million population per year. Men aged 15–35 years are affected most commonly. Common mechanisms of trauma are motor vehicle crashes (45%), falls (20%), sports injuries (15%) and physical violence (stabbing, gunshot wounds) (15%).

Injury to the cord can be expected in 1–3% of major trauma victims; the risk is approximately 8% if the victim is ejected from a vehicle. The majority of spinal injuries (55%) involve the cervical region. In adults, the commonest sites are C_5/C_6 and T_{12}/L_1.

Pathophysiology

Primary neural damage results directly from the initial insult.

Secondary neural injury may be caused by mechanical disruption after failure to immobilise, hypoxia (may be due to ventilatory impairment from cord damage or chest trauma), hypotension (hypovolaemia, sympathetic blockade, myocardial dysfunction), oedema, haemorrhage into the cord and hyper/hypoglycaemia.

Types of injury

1. Complete cord lesion. All motor function, sensation and reflexes are lost below the level of the lesion. Only 1% of patients who continue to have no cord function after 24 h will achieve functional recovery.

2. Incomplete cord lesion. There are four main clinical syndromes:

- Anterior cord syndrome. This is caused by ischaemic damage to the cord following aortic trauma or cross-clamping where blood supply from the anterior spinal artery is disrupted. There is damage to the corticospinal and spinothalamic tracts with paralysis and abnormal touch, pain and temperature sensation. The posterior columns are unaffected; joint position and vibration sense are preserved.
- Central cord syndrome. In this syndrome the central grey matter is damaged. Paralysis with variable sensory loss is greater in the upper limbs than the lower limbs because nerves to the upper limbs are located nearer to the centre of the cord. Bladder dysfunction presents as urinary retention.

- Brown-Séquard syndrome. This refers to hemisection of the cord, due usually to penetrating trauma. There is ipsilateral paralysis and loss of vibration and joint position sense with contralateral loss of pain and temperature sensation.
- Cauda equina syndrome. This presents with loss of bowel and bladder function with lower motor neurone signs in the legs following a lumbar fracture. Sensory changes are unpredictable.

Pattern of events

The initial injury causes immediate massive sympathetic activity with a sudden rise in systemic vascular resistance and blood pressure. Acute myocardial infarction, cerebrovascular accident or fatal arrhythmias may ensue. All voluntary and reflex activity ceases below the level of the lesion (spinal shock). Recovery to a chronic state with abnormal reflex activity occurs over several months.

Problems

1. Airway. There is increased risk of aspiration due to impaired upper airway reflexes and gastric stasis. Premonitory signs of vomiting may be absent.

2. Breathing. Cord injury above C_4 leads to loss of diaphragmatic function, apnoea and death if artificial ventilation is not commenced. Nerves from T_2–T_{12} innervate the intercostal muscles and patients with fractures above this level are reliant on diaphragmatic breathing with limited expansion, decreased tidal volumes and impaired cough. Residual volume is increased and the functional residual capacity (FRC) reduced. Muscle power is reduced, sputum clearance is poor, and pneumonia is common. Other respiratory problems include neurogenic pulmonary oedema, ARDS, Ondine's curse and pulmonary emboli. As spinal shock resolves, increasing muscle tone improves ventilation. Vital capacity may increase by 65–80%, enabling the patient to be weaned from mechanical ventilation.

3. Circulation. Loss of sympathetic vasoconstrictor tone causes neurogenic shock. Cord damage above T_2 disrupts the sympathetic innervation of the heart, causing loss of reflex tachycardia, impaired left ventricular function and the risk of severe bradycardia or asystole following unopposed vagal stimulation.

4. Neurology. Spinal shock refers to the muscle flaccidity and areflexia that occurs after spinal injury. It may last for 48 h to 9 weeks. Following the acute phase of spinal shock, 50–80% of patients with lesions above T_7 will demonstrate episodes of autonomic dysreflexia. Stimulation below the level of the lesion causes a mass spinal sympathetic reflex that would normally be inhibited from above. Patients develop a sudden, marked rise in blood pressure and compensatory severe bradycardia, with flushing and sweating above the level of the lesion. This may be so extreme as to cause seizures, cerebrovascular accidents or cardiac arrest. Triggering factors include distended bladder or bowel, cutaneous irritation from pressure sores and medical procedures.

5. Temperature. Hypothermia may be precipitated by heat loss due to peripheral vasodilatation.

6. Gastrointestinal tract. Paralytic ileus may last for several days.

7. Genitourinary. Bladder atony necessitates catheterisation.

8. Biochemical and endocrine. Increased ADH secretion leads to water retention with a dilutional hyponatraemia. Glucose intolerance may occur. This must be avoided as it causes worsening of the neurological injury by providing energy substrate, which, in the absence of sufficient oxygen delivery, is metabolised anaerobically. Nasogastric losses may cause hypokalaemic metabolic alkalosis. Hypoventilation causes respiratory acidosis. There is chronic loss of bone mass and osteoporosis, and there may be associated hypercalcaemia.

9. Skin. Prone to pressure sores.

10. Thromboembolism. High incidence of DVT and PE.

11. Musculoskeletal. May develop contractures and muscle spasms after resolution of spinal shock.

12. Psychological. Reactive depression is common.

Management

Primary survey and resuscitation
Fifty per cent of patients with damage to the spinal cord have other injuries. Secondary damage to the cord is reduced by immobilisation, minimising spinal hypoxia and hypoperfusion, and by ensuring the patient is fully resuscitated before transfer to a specialist centre.

Airway with cervical spine control
Manual in-line stabilisation of the neck is maintained until a correctly sized hard collar and lateral support and tape are fitted.

Early intubation should be undertaken if consciousness is depressed. Manual in-line stabilisation must be maintained throughout a rapid sequence induction of anaesthesia. The alternative is an awake fibreoptic intubation but it requires an experienced intubator and a cooperative patient.

Breathing
The patient is given sufficient oxygen to maintain $SpO_2 > 95\%$ and assisted ventilation instituted as required.

Circulation
An adequate blood pressure must be maintained to perfuse the damaged cord and decrease secondary injury. Most patients will stabilise with fluid loading alone but some may require vasopressors and inotropic support.

Secondary survey and diagnosis
Spinal injury must be suspected in all severely injured patients.

History – mechanism of injury
The risk of cervical spine injury is 10–15% if the patient is unconscious and injury is due to a fall or motor vehicle crash.

Examination
A careful neurological examination with meticulous documentation is essential. Spinal cord injury may occur without radiographic abnormality. It is important to determine the presence of any motor or sensory function below the level of a lesion, since this has important prognostic implications. Log-roll to assess for local tenderness and palpable 'step-off' deformity.
  Patients may demonstrate:

- Flaccid anal sphincter.
- Areflexia.
- Diaphragmatic breathing.
- Hypotension without tachycardia (if lesion above level of cardioaccelerator sympathetic outflow $\sim T_2$).
- Priapism.

Investigations/clearing the spine in trauma patients
- Patients who are alert, have no mental status changes, no neck pain, no distracting pain and no neurological deficits are considered to have a stable cervical spine and do not need radiological studies.
- All other trauma patients should have cervical spine X-rays: (lateral from occiput to the upper T_1 vertebral body, anteroposterior view showing the spinous processes of C_2–T_1 and an open mouth odontoid view showing the lateral masses of C_1 and entire odontoid process). Axial CT scans with sagittal reconstruction should be obtained for any questionable level of injury, or through the lower cervical spine if this area cannot be visualised on plain radiographs.
- All life-threatening haemodynamic and pulmonary problems should be addressed before a prolonged cervical spine evaluation is undertaken.
- Before removing spine immobilisation, all radiographs should be read by a clinician with expertise in interpreting these studies.
- If the cervical spine X-rays are normal but the patient complains of significant neck pain, flexion and extension views should be obtained.
- If the patient has a neurological deficit that may be referable to a cervical spine injury, they should have an immediate surgical subspecialty consultation and MRI scan of the cervical spine. MRI is the definitive investigation but it is difficult to use in the acute phase. MRI will demonstrate soft-tissue and ligamentous injury and give an indication of the severity of the cord injury.
- Trauma patients with an altered level of consciousness considered likely to leave the patient unable to complain of neck pain or neurologic deficits for 24 or more hours after their injury may be considered to have a stable cervical spine if adequate three-view plain X-rays (CT supplementation as necessary) and thin-cut axial CT images through C_1 and C_2 are read as normal by an experienced physician. With the advent of multi-slice helical CT scanners, it is becoming common

practice to scan the whole cervical spine and use 3D reconstruction instead of plain radiographs to screen for cervical injury in obtunded patients. If all of these studies are technically adequate and properly interpreted, the cervical spine should be considered stable and immobilisation devices removed.

- Thoracic and lumbar injuries are similarly excluded by examination, X-rays (AP and lateral) with targeted CT/MRI.

Definitive care

Most specialist centres advocate early fixation; therefore early referral to a spinal injuries unit is essential.

Airway

Tracheostomy is undertaken for long-term ventilation. This should be performed after any surgery to the cervical spine is completed.

Breathing

Close monitoring of ventilation is essential, as deterioration may occur insidiously over several days. Early intubation must be considered since respiratory complications account for the majority of deaths after spinal injury. Suxamethonium must be avoided after the first 24h for a year following injury since it may precipitate severe hyperkalaemia.

Circulation

Invasive blood pressure and central venous pressure monitoring are usually appropriate.

Minimising secondary injury

- Prevent hypotension and hypoxia.
- Steroids given within 8h of injury have a debatable effect on neurological outcome (statistically significant but possibly not clinically significant). An immediate loading dose of i.v. methylprednisolone $30 \, mg \, kg^{-1}$ i.v. over 15min is followed 45min later by a continuous infusion of $5.4 \, mg \, kg^{-1} h^{-1}$ for 23h. While popular in North America, this approach has varied support in other parts of the world.
- Treat hyper/hypothermia.

Autonomic dysreflexia

Management is preventive. Avoid precipitating stimuli and ensure good bowel and bladder care. Regional or general anaesthesia may be required to avoid crises precipitated by surgery.

Gastrointestinal tract

Early enteral feeding maintains gut mucosa integrity. Percutaneous gastrostomy (PEG) may be used for long-term feeding if swallowing is inadequate. Bowel management with laxatives is needed.

Genitourinary

Indwelling catheters are required at least initially.

Skin

Meticulous nursing and 2-hourly turning is needed to prevent pressure sores.

Thromboembolism
Prophylaxis with TED (thromboembolic deterrent) stockings, calf compression devices and s.c. low molecular weight heparin for minimum of 8 weeks.

Psychological
Multidisciplinary team support and guidance is essential. Clear advice and honesty are paramount. Support groups will help the relatives.

Spinal injuries in children
The low incidence of bony spinal injury (0.2% of all paediatric fractures and dislocations) is due to the mobility of the spine in children that can dissipate forces over a larger area. Treatment is similar to adults. Infants and children under 8 years old may require padding placed under the back to achieve the neutral position in which to immobilise the cervical spine.

SCIWORA (Spinal Cord Injury WithOut Radiological Abnormality)
There is no obvious injury to the spine in up to 55% of children with complete cord injuries. The upper cervical cord is usually affected where there is greatest mobility. It occurs almost exclusively in children under 8 years old.

Further reading

Bracken MB, Holford TR. Neurological and functional status 1 year after acute spinal cord injury: estimates of functional recovery in National Acute Spinal Cord Injury Study II from results modelled in National Acute Spinal Cord Injury Study III. *J Neurosurg* 2002; **96**: 259–66.

Ford P, Nolan JP. Cervical spine injury and airway management. *Curr Opin Anaesthesiol* 2002; **15**: 193–201.

Hoffman JR, Mower WR, Wolfson AB, *et al.* Validity of a set of clinical criteria to rule out injury to the cervical spine in patients with blunt trauma: National Emergency X-Radiography Utilization Study Group. *N Engl J Med* 2000; **343**: 94–9.

Hoffman JR, Wolfson AB, Todd K, Mower WR. Selective cervical spine radiography in blunt trauma: methodology of the National Emergency X-Radiography Utilization Study (NEXUS). *Ann Emerg Med* 1998; **32**: 461–9.

Nesathurai S. Steroids and spinal cord injury: revisiting the NASCIS 2 and NASCIS 3 trials. *J Trauma-Injury Infect Crit Care* 1998; **45**: 1088–93.

Tator CH. Biology of neurological recovery and functional restoration after spinal cord injury. *Neurosurgery* 1998; **42**: 696–707.

Trauma practice guidelines of the Eastern Association for the Surgery of Trauma (EAST). Identifying Cervical Spine Injuries Following Trauma: www.east.org

Related topics of interest

Status epilepticus

Status epilepticus describes prolonged or repetitive convulsive or non-convulsive seizures that continue without a period of recovery between attacks and last for longer than 30 min. Status epilepticus may arise in known epileptics (epilepsy has a prevalence of 1:200) or in non-epileptic individuals. Status epilepticus is an emergency during which the brain is at risk of secondary injury from hypoxia, hypotension, cerebral oedema and direct neuronal injury. The risk of permanent brain damage is proportional to the duration of seizures.

Status epilepticus may present as

- Generalised tonic/clonic seizures without full neurological recovery between attacks.
- Focal epileptic seizures without impaired consciousness.
- Non-convulsive seizures with impaired consciousness.

Causes of status epilepticus

- Idiopathic epilepsy (particularly associated with non-compliance with medication, changes in medication).
- Infection (meningitis, abscess, encephalitis, HIV).
- Head injury.
- Intracranial tumour (primary, secondary).
- Cerebrovascular disease (haemorrhage, thrombosis, embolism, eclampsia, cerebral vasculitis).
- Drug-induced/overdose (local anaesthetics, tricyclic antidepressants, theophylline, amphetamines, cocaine, LSD, insulin).
- Drug withdrawal (benzodiazepines, alcohol).
- Metabolic (hypoglycaemia, hyponatraemia, hypocalcaemia, hyperpyrexia, uraemia, hepatic failure, pyridoxine deficiency, porphyria).
- Non-epileptic status (known previously as pseudoepilepsy).

Investigation

- Blood biochemistry (glucose, sodium, calcium, magnesium, phosphate).
- Arterial blood gas.
- Drug screen for suspected drugs.
- Urinalysis.
- Anticonvulsant drug levels.
- Brain CT or MRI to identify structural brain lesions.
- Lumbar puncture (contraindicated if raised ICP or space-occupying lesion suspected).
- ECG and echocardiography to exclude cardiac embolism.
- EEG is required in all patients presenting with epilepsy. It will differentiate secondary generalised (focal seizures) from primary generalised seizures. It will occasionally detect subclinical epileptic activity in the absence of external signs of convulsions.

Clinical features

1. Airway compromise. During seizures the airway is compromised and there is risk of aspiration. Hypoxia is common because of inadequate ventilation combined with high oxygen requirements of continuous muscle activity. Hypercarbia occurs due to increased CO_2 production and reduced ventilation.

2. Metabolic changes. Hyperthermia, dehydration, acidosis, rhabdomyolysis, hyperkalaemia and, occasionally, renal impairment are caused by excessive muscle activity. Hypo- or hyperglycaemia can occur, both of which may result in secondary brain injury.

3. Cerebral consequences. Brain oedema may occur due to increased cerebral blood flow, hypercapnia, impaired venous drainage (position and raised venous pressure). Hypertension is common and may further add to cerebral oedema. Hypotension will usually signify hypovolaemia.

Management

Management follows the ABC priorities. Specific therapy should be directed to the underlying problem. Tracheal intubation may be required to enable airway protection in those who remain deeply comatose for a prolonged period. Ensure adequate ventilation, avoid excessive hyperventilation and maintain adequate circulating volume. Avoid hypotonic solutions, which will increase cerebral oedema. Hypoglycaemia is corrected with 50 ml of intravenous (i.v.) 50% glucose. If alcoholism is suspected, give thiamine 100 mg i.v.

Choice of anticonvulsant

1. Status epilepticus (grand mal)

- Initial (early) status epilepticus. Give lorazepam 4 mg i.v. over 2 min; this can be repeated after 15 min if seizures persist. Lorazepam is more effective than diazepam because therapeutic levels persist in the brain for a longer period (up to 24 h). In the prehospital environment or when intravenous access is unavailable rectal administration of diazepam will provide peak serum concentrations within 10–30 min. An alternative is buccal midazolam 5–10 mg.
- Established status epilepticus. If seizures persist despite lorazepam, give phenytoin 15–18 mg kg^{-1} i.v. at 50 mg h^{-1}. Alternatively, give fosphenytoin 15–20 mg phenytoin equivalent (PE) kg^{-1}. Fosphenytoin is a prodrug of phenytoin and is less likely to cause hypotension, arrhythmias and phlebitis.
- Refractory status epilepticus. If seizures persist 20 min after giving phenytoin, induce general anaesthesia with propofol or thiopental.

2. Tonic-clonic (grand mal). Drug options include sodium valproate, carbamazepine, phenytoin or thiopental.

3. Partial (focal)

- Psychomotor: carbamazepine, phenytoin.
- Absence (petit mal): sodium valproate, ethosuxamide.
- Myoclonic: clonazepam, sodium valproate.

Gabapentin, lamotrigine or vigabatrin may be added when control is difficult.

Check and correct anticonvulsant levels in known epileptics. Treat cerebral oedema with sedation, controlled hyperventilation and osmotic diuretics. Consider steroids for those with a known tumour, arteritis or parasitic infections. Consider surgery for space-occupying lesions (e.g. haemorrhage, abscess or tumour). Correct any hyperthermia. Maintain a brisk diuresis if there is any evidence of rhabdomyolysis. There is no role for long-acting muscle relaxants purely to control seizures. Continuing seizure activity implies inadequate anticonvulsant levels. Occasionally, paralysis may be required to facilitate ventilation if there is associated severe lung injury or for the control of ICP. If neuromuscular blockade is used, continuous EEG monitoring is mandatory to assess seizure activity.

Non-convulsive status

Status epilepticus will eventually burn itself out with resultant irreversible brain damage. Overt seizure activity may be markedly reduced or clinically absent in these later stages; however, the EEG will demonstrate continued seizure activity. The prognosis in this situation is extremely poor; anticonvulsant therapy must be used aggressively to avoid reaching this situation. Regardless of the initiating stimulus, status appears to enter a stage where seizures are perpetuated by excess excitatory amino acids, primarily glutamate. Ketamine, which has excitatory amino acid blocking activity, has been suggested as potentially useful in this situation but clear evidence to support its use is lacking. The importance of continuous EEG to enable continuous monitoring of status epilepticus is clear.

Non-epileptic status

Non-epileptic status is a diagnosis of exclusion. Simulated seizures may be differentiated from true epilepsy by features such as atypical movements (e.g. asynchronous limb and rolling movements), the presence of eye lash reflexes, resistance to eye opening, normal pupil responses during convulsion, retained awareness or vocalisation and normal tendon reflexes and plantar responses immediately after convulsion. They may be brought on by approaching the patient, are often recurrent and are seen in individuals who have some knowledge of what epilepsy looks like (health care workers or relatives of epileptics). Non-epileptic status is more common in females with a history of psychological disturbance. Occasionally, the diagnosis will become clear only on EEG monitoring.

Outcome

Outcome from status epilepticus is directly related to the duration of seizures, the incidence of secondary brain injury and the underlying pathology.

Further reading

Chapman MG, Smith M, Hirsch NP. Status epilepticus. *Anaesthesia* 2001; **56**: 648–59.
Delanty N, Vaughan CJ, French JA. Medical causes of seizures. *Lancet* 1998; **352**: 383–90.
Feely M. Fortnightly review: drug treatment of epilepsy. *BMJ* 1999; **318**: 106–9.
Lockey AS. Emergency department drug therapy for status epileptics in adults. *Emerg Med J* 2002; **19**: 96–100.
Walker MC. Status epilepticus on the intensive care unit. *J Neurol* 2003; **250**: 401–6.

Related topics of interest

Coma (p. 120)
Head injury (p. 164)

Stress ulceration

Stress ulceration or stress-related mucosal damage is distinct from peptic ulcer disease. Ulcers arising from critical illness are superficial, well demarcated, often multiple and not associated with surrounding oedema. They are usually located in the fundus of the stomach or the first part of the duodenum. Stress ulceration occurs in critically ill patients as a result of major physiological disturbances. The incidence of stress ulceration is poorly understood but has been quoted as ranging from 52 to 100% of all patients admitted to intensive care units (ICUs), depending on the diagnostic criteria used. The finding of occult blood on testing of either gastric aspirate or faecal material produces an unacceptably high incidence of false positive results when looking for stress ulceration. Adopting the stricter diagnostic criteria of overt bleeding or a decrease in haemoglobin of more than $2\,g\,dl^{-1}$, and complicated by either haemodynamic instability or the need for transfusion of red cells, produces an incidence <5%.

Upper gastrointestinal (GI) endoscopy remains the gold standard for the diagnosis of stress ulceration.

Pathogenesis

This was originally thought to be due to an excess of gastric acid production. It may be the explanation for those ulcers occurring in head-injured patients (Cushing's ulcer) or patients who have suffered burns (Curling's ulcer). Critically ill patients usually, however, suffer gastric exocrine failure and do not produce an excess of gastric acid. Reduced gastric mucosal defences may thus be more important. Gastric mucosal ischaemia occurs following shock or sepsis and may result in a failure of protective mucosal secretion. Damaging free radicals may also be formed. These mechanisms may be exacerbated by reperfusion injury following resuscitation. The mucosal barrier may also be disrupted by reflux of bile or pancreatic juice.

Complications

These are similar to those of peptic ulceration and include bleeding, perforation and obstruction, the latter two being rare from stress ulceration.

Risk factors for bleeding from stress ulceration

- Respiratory failure requiring mechanical ventilation.
- Coagulopathy.
- Multi-organ failure.
- Head injury.
- Severe burns.
- Sepsis.
- Anticoagulation therapy.
- Past history of peptic ulceration.

Management

Treatment of the underlying critical illness.

Enteral nutrition

This may decrease the incidence of stress ulceration by buffering gastric acid and improving the nutritional status of the catabolic patient.

Antacids

Antacids have been shown to decrease the incidence of both microscopic and macroscopic bleeding from the upper GI tract. The aim is to maintain the pH of the gastric content above 4.0. This is tedious to do, requiring regular measurement of pH by either aspiration of gastric content from a gastric tube or using a pH probe. Antacids must be given frequently (every 2–4 h). They may produce hypermagnesaemia, hyperaluminaemia, alkalosis, hypernatraemia, constipation or diarrhoea. Frequent administration of antacids may represent a large volume load to a non-functioning gut. For these reasons antacids are impractical in the ICU.

H_2-receptor antagonists

These include cimetidine, ranitidine, famotidine and nizatidine. They are as effective as antacids in reducing clinically significant bleeding compared with placebo. There is a wide range of potential side effects with each of these agents. The most important clinical side effect is the risk of nosocomial pneumonia due to the loss of the bacteriocidal effect of gastric acid. This promotes colonisation of the stomach and subsequently the nasopharynx, followed by aspiration into the trachea. Strategies to reduce the incidence of nosocomial pneumonia include nursing the patient with the head of the bed elevated and the use of subglottic suction devices in intubated patients.

There is no logic in giving H_2-receptor antagonists to patients with gastric exocrine failure and an already elevated gastric pH.

Sucralfate

This is the basic aluminium salt of sucrose octasulphate. It is given via a nasogastric tube. It does not raise intragastric pH, but polymerises and adheres to damaged ulcerated mucosa. It also binds bile salts and increases mucosal production of mucus and bicarbonate. Sucralfate is less effective than H_2-receptor antagonists in preventing stress ulceration. It may be associated with a lower incidence of nosocomial pneumonia, but this is controversial.

Omeprazole

This is a hydrogen–potassium ATPase receptor antagonist. It binds irreversibly to the gastric parietal cell proton pump, markedly reducing the secretion of hydrogen ions. It may be less effective in fasting patients but in critically ill patients it maintains the gastric pH above 4.0. Omeprazole is probably the drug of choice for secondary prevention following a GI bleed.

Misoprostol

An analogue of prostaglandin E_1 that inhibits basal and stimulated gastric acid secretions and increases gastric mucus and bicarbonate production, the role of misoprostol in the prevention of stress ulceration has yet to be established.

Further reading

Cook DJ, *et al*. Stress ulcer prophylaxis in critically ill patients: resolving discordant metanalysis. *JAMA* 1996; **275**: 308–14.
Cook DJ, *et al*. A comparison of sucralfate and ranitidine for the prevention of upper gastrointestinal bleeding in patients requiring mechanical ventilation. *N Engl J Med* 1998; **338**: 791–7.
Messori A, Trippoli S, Vaiani M, Gorini M, Corrado A. Bleeding and pneumonia in intensive care patients given ranitidine and sucralfate for prevention of stress ulcer: meta-analysis of randomised controlled trials. *BMJ* 2000; **321**: 1–7.

Related topics of interest

Stroke

A stroke is defined as a focal (or global, as in subarachnoid haemorrhage) neurological deficit of abrupt onset, of non-traumatic origin which lasts more than 24 h or which leads to death. A transient ischaemic attack (TIA) is qualitatively the same but signs and symptoms resolve within 24 h. Stroke is the leading cause of brain injury in adults. It has an incidence of 400 per 100000 population per annum. The incidence shows marked age variation, being 2000 per 100000 in those aged over 85 years. Early death after stroke is usually due to complications of the cerebral injury itself. Around 30% of stroke patients die within a year of the onset of their symptoms. Nearly 50% of stroke survivors are left dependent, though the degree of dependency varies greatly.

Pathogenesis

1. Ischaemic stroke. This comprises thrombotic and embolic disease and accounts for > 80% of cases. Mechanisms of injury include:

- Atherothrombosis of large and medium-sized cerebral vessels (50%).
- Intracranial small vessel disease (25%).
- Cardiac embolism (20%).

2. Haemorrhagic stroke. 20% of all strokes, divided between primary intracranial haemorrhage (15%) and subarachnoid haemorrhage (5%).

Investigation

The physical signs of the stroke should be documented. Serial blood pressure measurements should be made and a cardiac rhythm other than sinus rhythm sought. Stroke following an ischaemic event and that following haemorrhage cannot be differentiated clinically. A CT scan of the brain will help differentiate them and exclude stroke from other causes such as tumour or abscess. It should be performed as soon as possible. If it is greater than 7 days since the onset of symptoms an MRI may be required to exclude intracerebral haemorrhage. This is because the CT appearance of smaller haemorrhages changes over time with loss of the characteristic white hyperdensity, resulting in possible confusion with infarction.

Management

The aims of the acute management of stroke are to maintain cerebral perfusion and restore blood flow to cerebral tissue at risk from infarction.

1. Maintain cerebral perfusion. The blood pressure should not be allowed to fall or be actively lowered except in the presence of severe hypertension. A low cardiac output state (e.g. heart failure, atrial fibrillation) should be treated. Additional oxygen should be given by facemask. The patient should be nursed with 30° of head-up tilt (aids cerebral venous drainage).

2. Restore blood flow to cerebral tissue at risk of infarction. Thrombolysis with recombinant tissue plasminogen activator (rt-PA) (alteplase given at $0.9\,mg\,kg^{-1}$ over 1 h) increases the chance of surviving without disability in a highly selected group of patients with ischaemic stroke who can be treated within 3 h of the onset of their symptoms. Thrombolysis, however, carries a risk of death of about 1 in 20 (secondary to intracranial haemorrhage).

3. Anticoagulation. Aspirin 300 mg given as soon as a CT scan has excluded intracranial haemorrhage results in a small but significant improvement in neurological outcome. This initial dose should then be reduced to a maintenance dose of 75–150 mg daily. The use of heparin in acute stroke in patients in sinus rhythm has not been shown to produce benefit. Patients found to be in atrial fibrillation should be considered for cardioversion (pharmacological, or electrical if there is acute haemodynamic disturbance). If it is not contraindicated, warfarin should be started 1–2 weeks after the stroke to maintain the international normalised ratio (INR) at 2–3 times normal if the patient remains in atrial fibrillation.

4. Commence acute stroke rehabilitation

Outcome

Outcome from acute stroke is improved if the patient is admitted to and managed in a stroke unit rather than a general ward.

Further reading

SIGN guideline on managing patients with stroke – summary of the main recommendations:
  http://www.sign.ac.uk/pdf/qrg64.pdf
Stroke Trials Directory, a continuously updated registry of randomised clinical trials in stroke research. The web address is:
  http://www.strokecenter.org/trials/
Wardlow C, Sudlow C, Dennis M, Wardlow J, Sandercock P. Stroke. *The Lancet* 2003; **362**: 1211–24.

Related topics of interest

Head injury (p. 164)
Subarachnoid haemorrhage (p. 300)

Subarachnoid haemorrhage

Kim Gupta

Epidemiology

Blood can be found in the subarachnoid space following intracranial haemorrhage of any cause (most commonly trauma). The term subarachnoid haemorrhage (SAH) is generally applied to a spontaneous haemorrhage, usually from a ruptured intracranial aneurysm (85%) or arteriovenous malformation (AVM).

Aneurysmal subarachnoid haemorrhage
The prevalence of intracranial aneurysms in the general population is high (ranging from 0.4% for retrospective autopsy studies to 6% for prospective angiography studies). The incidence of rupture is 6–8 per 100000 population per year. Most aneurysms occur sporadically. Risk factors include hypertension, cigarette smoking and positive family history. Disease associations include Ehlers–Danlos syndrome, Marfan's syndrome, neurofibromatosis and polycystic kidney disease. Approximately 80% of aneurysms occur on the anterior cerebral circulation and 20% on the posterior circulation.

Ruptured cerebral arteriovenous malformation
Ruptured AVM presents more commonly with intraparenchymal or intraventricular haemorrhage than SAH. Arteriovenous malformation rupture generally occurs at a younger age (peak age mid-twenties) than aneurysm rupture (peak age mid-fifties). Up to 20% of patients with an AVM will also have one or multiple associated intracranial aneurysms.

Idiopathic subarachnoid haemorrhage
Approximately 10% of patients presenting with spontaneous SAH will have no aneurysm or AVM on initial angiogram. Although 20% of these will have an aneurysm on repeat angiogram, in the remainder no vascular cause of the SAH is ever found. These patients have a good prognosis.

Clinical features

Aneurysms are clinically silent until they rupture. SAH classically presents as a sudden-onset severe headache with nausea and vomiting. This is followed by signs of meningeal irritation (neck stiffness, photophobia). Neurological abnormalities, when present, may include decreased conscious level, cranial nerve palsy, seizures or lateralising signs depending on the site and nature of the bleed. The prognosis following SAH correlates closely with the clinical state on admission. Clinical grading scores

– e.g. Hunt and Hess Scale and World Federation of Neurological Surgeons (WFNS) Scale – are commonly used to quantify this (Table 17). Abnormal S-T segments or T waves exist on the electrocardiograph (ECG) of 25% of patients, and may easily be misdiagnosed as myocardial infarction.

Table 17 Clinical grading scales for aneurysmal subarachnoid haemorrhage (SAH)

Grade	Hunt and Hess Scale	WFNS[a] Scale
I	Asymptomatic or mild headache	GCS[b] 15
II	Moderate to severe headache, nuchal rigidity, cranial nerve palsy	GCS 13–14, without focal deficit
III	Lethargy, confusion, mild focal deficit	GCS 13–14, with focal deficit
IV	Stupor, moderate to severe hemiparesis, early decerebrate rigidity	GCS 7–12
V	Deep coma, decerebrate rigidity, moribund	GCS 3–6

[a] WFNS, World Federation of Neurological Surgeons.
[b] GCS, Glasgow Coma Scale.

Investigations

Detection of subarachnoid blood

A non-contrast computed tomographic (CT) scan of the brain is the investigation of choice. This detects blood in 95% of patients scanned within 24h. The volume of blood on CT scan is also prognostic, and correlates with the incidence of vasospasm (see below Table 18). CT sensitivity decreases to 80% at 3 days and 50% at 1 week post-SAH. Lumbar puncture (LP) can be performed if the CT scan is normal and SAH is clinically suspected. Xanthochromia (yellow discoloration) after cerebrospinal fluid (CSF) centrifugation is diagnostic but takes several hours to form.

Table 18 Fisher Scale for grading subarachnoid haemorrhage (SAH) using computed tomography (CT)

Grade	CT appearance
1	No SAH on CT
2	Thin SAH (<1mm)
3	Thick SAH (>1mm)
4	Intracerebral or intraventricular haemorrhage, with no or thin SAH (<1mm)

Location of aneurysm

Four-vessel (bilateral carotid and vertebral) digital subtraction angiography is the investigation of choice and is more sensitive than magnetic resonance imaging (MRI) or CT angiography. It can cause neurological morbidity in 0.3% and has a mortality rate of 0.1%.

Management of aneurysmal subarachnoid haemorrhage

Initial resuscitation and stabilisation according to ABC are essential. Subsequent care should ideally occur in a neurosurgical centre and concentrates on the following areas:

Prevention of re-bleeding

Further bleeding from a ruptured aneurysm carries an immediate mortality up to 50%. The risk of this occurring is 4% in the first 24 h and 1–2% per day for the next 12 days. The cumulative risk is 20% over the first 2 weeks.

The risk of re-bleeding is reduced by strict control of elevated blood pressure (maintain systolic pressure 120–150 mmHg) prior to repair of the aneurysm. Repair can be surgical or endovascular. Surgery aims to place a clip across the aneurysm neck. Endovascular repair involves radiologically guided placement of soft metallic coils into the aneurysm lumen, which thrombose and obliterate the aneurysm. In experienced hands the mortality of endovascular repair is approximately 1% and the procedural complication rate is 3–9%.

Treatment of hydrocephalus

Hydrocephalus is present in 19% of patients with SAH on presentation and develops in an additional 3% within the first week. It usually presents as an acute neurological deterioration and requires urgent surgical CSF drainage.

Prevention and treatment of cerebral artery vasospasm

Angiography demonstrates vasospasm in 67% of patients following aneurysmal SAH. In approximately half of these, delayed ischaemic deficit results in neurological symptoms (ranging from confusion to hemiparesis and coma). Risk of vasospasm increases with increased severity grading of SAH (clinical and CT). It typically presents around day 3 post-SAH and peaks at day 7. It may be diagnosed angiographically or using transcranial Doppler sonography.

Nimodipine is a calcium channel blocker that improves clinical vasospasm, and overall outcome following aneurysmal SAH. It should be given to all such patients for 21 days. 'HHH' (triple H) therapy refers to the induction of hypertension, hypervolaemia and haemodilution. It is advocated in many units for the prevention and treatment of delayed ischaemic deficit secondary to vasospasm. Some centres treat vasospasm using chemical angioplasty with vasodilator (papaverine) infused under radiological control, or with balloon angioplasty.

Medical complications

Medical complications contribute to significant morbidity and may account for up to 23% of deaths after SAH. The main complications are arrhythmias (35%), pulmonary oedema (23%), hepatic dysfunction (24%), renal dysfunction (7%) and thrombocytopenia (4%). Water and sodium imbalance occurs in 30% of patients after SAH. Causes include inappropriate antidiuretic hormone (ADH) secretion, a diuretic and natriuretic state referred to as 'cerebral salt wasting' and diabetes insipidus. Fluid and electrolyte replacement therapy to avoid hypovolaemia is required.

Outcome after aneurysmal subarachnoid haemorrhage

Outcome after aneurysmal SAH has improved over the past six decades. Mortality in the 1950s was approximately 46%. Mortality today averages 33%, with some specialist centres attaining 20% or lower. Up to 40% of survivors will remain dependent or suffer a significant restriction in lifestyle.

Further reading

de Gans K, Nieuwkamp DJ, Rinkel GJE, Algra A. Timing of aneurysm surgery in SAH: a systematic review of the literature. *Neurosurgery* 2002; **50**: 336–40.

Dorsch NWC. Therapeutic approaches to vasospasm in subarachnoid hemorrhage. *Curr Opin Crit Care* 2002; **8**: 128–33.

Feigin VL, Rinkel GJE, Algra A, van Gijn J. Circulatory volume expansion for aneurysmal subarachnoid hemorrhage (Cochrane Review). In: *The Cochrane Library*, Issue 3. Oxford: Update Software, 2003.

Fleetwood IG, Steinberg GK. Arteriovenous malformations. *Lancet* 2002; **359**: 863–73.

International Subarachnoid Aneurysm Trial (ISAT) Collaborative Group. International Subarachnoid Aneurysm Trial (ISAT) of neurosurgical clipping versus endovascular coiling in 2143 patients with ruptured intracranial aneurysms: a randomised trial. *Lancet* 2002; **360**: 1267–74.

Lozier AP, Sander Connolly Jr E, Lavine SD, Solomon RA. Guglielmi detachable coil embolization of posterior circulation aneurysms: a systematic review of the literature. *Stroke* 2002; **33**: 2509–18.

Rinkel GJE, Feigin VL, Algra A, Vermeulen M, van Gijn J. Calcium antagonists for aneurysmal subarachnoid haemorrhage (Cochrane Review). In: *The Cochrane Library*, Issue 3. Oxford: Update Software, 2003.

Related topics of interest

Brain death and organ donation (p. 55)
Coma (p. 120)
Head injury (p. 164)
Status epilepticus (p. 291)

Thyroid emergencies

The thyroid gland concentrates iodide and produces tetraiodothyronine (T4) and tri-iodothyronine (T3). Triiodothyronine has more metabolic activity than T4. Thyroid gland function is regulated by thyroid-stimulating hormone (TSH), which is secreted by the anterior pituitary gland. The secretion of TSH is controlled partly by higher centres such as the hypothalamus via thyrotrophin-releasing hormone (TRH).

Thyroid crisis

Pathogenesis
Thyroid crises occur more commonly in women than men. In patients with poorly controlled hyperthyroidism they may be precipitated by an intercurrent illness, especially an infection, trauma, thyroid surgery, poorly controlled diabetes mellitus or labour. A thyroid crisis may also occur in eclamptic patients with otherwise well-controlled thyroid function.

Clinical features
These are those of extreme hyperthyroidism and may be confused in the critically ill with sepsis or malignant hyperthermia. The signs include:

- Pyrexia.
- Confusion, restlessness and delirium.
- Tachycardia, atrial fibrillation and high output cardiac failure. Flushing, sweating and abdominal pain.
- Dehydration and ketosis.

Even with appropriate treatment, the risk of death remains high.

Management
This should be both supportive and specific. Supportive measures include supplementary oxygen (the metabolic rate is high) and treatment of the precipitating cause of the crisis. Attention to hydration is essential and the patient may require cooling and sedating. Assisted ventilation may be required and dantrolene has been used to good effect in those cases characterised by extreme muscle activity. Specific therapy aims at reducing the synthesis, release and peripheral effects of thyroid hormones.

1. Beta-blockade. Intravenous (i.v.) propranolol remains the drug of choice providing there are no contraindications to a poorly selective beta-blocker (e.g. reactive airways, heart failure). Beta-blockade will reduce the heart rate, fever, tremor and agitation. Propranolol also reduces the peripheral conversion of T4 to T3.

2. Thiourea derivatives. Propylthiouracil must be given enterally. It blocks the iodination of tyrosine and partially inhibits the peripheral conversion of T4 to T3. Carbimazole is metabolised to methimazole and is slower in onset, though longer acting. It is often associated with a temporary reduction in the white cell count.

3. Iodine and lithium. Both these substances inhibit the synthesis and release of thyroid hormones.

4. Digoxin. Digoxin may be required to treat atrial fibrillation once any hypokalaemia has been corrected. Amiodarone is an alternative, though may itself alter thyroid function.

Myxoedema coma

Pathogenesis
This occurs more frequently in the winter and typically in elderly female patients. It is the end stage of untreated hypothyroidism and is associated with a high mortality. It may occur secondary to autoimmune thyroiditis, radioiodine therapy, following the administration of antithyroid drugs, iodine, lithium or amiodarone, or after thyroidectomy. The following laboratory results are indicative of the associated conditions:

Primary hypothyroidism	↑TSH and ↓T3/T4
Secondary hypothyroidism	↓TSH and ↓T3/T4
Tertiary (hypothalamic)	↓TRH

Clinical features
The clinical presentation is that of coma associated with depressed thyroid function. Coma may be precipitated by a low body temperature, CNS depressants, infection, trauma or heart failure. The coma is often associated with seizures as well as the following features:

* Hypothermia.
* Hypoventilation (causing hypercarbia and hypoxia).
* Hypotension.
* Constipation.
* ECG changes – low heart rate, low voltage recording, prolonged QT interval, flat or inverted T waves.
* Hypoglycaemia.
* Hyponatraemia, with increased total body water (TBW) but low circulating volume.
* Hypophosphataemia.
* Hypercholesterolaemia (primary hypothyroidism).
* Raised CPK (creatine phosphokinase), AST (aspartate amino-transferase) and LDH (lactate dehydrogenase).

Management
The management is both supportive and specific. Supportive measures include control of the airway and assisted ventilation with warmed, humidified gases. External warming may also be required. Correct hypoglycaemia and give fluid under CVP guidance to restore normovolaemia. Patients with hyponatraemia will require water restriction.

The underlying cause of the hypothyroidism requires specific treatment. Thyroid hormones may be given in small incremental doses. Some advocate the use of steroids, as there may be a reduced adrenal glucocorticoid response.

The thyroid gland in critical illness

Serum thyroid hormone levels reduce during severe illness. In mild illness, this involves only a decrease in serum T3 levels. However, as the severity of the illness increases, there is a fall in both serum T3 and T4. This decrease in serum thyroid hormone levels has been reported in starvation, sepsis, after surgery, myocardial infarction, following coronary pulmonary bypass and in bone marrow transplant recipients. Although these patients have abnormally low circulating thyroid hormones they are not hypothyroid and usually have low or normal TSH levels. The condition has been called the euthyroid sick syndrome.

Proposed mechanisms include impaired responsiveness of the thyroid to TSH, reduced serum binding of thyroid hormones, or reduced peripheral conversion of T4 to T3. It has been postulated that endogenous cortisol has an inhibitory effect on TSH concentrations in patients with euthyroid sick syndrome. In low T4 and T3 syndromes, those with the lowest plasma T4 levels have the highest mortality, but giving T3 or T4 to these patients does not improve outcome. Current recommendations are therefore to not attempt to correct low serum thyroid hormone levels in critical illness.

Further reading

Lavery GG, Glover P. The metabolic and nutritional response to critical illness. *Curr Opin Crit Care* 2000; **6**: 233–8.

Vasa FR, Molitch ME. Endocrine problems in the chronically critically ill patient. *Clin Chest Med* 2001; **22**: 193–208.

Related topics of interest

Diabetes mellitus (p. 129)
Hyperthermia (p. 170)
Hypothermia (p. 174)

Tracheostomy

Tracheostomy has always been fundamental to the airway management of patients requiring long-term mechanical ventilation on the critical care unit. However, the widespread introduction of percutaneous dilatational tracheostomy (PDT) techniques over the last decade has dramatically increased the use of tracheostomy in the critically ill patient.

Indications

The main indications for tracheostomy are prolonged ventilation, weaning from ventilatory support, bronchial toilet and upper airway obstruction. Translaryngeal tracheal intubation may cause laryngeal damage in two ways: (a) abrasion of the laryngeal mucosa from tube movement during coughing, etc; (b) pressure necrosis from the round tracheal tube as it passes through the pentagonal-shaped larynx. Whether early conversion of tracheal tube to tracheostomy reduces the incidence of laryngotracheal damage is controversial. In the past, a tracheostomy was undertaken only when it was estimated that the patient would be ventilator-dependent for at least 2–3 weeks. Percutaneous techniques have reduced considerably the threshold for performing tracheostomies. The advantages of tracheostomy over prolonged translaryngeal tracheal intubation include:

- Less sedation required.
- Better oral hygiene.
- Enables patient to eat and speak.
- Airway fixed more securely enabling greater patient mobility.
- Less dead space and work of breathing.
- Improved efficiency of airway suctioning.
- Faster weaning from mechanical ventilation.
- Reduced length of stay in the critical care unit.

Modern mechanical ventilators have very sensitive flow triggers. In combination with tracheostomy, the need for sedation is virtually eliminated and weaning is much more efficient. The removal of sedation improves the success of enteral feeding.

Percutaneous dilatational tracheostomy

PDT has been popularised by Ciaglia, who described his technique of serial dilatation over a wire in 1985. The Ciaglia technique has evolved into a single dilator system, which is more convenient and faster. Other existing techniques for percutaneous tracheostomy include a single forceps dilatation (Griggs), a single dilator with a screw thread (PercuTwist) and translaryngeal tracheostomy (Fantoni). In comparison with surgical tracheostomy, PDT has many advantages and relatively few disadvantages.

Advantages of PDT
- No need for the patient to go to the operating theatre.
- Short operating time.

- Lower cost.
- Low incidence of wound infection.
- Small, cosmetically more acceptable scar.
- Low incidence of tracheal stenosis.
- Less bleeding.

Disadvantages of PDT
- More difficult to replace in an emergency.
- Loss of airway during procedure.
- De-skills surgeons.

The list of absolute contraindications to PDT has become shorter with increasing experience of the technique. The addition of fibreoptic guidance improves safety and is essential in patients with more difficult anatomy. Many clinicians recommend routine bronchoscopy during PDT.

Contraindications to PDT
- Absolute:
  - The need for immediate airway access (where intubation is impossible in an emergency, cricothyroidotomy remains the technique of choice).
  - Children – this may change as more data become available.
- Relative:
  - Ill-defined anatomy (inability to feel cricoid, obesity, thyroid enlargement).
  - Coagulopathy.
  - Haemodynamic instability.
  - Neck extension contraindicated.
  - High oxygen, positive end-expiratory pressure (PEEP) and ventilatory requirement.

Complications of PDT
Comparative studies have shown that the incidence of early complications with PDT is lower than those with surgical tracheostomy. The minimal tissue damage makes infection (0–4 versus 10–30%) and secondary haemorrhage less likely. The limited data available on long-term complications also suggest that PDT is less likely to cause tracheal stenosis than conventional, surgical tracheostomy.

- Immediate complications:
  - Hypoxia due to failure of ventilation during procedure (accidental extubation or puncture of the tracheal tube cuff).
  - Misplacement: too high, paratracheal, through posterior wall of trachea, into oesophagus.
  - Bleeding: minor, common; major, rare.
- Intermediate complications:
  - Early displacement of the tracheostomy tube – very small tracheal stoma makes replacement very difficult without dilators.
  - Obstruction from blood or secretions.
  - Infection.
  - Secondary haemorrhage.

- Late complications:
  - Tracheal stenosis (26% when defined by a tracheal stenosis of $>10\%$).
  - Subglottic stenosis – rare.

The technique of PDT

The single dilator modification of the Ciaglia technique is described. The infusion rates of sedative drugs are increased and a neuromuscular blocker is given. The patient's head and neck are extended by placing a pillow under the shoulders. The inspired oxygen concentration is set to 100% and the tracheal tube is withdrawn until the top of the cuff is across the cords. Alternatively, the tracheal tube can be replaced with a laryngeal mask airway (LMA) or, better, a ProSeal laryngeal mask airway (PLMA).

1. Clean the anterior neck with antiseptic solution and drape the area. Infiltrate the skin and subcutaneous tissues with 1% lidocaine and adrenaline (epinephrine) over the space between the first and second or second and third tracheal rings.
2. A second operator inserts a bronchoscope through the tracheal tube, or through the LMA and glottis, so that upper trachea can be seen.
3. Puncture of the trachea while infiltrating with local anaesthetic will enable bronchoscopic confirmation of the correct position in the midline of the appropriate level.
4. The local anaesthetic needle is removed and the cannula from the PDT kit is inserted at right angles to the trachea between the first and second or second and third rings. It is advanced until air is aspirated freely and the correct location is confirmed through the bronchoscope. Slide the cannula off into the trachea and confirm free aspiration of air.
5. Insert the 'J' wire through the cannula and feed 5–8 cm into the trachea before carefully removing the cannula. There should be no resistance to wire insertion and its advancement toward the carina is confirmed through the bronchoscope.
6. Advance the short introducing dilator over the wire and into the access site. Remove the dilator, leaving the wire in position.
7. Make a small vertical incision (2–3 mm) through the skin and subcutaneous tissues either side of the wire.
8. Load the tracheostomy tube (an 8.0 mm ID tracheostomy tube will be adequate for most patients) on its obturator or the correct-sized dilator.
9. Dip the horn-shaped dilator in water to lubricate the hydrophilic coating. Place the dilator over the guiding catheter and advance both over the wire and into the trachea, aligning the proximal end of the guiding catheter with the solder mark on the wire.
10. Advance the dilator, guiding catheter and wire as a single unit into the trachea, as far as the skin level mark on the dilator.
11. Remove the dilator and guiding catheter, leaving the wire in position.
12. Advance the preloaded tracheostomy tube over the wire into the trachea.
13. Remove the dilator, guiding catheter and wire, inflate the cuff and connect the catheter mount and ventilator. Confirm adequate ventilation and secure the tracheostomy tube.

Further reading

Beiderlinden M, Walz MK, Sander A, Groeben H, Peters J. Complications of bronchoscopically guided percutaneous dilatational tracheostomy: beyond the learning curve. *Intensive Care Med* 2002; **28**: 59–62.

Related topics of interest

Transfer of the critically ill

N Weale

As hospital specialist services become more centralised, the transfer of critically ill patients between hospitals becomes more frequent. Transfers may be primary (to hospital from the site of the incident/accident) or secondary (between hospitals). Patients are also frequently transferred within a hospital. Since relatively few doctors practice prehospital care, most medically supervised transfers are secondary. Transfer can be hazardous for the patient and rarely for accompanying personnel. Attention is increasingly being given to designated transfer teams, the development of transfer guidelines and training of staff. Key points to consider when transferring the critically ill include:

- Communication between hospitals.
- Detailed patient assessment.
- Pretransfer physiological stabilisation.
- Anticipation of likely problems during transfer.
- Pretransfer interventions.
- Equipment checks.
- Comprehensive handover.

General principles

Before transferring any critically ill patient the risks of transfer should be weighed against the potential benefits of treatment at the receiving unit. Transfer should be arranged if the appropriate level of care is not available at the original location. Early communication between senior clinical staff at the referring and the receiving hospital is essential. Ideally, the receiving hospital should take responsibility for the transfer and provide a team to undertake it. Patients should be resuscitated and physiologically stable (unless the patient has a condition which can only be stabilised at the receiving hospital).

Potential hazards of transfer

- Removal of patient from secure hospital environment.
- Reduced number of carers who may lack experience.
- Reduced or less effective monitoring.
- Reduced access to patient.
- No access to additional equipment.
- Difficulty in performing resuscitation or other practical procedures.
- Hostile environment: limited space, noise, motion sickness, fatigue.

The clinician supervising the transfer is responsible for assessment of the patient at the referring hospital. This must include a primary survey and a review of the history. When it is decided to sedate a patient with a head injury, record the neurological status before sedation is given. Record the neurological status of patients with suspected spinal injuries before and after the transfer.

Unconscious patients should be intubated before transfer. Most head-injured patients with an altered level of consciousness will require intubation. Record the inspired oxygen concentration and undertake an arterial blood gas analysis. If a transfer ventilator is to be used, check an arterial blood gas 10–20 min after connecting the patient to it. Achieve haemodynamic normality and stability before the transfer. Insert and secure adequate intravenous lines. Use warm intravenous fluids and ensure blood and blood products are available if required. If infusions of inotropes are required, draw up and label spare infusions. Splint fractures to prevent neurovascular damage.

A comprehensive written referral must accompany the patient. On departure, contact the receiving hospital and give an estimated time of arrival.

Personnel

Personnel accompanying a critically ill patient should be able to cope with all common problems. Ideally, a transfer team should retrieve the patient from the referring hospital. Such teams are well established for children but are not always available for adult patients. A doctor skilled in resuscitation and support of organ systems must accompany the patient, along with at least one appropriately trained assistant. The doctor supervising the transfer will often be an anaesthetist or intensive care doctor. Adequate death and injury insurance must be provided for the transfer team.

Equipment

All equipment should be checked before collecting the patient; it should be reliable, simple and durable.

The following basic equipment must accompany all critically ill patients.

- Mechanical ventilator (with facility for airway pressure monitoring, minute volume measurement and disconnect alarm).
- Oxygen – enough for the transfer plus enough for unforeseen delays, preferably with an independent alternative supply.
- Airway equipment – intubation and surgical airway equipment.
- Self-inflating bag-valve-mask device.
- Effective suction apparatus.
- Intravenous access and infusion equipment and a stock of intravenous fluids.
- Syringe pumps (with fully charged batteries).
- Volumatic intravenous fluid pumps (infusion by gravity is unreliable during transfer).
- Defibrillator.
- Spare batteries.

Drugs

The following must be carried:

- Resuscitation drugs – adrenaline (epinephrine) and atropine.
- Cardiovascular drugs, e.g. nitrates, antiarrhythmics, inotropes.
- Anticonvulsants, e.g. diazepam, thiopental.
- Analgesics.
- Hypnotics, e.g. midazolam, propofol.
- Muscle relaxants.
- Respiratory drugs, e.g. salbutamol.
- Other drugs such as naloxone, mannitol, glucose.

Monitoring

The ideal monitoring for critically ill patients during transfer is the same as would be used on the intensive care unit. This may not always be possible but modern multi-function monitors enable several pressure waves to be displayed, in addition to standard functions.

Non-invasive blood pressure monitoring is susceptible to vibration artefact as well as inaccuracy due to arrhythmias (e.g. atrial fibrillation). Where haemodynamic instability is a possibility, intra-arterial pressure monitoring is the only reliable method of measurement. Pulse oximetry is mandatory, as is capnometry in ventilated patients. Temperature should be measured, particularly in children. Catheterise and record hourly urine output in all critically ill patients. Monitor central venous pressure as necessary.

Modes of transport

The majority of interhospital transfers are undertaken by ground ambulance. The problems of ground ambulance transfers are excessive movement, noise, lack of space, motion sickness and occasionally extended transfer times (either due to long distances or traffic congestion). If the patient deteriorates en route, the ambulance should be stopped to enable effective resuscitation, intervention or examination of the patient.

Air ambulance transfers may be appropriate in certain circumstances. The usual indications are that the patient needs to be transferred a long distance or in a short period of time. Transfer may be by fixed wing aircraft or by helicopter. Fixed wing aircraft are used for long distances. Helicopters can travel moderate distances quickly and often land at, or very close to, the receiving hospital.

Air transfers are expensive. Problems en route include poor patient access, limited space, motion sickness, high noise levels and vibration. In fixed wing transfers, cabins are pressurised only to the equivalent of approximately 2000 m above sea level so supplementary oxygen should always be administered. The expansion of gases at altitude can be a problem if a patient has a pneumothorax or excessive gas in the bowel (e.g. in bowel obstruction) and where a tracheal tube is filled with air (saline should be substituted).

Transfers within hospitals

The general principles of transfers between hospitals are equally applicable to transfers within hospitals. The patient should not be moved until the receiving department is ready to commence the investigation or procedure. At least two people, usually a doctor and a nurse, should accompany the patient on the transfer.

Further reading

Guidelines for the Transport of the Critically Ill Adult. The Intensive Care Society, 2002.
Safe Transfer and Retrieval – The Practical Approach. Advanced Life Support Group, 2002.
The Neuroanaesthesia Society of Great Britain and Ireland and The Association of Anaesthetists of Great Britain and Ireland. *Recommendations for the Transfer of Patients with Acute Head Injuries to Neurosurgical Units.* The Association of Anaesthetists of Great Britain and Ireland, 1996.

Related topics of interest

Trauma – primary survey (p. 315)
Trauma – secondary survey (p. 318)
Trauma – anaesthesia and critical care (p. 322)

Trauma – primary survey

Trauma is the leading cause of death in the first four decades of life. Hypoxia and hypovolaemia are common causes of preventable trauma deaths. The Advanced Trauma Life Support (ATLS) course teaches a structured approach to the management of trauma. Severely injured patients admitted to an emergency department (ED) will require the immediate attention of the critical care team.

Prehospital management

Time spent at the scene must be minimised. Treatment at the scene should be limited to stabilising the airway and spine and ensuring adequate ventilation. Unless the patient is trapped, attempts at intravenous cannulation should be deferred until en route to hospital.

Communication

Wherever possible, ambulance personnel should warn ED staff of the impending arrival of a seriously injured patient. Emergency department staff can prepare the resuscitation room and call the trauma team. The appropriate drugs, fluids and airway equipment should be prepared before the patient's arrival.

The trauma team

Trauma patient resuscitation is best undertaken by a team of medical and nursing staff coordinated by an experienced leader. Resuscitative procedures can be undertaken simultaneously. The initial management of the trauma patient is divided into four phases:

- Primary survey.
- Resuscitation.
- Secondary survey.
- Definitive care.

The primary survey

1. Airway and cervical spine control. High-concentration oxygen is given by facemask with a reservoir bag. The cervical spine is stabilised with manual in-line cervical stabilisation (MILS) or a rigid cervical collar with lateral blocks. Tracheal intubation will be required if the airway is at risk (comatose, haemorrhage or oedema). Unless the patient is in extremis, intubation will necessitate rapid sequence induction of anaesthesia, MILS and cricoid pressure. Induction of general anaesthesia will cause profound hypotension in the presence of hypovolaemia.

2. Breathing. Immediately life-threatening chest injuries require urgent treatment at this stage:

- **Tension pneumothorax.** Reduced chest movement, reduced breath sounds and a resonant percussion note on the affected side, along with respiratory distress, hypotension and tachycardia, indicate a tension pneumothorax. Deviation of the trachea to the opposite side is a late sign, and neck veins may not be distended in the presence of hypovolaemia. Treatment is immediate decompression with a large cannula placed in the 2nd intercostal space, in the mid-clavicular line on the affected side. Once intravenous access has been obtained, a large chest drain (36F) is placed in the 5th intercostal space in the anterior axillary line, and connected to an under-water seal drain.
- **Open pneumothorax.** Any open pneumothorax should be covered with an occlusive dressing and sealed on three sides.
- **Flail chest.** The underlying pulmonary contusion may cause immediately life-threatening hypoxia, which will require intubation and mechanical ventilation.
- **Massive haemothorax.** This is defined by greater than 1500 ml of blood in a hemithorax and will result in reduced chest movement and dull percussion note, in the presence of hypoxaemia and hypovolaemia. A chest drain is placed once volume resuscitation has been started.
- **Cardiac tamponade.** Distended neck veins in the presence of hypotension are suggestive of cardiac tamponade, although after rapid volume resuscitation myocardial contusion will also present in this way. If cardiac tamponade is suspected, and the patient is deteriorating despite all resuscitative efforts, thoracotomy, or sternotomy and pericardiotomy is indicated. Pericardiocentesis should be performed only if there is no available surgeon and the patient is in extremis – it is associated with serious complications and may not relieve tamponade because the blood is often clotted.

3. Circulation. Control any major external haemorrhage with direct pressure. Rapidly assess the patient's haemodynamic state and attach ECG leads. Until proven otherwise, hypotension is caused by hypovolaemia. Less likely causes include myocardial contusion, cardiac tamponade, tension pneumothorax, neurogenic shock and sepsis. Although not entirely reliable, the degree of hypovolaemic shock can be divided into four classes according to the percentage of the total blood volume lost, and the associated symptoms and signs:

- Class 1   15%   Minimal signs.
- Class 2   30%   Narrowed pulse pressure and tachycardia.
- Class 3   30–40%   Fall in systolic pressure and oliguria.
- Class 4   >40%   Preterminal.

Intravenous access is best obtained with two large-bore peripheral cannulae. Alternatives include the subclavian, internal jugular or femoral veins. The response to an initial fluid challenge (2 l of crystalloid or 1 l colloid) will indicate the degree of hypovolaemia. All fluid must be warmed. Hypothermia will increase bleeding, and independently increases mortality. In the seriously injured a transfusion trigger of 10 g dl^{-1} is appropriate. Failure to respond to the initial 2 l fluid challenge indicates the need for blood as well as the need for immediate surgery to control bleeding.

In the presence of uncontrolled bleeding, aggressive fluid resuscitation in an attempt to restore a 'normal' blood pressure will increase the bleeding and may increase mortality. Until bleeding has been controlled surgically, a blood pressure of about 80 mmHg systolic may be the best compromise between minimising blood loss and avoiding organ ischaemia. This strategy should not be applied to the head-injured patient, who requires an adequate cerebral perfusion pressure.

The presence of coagulopathy, acidosis and hypothermia may indicate the need for 'damage control' surgery. This is undertaken during the resuscitation phase – bleeding is controlled, by packing if necessary, contamination from perforated bowel is controlled and the abdomen is rapidly closed using some form of temporary technique. Definitive surgery and formal abdominal closure is undertaken only after the patient has been adequately resuscitated with full resolution of any coagulopathy or metabolic acidosis.

4. Disability. The size of the pupils and their reaction to light is checked and the Glasgow Coma Scale (GCS) is assessed rapidly.

5. Exposure/environment. The patient should be undressed completely and then protected from hypothermia with warm blankets.

X-rays

The chest X-ray and pelvic X-ray are obtained immediately after the primary survey. Cervical spine X-rays can be deferred until the secondary survey. A cervical spine injury is assumed in all trauma patients until a reliable clinical examination and radiological clearance have been obtained.

Tubes

A urinary catheter is inserted – urine output is a guide to renal blood flow. A nasogastric tube will decompress the stomach. If there is any suspicion of a basal skull fracture, use the orogastric route.

Further reading

Nolan JP, Parr MJA. Aspects of resuscitation in trauma. *Br J Anaesthesia* 1997; **79**: 226–40.
Shapiro MB, Jenkins DH, Schwab CW, Rotondo MF. Damage control: collective review. *J Trauma* 2000; **49**: 969–78.

Related topics of interest

Acute respiratory distress syndrome (p. 5)
Burns (p. 59)
Head injury (p. 164)
Hypothermia (p. 174)

Trauma – secondary survey

The detailed head-to-toe examination is not undertaken until resuscitation is well underway and the patient's vital signs are relatively stable. Continual re-evaluation is essential. Those patients with exsanguinating haemorrhage may need a laparotomy as part of the resuscitation phase.

Head and neck

1. The head. The head is inspected for lacerations, haematomas or depressed fractures. Check for signs of a basal skull fracture:

- Racoon eyes.
- Battle's sign (bruising over the mastoid process).
- Haemotympanum.
- Cerebrospinal fluid rhinorrhoea and otorrhoea.

Brain injury is discussed elsewhere.

2. Face and neck. The orbital margins and zygoma are inspected. Check for mobile segments in the mid-face or mandible. While an assistant maintains the head and neck in neutral alignment, the neck is inspected for swelling, lacerations, tenderness or deformities.

Thorax

There are six potentially life-threatening injuries that may be identified by careful examination and investigation of the chest during the secondary survey. In addition to a chest X-ray (CXR), helical CT scanning with contrast or angiography may be indicated in patients with severe chest trauma.

1. Pulmonary contusion. Even in the absence of rib fractures, pulmonary contusion is the commonest potentially lethal chest injury. The earliest indication of pulmonary contusion is hypoxaemia (reduced PaO_2/FiO_2 ratio). Patchy infiltrates may not develop until later. Increasing the FiO_2 alone may be insufficient. Mask CPAP or tracheal intubation and positive pressure ventilation may be required to maintain adequate oxygenation.

2. Cardiac contusion. Cardiac contusion must be considered in any patient with severe blunt chest trauma, particularly those with sternal fractures. Cardiac arrhythmias, ST changes and elevated troponin may indicate contusion but these signs are non-specific. Echocardiography is the most useful investigation. The right ventricle is most frequently injured, as it is predominantly an anterior structure. The severely contused myocardium is likely to require inotropic and/or mechanical support.

3. Blunt aortic injury (BAI). The thoracic aorta is at risk in any patient sustaining a significant decelerating injury. Only 10–15% of these patients will reach hospital alive.

The commonest site for aortic injury is just distal to the origin of the left subclavian artery at the level of the ligamentum arteriosum. In survivors, the haematoma is contained by an intact aortic adventitia and mediastinal pleura. Patients sustaining BAI usually have multiple injuries and may be hypotensive at presentation. However, upper extremity hypertension is present in 40% of cases. The supine chest radiograph will show a widened mediastinum in the vast majority of cases. However, in 90% of cases a widened mediastinum is due to venous bleeding. An erect CXR will provide a clearer view of the thoracic aorta. Other signs suggesting possible rupture of the aorta are:

- Wide mediastinum.
- Pleural capping.
- Left haemothorax.
- Deviation of the trachea to the right.
- Depression of the left mainstem bronchus.
- Loss of the aortic knob.
- Deviation of the nasogastric tube to the right.
- Fractures of the upper three ribs.
- Fracture of the thoracic spine.

Helical CT scanning with contrast is the standard screening investigation but angiography is used for indeterminate scans. If BAI is suspected or confirmed, the patient's blood pressure should be maintained at 80–100 mmHg systolic using a beta-blocker such as esmolol, which will reduce aortic wall shear stress. Having controlled any other sources of bleeding, the patient must be transferred to the nearest cardiothoracic unit. Thirty per cent of patients with blunt aortic injury reaching hospital alive may die.

4. Diaphragmatic rupture. Rupture of the diaphragm occurs in about 5% of patients sustaining severe blunt trauma to the trunk. The diagnosis is often made late. Approximately 75% of ruptures occur on the left side. The stomach or colon commonly herniates into the chest and strangulation of these organs is a significant complication. Plain X-ray may reveal an elevated hemidiaphragm, gas bubbles above the diaphragm, shift of the mediastinum to the opposite side, or the nasogastric tube in the chest.

5. Oesophageal rupture. A severe blow to the upper abdomen may result in a torn lower oesophagus as gastric contents are forcefully ejected. The conscious patient will complain of severe chest and abdominal pain and mediastinal air may be visible on the CXR. Gastric contents may appear in the chest drain. The diagnosis is confirmed by contrast study of the oesophagus or endoscopy. Urgent surgery is essential since accompanying mediastinitis carries a high mortality.

6. Rupture of the tracheobronchial tree. Laryngeal fractures are rare. Signs of laryngeal injury include hoarseness, subcutaneous emphysema and palpable fracture crepitus. Tracheostomy, rather than cricothyroidotomy, may be indicated. Transections of the trachea or bronchi proximal to the pleural reflection cause massive mediastinal and cervical emphysema. Injuries distal to the pleural sheath lead to pneumothoraces.

The bronchopleural fistula causes a large air leak. Most bronchial injuries occur within 2.5 cm of the carina and the diagnosis is confirmed by bronchoscopy. Tracheobronchial injuries will require urgent repair through a thoracotomy.

Abdomen

The priority is to determine the need for laparotomy and not to spend considerable time trying to define precisely which viscus is injured. The abdomen is inspected for bruising, lacerations and distension. Careful palpation may reveal tenderness. A rectal examination is performed to assess sphincter tone, a high prostate and to exclude the presence of a perforating pelvic fracture. Diagnostic peritoneal lavage (DPL), ultrasound or CT is indicated whenever abdominal examination is unreliable:

- Patients with a depressed level of consciousness (head injury, drugs or alcohol).
- In the presence of lower rib or pelvic fractures.
- When the examination is equivocal, particularly if prolonged general anaesthesia for other injuries will make reassessment impossible.
- The surgeon who will be responsible for any subsequent laparotomy should perform the DPL.

CT scanning and ultrasound have virtually replaced DPL for assessing the abdomen. Modern multi-slice helical CT scanners are very fast and provide superior image quality compared with their older counterparts. Major pelvic trauma resulting in exsanguinating haemorrhage should be dealt with during the resuscitative phase as part of damage control surgery.

Extremities

All limbs must be inspected for bruising, wounds and deformities, and examined for vascular and neurological defects. Neurovascular impairment may be corrected by realignment of any deformity and splintage of the limb.

Spinal column

A detailed neurological examination at this stage should detect any motor or sensory deficits. The patient will need to be log-rolled to enable a thorough inspection and palpation of the whole length of the spine. A safe log-roll requires a total of five people: three to control and turn the patient's body, one to maintain the cervical spine in neutral alignment with the rest of the body and one to examine the spine. Patients with impaired consciousness, distracting injuries, pain and tenderness in the spine or neurological deficit require radiological investigation of their whole spine. Three X-rays (antero-posterior (AP), lateral and open-mouth) of the cervical spine and AP and lateral views of the thoracolumbar spine are required. Failure to achieve adequate views will necessitate targeted CT scanning. Using helical multi-slice CT scanners, a patient who requires head, chest and abdominal scans can have radiological clearance of their spine achieved more easily by CT scanning. Reconstruction views of the cervical spine, combined with scanograms (scout views obtained when scanning the chest and abdomen) of the thoracolumbar spine, can be obtained far more rapidly than radiographs.

Analgesia

Effective analgesia should be given to the patient as soon as practically possible. Intravenous opioid (e.g. fentanyl or morphine) is titrated to the desired effect. If the patient needs surgery imminently, then immediate induction of general anaesthesia is a logical and very effective solution to the patient's pain. A thoracic epidural will provide excellent analgesia for multiple rib fractures and will help the patient to tolerate physiotherapy and reduce the requirement for intubation and mechanical ventilation.

Further reading

Ford P, Nolan J. Cervical spine injury and airway management. *Curr Opin Anaesthesiol* 2002; **15**: 193–201.

Marion D, Domeier R, Dunham CM, Luchette F, Haid R. Determination of cervical spine stability in trauma patients (update of the 1997 EAST cervical spine clearance document). Eastern Association for the Surgery of Trauma, 2000. www.east.org

Nagy K, Fabian T, Rodman G, *et al*. Guidelines for the diagnosis and management of blunt aortic injury. Eastern Association for the Surgery of Trauma, 2000. www.east.org

Nolan JP, Parr MJA. Aspects of resuscitation in trauma. *Br J Anaesthesia* 1997; **79**: 226–40.

Related topics of interest

Acute respiratory distress syndrome (p. 5)
Burns (p. 59)
Head injury (p. 164)
Hypothermia (p. 174)
Trauma – anaesthesia and critical care (p. 315)
Trauma – primary survey (p. 318)

Trauma – anaesthesia and critical care

Induction of anaesthesia

A smooth induction of anaesthesia and neuromuscular blockade provides optimal conditions for intubation in high-risk trauma patients. All anaesthetic induction agents are vasodepressors and respiratory depressants and have the potential to produce or worsen hypotension. There is no evidence that the choice of induction agent alters survival in major trauma patients. Their appropriate use during resuscitation involves a careful assessment of the clinical situation and a thorough knowledge of their clinical pharmacology. Severely injured patients requiring intubation generally fall into three groups:

1. Patients who are stable and adequately resuscitated; they should receive a standard or slightly reduced dose of induction agent.
2. Patients who are unstable or inadequately resuscitated but require immediate intubation; they should receive a reduced, titrated dose of induction agent.
3. Patients who are in extremis, and are severely obtunded and hypotensive; here induction agents can be omitted but muscle relaxants may be used to facilitate intubation. As soon as adequate cerebral perfusion is achieved anaesthetic and analgesic drugs should be administered.

Suxamethonium remains the neuromuscular blocker with the fastest onset of action, and is usually the first-choice relaxant for intubation of the acute trauma patient. Some experienced clinicians prefer to use rocuronium.

Intraoperative management

The following considerations are of relevance to the anaesthetist during surgery for the severely injured patient:

1. Prolonged surgery. The patient will be at risk from heat loss and the development of pressure sores. Anaesthetists (and surgeons) should rotate to avoid exhaustion. Avoid nitrous oxide in those cases expected to last more than 6 h.

2. Fluid loss. Be prepared for heavy blood and 'third space' losses. The combination of hypothermia and massive transfusion will result in profound coagulopathy. Expect to see a significant metabolic acidosis in patients with major injuries. This needs frequent monitoring (arterial blood gases) and correction with fluids and inotropes, as appropriate.

3. Multiple surgical teams. It is more efficient if surgical teams from different specialties are able to work simultaneously. However, this may severely restrict the amount of space available to the anaesthetist.

4. Acute lung injury. Trauma patients are at significant risk of hypoxia caused by acute lung injury. This may be secondary to direct pulmonary contusion or due to fat embolism from orthopaedic injuries. Advanced ventilatory modes may be required to maintain appropriate oxygenation. The ability to provide positive end-expiratory pressure (PEEP) is essential.

Management of the trauma patient on the critical care unit

The initial management of the trauma patient on the critical care unit comprises continuation of resuscitation and correction of metabolic acidosis. Once haemodynamic stability has been achieved, the focus shifts to the prevention of complications and exclusion of injuries missed in the emergency department ('tertiary survey').

Major trauma patients will develop the systemic inflammatory response syndrome (SIRS). Secondary infection will compound the risk of developing multiple organ failure and some units give topical antibiotics to reduce the risk of infection from the patient's own gut. This strategy of selective decontamination of the digestive tract (SDD) remains controversial because of concerns about creating resistant organisms and because it has not been shown to reduce mortality.

Ventilation strategies aim to minimise barotrauma and volutrauma (see Acute respiratory distress syndrome (ARDS) p.5). Early long bone fracture fixation enables the patient to be mobilised and reduces respiratory complications. It may reduce the risk of developing fat embolism syndrome, although this has not been proven.

Enteral feeding reduces the incidence of septic complications.

Fat embolism syndrome

Fat embolism syndrome is associated typically with a fracture of a long bone or the pelvis. The pathogenesis of fat embolism syndrome is not absolutely certain but the most likely mechanism is that intramedullary fat and other particulate matter (microemboli) enters the circulation through venous sinusoids that have been disrupted by the fracture. This material lodges in the small blood vessels in the lung. This phenomenon is extremely common after long bone fractures and occurs routinely during the course of hip replacement surgery. In the majority of cases it produces no clinically significant effect. However, in some cases, the fat provokes a significant inflammatory response causing lung injury and hypoxia. This process takes several hours to develop and probably accounts for the typical delay of at least 6–12h after injury before the onset of fat embolism syndrome.

The cerebral manifestations of fat embolism syndrome may be secondary to hypoxia or to the effects of fat emboli in the cerebral circulation or, more likely, a combination of both. Fat emboli can gain access to the cerebral circulation by passing through the pulmonary capillaries, or through shunts in the lungs, or through a potentially patent foramen ovale. The latter occurs in more than 20% of the population. Cerebral fat emboli cause perivascular oedema or may provoke local platelet aggregation, which then produces microvascular thrombosis. This, along with any accompanying hypoxia, is responsible for the reduction in conscious level. Cerebral fat embolism can be identified by magnetic resonance (MR) scanning.

A petechial rash on the anterior part of the thorax and neck, mucous membranes and conjunctiva is seen in about 50% of patients with fat embolism syndrome.

The diagnosis of fat embolism depends on the presence of at least two of the three main signs of hypoxia, reduced conscious level and petechial rash. In addition, fever is often present. A chest X-ray will usually show infiltrates consistent with ARDS, but it may be normal initially. Treatment of fat embolism syndrome is supportive. Some patients can be managed with high-flow oxygen or continuous positive airway pressure (CPAP), but more severe cases will require tracheal intubation and positive pressure ventilation using a protective strategy (see Respiratory support – invasive, p. 260)

Further reading

Dunham CM, Bosse MJ, Clancy TV, *et al.* Practice management guidelines for the optimal timing of long bone fracture stabilization in polytrauma patients: The EAST Practice Management Guidelines Work Group, 2000:
www.east.org.
Nolan JP. Care for trauma patients in the intensive care unit. *Curr Anaesthesia Crit Care* 1996; **7**: 139–45.
Nolan JP, Parr MJA. Aspects of resuscitation in trauma. *Br J Anaesthesia* 1997; **79**: 226–40.
Ten Duis HJ. The fat embolism syndrome. *Injury* 1997; **28**: 77–85.

Related topics of interest

Acute respiratory distress syndrome (p. 5)
Burns (p. 59)
Head injury (p. 164)
Hypothermia (p. 174)
Trauma – primary survey (p. 315)
Trauma – secondary survey (p. 318)

Venous thromboembolism

Victor Tam

Venous thromboembolism (VTE) is responsible for significant morbidity and mortality. Effective and safe prophylactic strategies exist, but their implementation is often suboptimal.

In the absence of prophylaxis, there is a high risk that up to 50% of hospital inpatients will develop deep venous thrombosis (DVT). Venous thrombosis starts usually in the calf veins of the lower limb and extends proximally: 1–5% may progress to fatal pulmonary embolism. The propagation of VTE depends on a thrombophilic state, which is defined by Virchow's triad (changes of blood flow, blood vessel wall and blood contents). The risk of VTE is increased by immobility, obesity, smoking, previous VTE, increasing age and varicose veins. There are also numerous acquired and inherited thrombophilia conditions that predispose to the development of VTE. Patients should therefore be assessed individually for optimal choice of VTE prophylaxis.

Predisposing thrombophilic conditions

Acquired
- Serious medical illness – acute myocardial infarction, ischaemic stroke, cardiac failure, respiratory failure, shock, multiorgan failure.
- Major surgery – hip replacement, knee replacement, pelvic/abdominal surgery.
- Underlying malignancy – myeloproliferative disorders, adenocarcinoma, metastatic disease.
- Hyperviscosity – Waldenström's macroglobulinaemia, myeloma.
- Nephrotic syndrome.
- Antiphospholipid syndrome.
- Oestrogen therapy – hormone replacement therapy, tamoxifen, oral contraceptives.
- Multiple trauma.

Inherited
- Factor V Leiden/Activated protein C resistance.
- Antithrombin III deficiency.
- Protein C deficiency.
- Protein S deficiency.
- Prothrombin gene mutation 20210A.
- Hyperhomocysteinaemia.
- ↑ Factor VIII activities, dysfibrinogenaemia, factor XII deficiency, plasminogen deficiency/heparin cofactor II deficiency.

Clinical presentation of VTE

Extensive DVT may be associated with minimal signs or symptoms, and typical features including pain, erythema, swelling and tenderness of the involved limb can be caused by non-thrombotic disorders. Homan's sign (pain on forced dorsiflexion of the foot) does not help diagnose or exclude DVT.

The three most common symptoms of pulmonary embolism (PE) are dyspnoea, tachypnoea and pleuritic chest pain. Clinical signs are usually non-specific and at best support the diagnosis. They include haemoptysis, hypoxia, pleural rub, pulmonary hypertension, DVT and sign of right heart failure. The ECG may show tachyarrhythmia, non-specific ST segment changes, axis changes or, rarely, and only in the case of a large PE, an S wave in lead I, a Q wave and T wave inversion in lead III ('S1, Q3, T3'). The chest X-ray features are non-diagnostic and often show non-specific changes (e.g. atelectasis, pleural effusion). There may also be an elevated hemidiaphragm. The patient may have a mild pyrexia and elevated white cell count.

PE may present with one of three clinical syndromes:

1. Pulmonary infarction/haemorrhage (60% of diagnosed cases of PE).
2. Isolated shortness of breath (25% of diagnosed cases of PE).
3. Sudden circulatory collapse (10% of diagnosed cases of PE). One-third of these patients die within a few hours of presentation.

Diagnosis of VTE

VTE cannot be diagnosed or excluded on history and physical examination alone. An assessment of clinical probability for VTE must be undertaken before determining the appropriate diagnostic pathway. A negative D-dimer assay rules out VTE only in the low and intermediate clinical probability groups; it should not be undertaken in those patients with a high clinical probability of PE. Elevated D-dimers are present in nearly all patients with VTE, but are also associated with inflammatory states, trauma, the postoperative period, peripheral vascular disease and cancer. Thus, D-dimer testing has no role in the critically ill and, in any event, a positive result will necessitate further investigation.

Suspected DVT

Venous Doppler ultrasonography is the investigation currently recommended, although venography is still the gold standard. Impedance plethysmography is slightly inferior to ultrasonography but its accuracy is improved when combined with a D-dimer test. The role of MRI has not yet been established.

Suspected PE

Computed tomographic pulmonary angiography (CTPA) has revolutionised the investigation of PE and is now the investigation of choice in patients with high and intermediate clinical probability of PE. This includes critically ill patients with suspected PE. Although subsegmental clot can be missed with CTPA, in the vast majority of cases the concurrent presence of more proximal clot supports the concept that anticoagulation can be withheld when PE is excluded on CTPA. The latest British

Thoracic Society guidelines indicate that patients with a good-quality negative CTPA do not require further investigation or treatment for PE. Isotope lung scanning has limitations:

- A low probability result excludes PE, but an intermediate result is common in those with symptomatic cardiopulmonary disease and conditions causing intrapulmonary shadowing on the chest radiograph (a significant proportion of critically ill patients).
- A significant minority of high probability results are false-positive.

Treatment of VTE

VTE should be treated promptly to avoid thrombus extension, fatal PE and the development of the post-thrombotic syndrome.

1. Anticoagulation. Patients diagnosed with VTE should be treated with subcutaneous low molecular weight heparin (LMWH) or intravenous unfractionated heparin (UFH). LMWH dose is based on body weight without the need for monitoring. UFH is titrated to an activated partial thromboplastin time (APTT) of 1.5–2 times the control. Oral anticoagulation may be commenced at the same time or shortly after starting heparin or LMWH. There should be a 5-day overlap with both therapies and the international normalised ratio (INR) maintained at approximately 2–3 times normal before the heparin is stopped. Many centres now manage uncomplicated DVT and PE with administration of LMWH and commencement of oral anticoagulation at home, thus avoiding hospital admission altogether. Early follow-up of patients managed in this way has shown comparable rates of fatal and non-fatal PE compared with patients treated with UFH. The duration of anticoagulation is dependent on several factors:

- 4–6 weeks for PE associated with temporary risk factors.
- 3 months for the first idiopathic PE.
- 6 months for a first proximal DVT.

2. Inferior vena cava (IVC) filters. IVC filters should be inserted in patients with a proximal DVT or PE when anticoagulation is contraindicated or if PE has recurred despite adequate anticoagulation. An IVC filter may also be inserted if the PE is major (hypotension or right ventricular failure) or if recurrent PE is likely to be fatal.

3. Thrombolytic therapy. Lysis of PE is achieved more rapidly with a thrombolytic than with anticoagulation alone; however, with the exception of patients with a massive PE, long-term survival is no different. After massive PE, thrombolysis resulted in lower in-hospital mortality and PE recurrence, but a higher incidence of major haemorrhage, compared with anticoagulation alone.

4. Pulmonary embolectomy. Patients who have suffered a massive PE, and are shocked despite resuscitative measures or thrombolysis, may benefit from open embolectomy. Mortality remains high, even in patients offered surgery.

Prophylaxis modalities

Physical

1. Adequate hydration, early mobilisation, frequent positioning of immobile patient.

2. Compression elastic stockings (CES). CES reduce venous stasis and the incidence of DVT. They are used in lower-risk patients and selected moderate-risk patients when anticoagulation is contraindicated (e.g. neurosurgical). CES are often used in combination with other forms of prophylaxis in high-risk patients, although evidence of additional benefit is unclear in this setting. There is some evidence to suggest long-term use of CES reduces the incidence of post-thrombotic syndrome following a DVT.

3. Intermittent pneumatic compression (IPC). Sequential compression of calves enhances blood flow in the deep veins and reduces plasminogen activator inhibitor (mechanism unknown). This local and systemic effect reduces the incidence of DVT and is more effective than CES in high-risk patients in combination with anticoagulants or when anticoagulants are contraindicated.

Both CES and IPC should be used early from the times of immobility until full ambulation but should not be used in limbs with critical ischaemia.

4. Regional anaesthesia. Regional anaesthesia techniques (spinal/epidural) are associated with reduced perioperative venous thromboembolism.

Pharmacological

1. Unfractionated heparin. Extensive studies and meta-analyses have confirmed the efficacy of low-dose UFH to prevent VTE in both surgical and non-surgical patients with no increase in major haemorrhage. However, platelet count should be monitored for the development of heparin-induced thrombocytopenia and associated thrombosis syndrome (HITTS).

2. Low molecular weight heparin. LMWH given subcutaneously is at least as effective or superior to low-dose UFH or warfarin. LMWH also has the advantage of a lower dosing frequency without routine laboratory monitoring and a lower incidence of thrombocytopenia than UFH. However, LMWH tends to accumulate in renal failure, which may necessitate dose adjustment.

3. Warfarin. Warfarin is not the first-line prophylaxis; it requires laboratory monitoring and oral administration, making it inappropriate for the critically ill and for most major surgical patients.

4. Thrombin inhibitor. Hirudin is a thrombin inhibitor derived from the saliva of the leech. Recombinant hirudin has been shown to be more effective than LMWH in VTE prophylaxis with no difference in bleeding. It is currently the drug of choice in HITTS syndrome.

5. Specific factor Xa inhibitor. Fondaparinux is a synthetic heparin pentasaccharide that inhibits factor Xa via AT III without inhibiting thrombin. When given to patients undergoing major orthopaedic surgery, in comparison with LMHW, fondaparinux was associated with a 50–60% relative reduction in VTE risk. It is not yet universally available.

Insertion of IVC filter
Placement of an IVC filter in patients with DVT reduces the immediate risk of PE. However, they tend to have a higher rate of recurrent DVT in the long term. While there is little indication for their use in primary prevention of DVT, they are indicated in patients with VTE in whom conventional anticoagulation is contraindicated or ineffective.

Prophylaxis recommendations

Surgical
- Surgical patients are stratified into low, moderate or high-risk group according to duration, type of operation and additional risk factors.
- Low-risk patients who are < 40 years old, undergoing minor procedures and have no additional risk factors do not need specific prophylaxis other than early mobilisation.
- High-risk patients who are > 60 years old, undergoing major surgery, or 40–60 years old having major surgery with additional risk factors, or associated with thrombophilia or a past history of VTE, should receive LMWH or low-dose UFH and IPC or CES.
- Prophylaxis for other moderate risk patients is either LMWH or low-dose UFH or IPC/CES if heparin is contraindicated.

Medical
1. Cardiac. Both UFH and LMWH have been shown to be effective in preventing VTE in cardiac failure. After acute myocardial infarction, full-dose therapeutic anticoagulation with UFH or LMWH is given initially, followed later by prophylactic doses.

2. Ischaemic stroke. Up to 55% of stroke patients developed VTE. All ischaemic stroke patients should receive either LMWH or low-dose UFH for 10–14 days. Currently, there are no data on VTE prophylaxis in haemorrhagic stroke patients.

3. Malignancy. Cancer patients have a hypercoagulable state due to tissue factor and cancer procoagulant and those who are immobile should be given VTE prophylaxis. Patients receiving chemotherapy with a long-term central venous catheter should receive either low-dose warfarin or LMWH to avoid VTE.

4. Others medical conditions. General medical patients have a 15% incidence of DVT without prophylaxis. Both low-dose UFH and LMWH have been shown to reduce VTE in patients with acute medical illness.

Orthopaedic surgery
Patients with hip fracture and those who undergoing major elective orthopaedic

surgery, such as hip or knee replacement, are at high risk (up to 50%) of developing VTE. Prophylaxis is achieved with LMWH, UFH, hirudin, factor Xa inhibitor or adjusted-dose warfarin. LMWH is more effective than low-dose UFH or warfarin. Hirudin or fondaparinux is more effective than LMWH.

Neurosurgical/trauma

Intermittent pneumatic compression is the best form of prophylaxis when CNS haemorrhage is a major concern in neurosurgical patients. Enoxaparin (an LMWH) 30 mg twice daily has been shown to reduce VTE safely after elective neurosurgery, multiple trauma and spinal cord injuries, although most clinicians do not give it until 12–24 h after surgery.

Critical care patient

Medical patients in critical care units generally have multiple risks of VTE. The incidence of DVT is 25–30%. The recommended prophylaxis is LMWH or low-dose UFH. Patients should receive IPC or CES when bleeding is a concern.

Pregnancy

Several factors, including prior VTE, history of thrombophilia, Caesarean section, obesity and advanced age, increase the risk of VTE in pregnancy. High-risk patients should receive VTE prophylaxis using UFH or LMWH during their pregnancy and in the postpartum period.

Further reading

ABC of antithrombotic therapy. Venous thromboembolism, pathophysiology, clinical features and prevention. *BMJ* 2002; **325**: 887–90.

British Thoracic Society Standards of Care Committee Pulmonary Embolism Guideline Development Group. British Thoracic Society guidelines for the management of suspected acute pulmonary embolism. *Thorax* 2003; **58**: 470–84.

Fedullo PF, Tapson VF. The evaluation of suspected pulmonary embolism. *N Engl J Med* 2003; **349**: 1247–56.

Tovey C, Wyatt S. Diagnosis, investigation, and management of deep vein thrombosis. *BMJ* 2003; **326**: 1180–4.

Related topics of interest

Obstetric emergencies – medical (p. 214)

Weaning from ventilation

Jonathan Hadfield

Mechanical ventilation is associated with complications, which makes it important to discontinue ventilator support at the earliest opportunity. More than 40% of the time that a patient receives mechanical ventilation in a critical care unit is spent trying to wean the patient from the ventilator.

Once the underlying pathological process inducing the need for mechanical ventilation has resolved, the patient gradually resumes the full ventilatory workload to enable discontinuation of mechanical support. Weaning enables gradual exercise and reconditioning of the respiratory muscles and return of coordinated activity.

The speed with which a patient may be weaned from ventilatory support is dependent on the duration of ventilation. Rapid weaning and early extubation can be expected in postoperative patients, acute asthma exacerbations and drug overdoses, whereas longer weaning periods are predicted for those with more extensive dysfunction such as chronic obstructive pulmonary disease (COPD) and acute respiratory distress syndrome (ARDS). The use of assist modes of ventilation at the earliest opportunity will help maintain respiratory muscle function.

Considerations

- Prerequisites – is the patient ready for weaning?
- Predictors – will the patient manage to self-ventilate?
- Preparation of the patient for weaning.
- Methods or techniques of weaning.

Prerequisites

Weaning is unlikely to be successful if:

- There is persistent hypoxia (common criteria for acceptable oxygenation are $PaO_2 > 8\,kPa$, $FiO_2 \leq 0.4–0.5$, and $PEEP \leq 5–8\,cmH_2O$)
- The patient's psychological status is poor (e.g. confusion, agitation, depression).
- The original disease is still active.
- There is haemodynamic instability or a continued requirement for high-dose pressor support.
- Significant sepsis is present (increased O_2 consumption and CO_2 production, increasing respiratory demand).
- There is severe abdominal distension producing diaphragmatic tamponade.

Predictors

Successful weaning may be predicted by:

- Vital capacity $>10\text{--}15\,\text{ml}\,\text{kg}^{-1}$.
- Tidal volume $>5\,\text{ml}\,\text{kg}^{-1}$.
- Minute volume $<10\,\text{l}\,\text{min}^{-1}$.
- Respiratory rate <35 breaths min^{-1}.
- Maximum negative inspiratory pressure $>20\,\text{cmH}_2\text{O}$.

More complex means of assessment include:

- Work of breathing (computed from transpulmonary pressure and volume).
- Measurement of respiratory muscle oxygen consumption.
- Assessment of respiratory muscle function (electromyograms of diaphragm, trans-diaphragmatic pressures).
- Ultrasound assessment of intercostal muscle bulk.
- Assessment of ventilatory drive using airway occlusion pressure measured at the mouth or tracheal tube in the first 0.1 s of inspiratory effort against an occluded airway.

Preparation

Stop giving neuromuscular blocking drugs. If appropriate, control pain using a regional technique, such as an epidural infusion of local anaesthetic, to minimise the requirement for systemic opioids, which cause respiratory depression. Nutrition must be optimised to fuel the respiratory muscles and anabolic processes of the body. Malnutrition will cause atrophy and weakness of the respiratory muscles. Excessive calorific intake, especially of carbohydrate, will increase CO_2 production and exert greater demands on the respiratory muscles. Maintain electrolytes essential to muscle function (Ca^{2+}, Mg^{2+}, K^+, PO_4^{2-}) within the normal ranges. Explain the weaning process to the patient and provide continuous support and encouragement to maintain motivation and cooperation.

Method

Using assist modes of ventilation (e.g. pressure support) it is possible to adjust the level of support to meet the patient's demands, while still allowing gradual exercise of the respiratory muscles. From the outset, the ventilator settings are matched continually to the requirements of each patient. Weaning thus becomes a continuous process beginning from the time the initial pathology begins to resolve.

1. Pressure support weaning. In this mode, all breaths are initiated by the patient, following which the ventilator generates an inspiratory pressure in the breathing circuit to assist each breath. The inspiratory phase is terminated when the inspiratory flow reaches a threshold value (e.g. 25% of peak flow). In its simplest form, there is no backup ventilation should the patient become apnoeic; however, some ventilators include a backup mode as the default setting. The pressure support is gradually reduced, usually to a level of $5\text{--}10\,\text{cmH}_2\text{O}$ (a minimum necessary to eliminate work done against resistance to airflow through a tracheal tube and ventilator breathing system), at which point a trial of continuous positive airway pressure (CPAP) may be initiated or the patient extubated.

2. CPAP/T-piece weaning. A CPAP/T-piece circuit is used intermittently for progressively extended periods, enabling the patient to take over all the work of breathing with shortening periods of rest on the ventilator. This technique is simple but requires close observation of the patient to avoid exhaustion.

3. Intermittent mandatory ventilation (IMV) weaning. The ventilator delivers a preset tidal volume at a preset rate ensuring a minimum minute volume is delivered to the patient irrespective of his/her own effort. Patient-generated breaths are then permitted in between. These breaths can also be delivered in a pressure mode. The number of ventilator-delivered breaths is reduced gradually, enabling the patient to take on the full work of breathing. Ventilator breaths are usually synchronised to the patient's own efforts (SIMV). The ventilator will deliver a mandatory breath independent of respiratory effort only if a patient-initiated breath does not occur within a specified time period. Recent data suggest that SIMV and IMV are not as effective at reducing respiratory work as pressure support.

Patients who are easy to wean from mechanical ventilation will progress successfully, irrespective of the technique used. Prospective randomised trials of weaning modes have reached conflicting conclusions; however, there is consensus that SIMV is the least-efficient method of weaning from ventilation.

4. Adjunctive treatments
- Salbutamol: inhaled β_2 agonists may reduce work of breathing by 25%, even if there is no evidence of bronchospasm.
- Aminophylline may improve diaphragmatic contractility and may be beneficial in counteracting respiratory muscle fatigue in patients whose work of breathing is normally increased (e.g. COPD).

Failure to wean

Close observation of the patient for early signs of failure to wean is essential to avoid distress, fatigue and haemodynamic compromise. Subjective symptoms of fatigue and dyspnoea will often be the first indicators, followed by evident exhaustion accompanied by a falling tidal volume and rising respiratory rate. An f/VT ratio of $>100\,1^{-1}$ predicts weaning failure. At this point the level of support must be increased to assist the respiratory muscles and avoid fatigue. Respiratory muscles once fatigued to a state of exhaustion take many hours to recover.

It is sensible to initiate weaning early on in the day, so that progress can be closely monitored, possibly with planned periods of rest overnight.

Non-invasive ventilation can be used to facilitate early extubation in some patients, particularly those with COPD, who would otherwise fail to wean.

Further Reading

Esteban A, Alia I. Clinical management of weaning from mechanical ventilation. *Intensive Care Med* 1998; **24**: 999–1008.

MacIntyre NR. Evidence-based guidelines for weaning and discontinuing ventilatory support. *Chest* 2001; **120**: 375S–95S.

Related topics of interest

Index

Page numbers in *italics* indicate figures or tables.